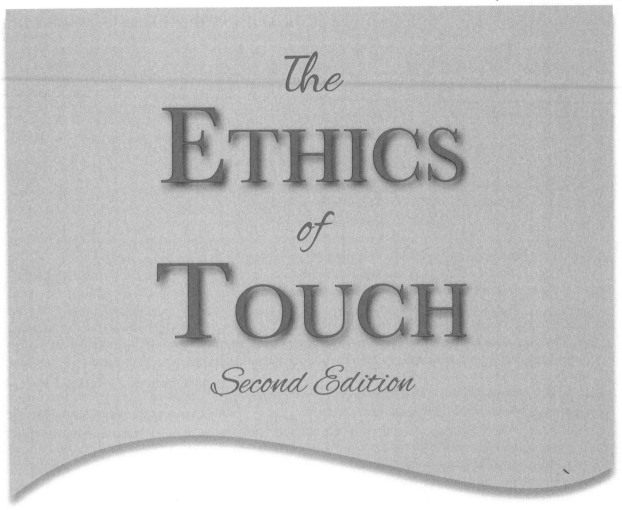

The
ETHICS
of
TOUCH
Second Edition

The Hands-on Practitioner's Guide To Creating a Professional, Safe, and Enduring Practice

Ben E. Benjamin, Ph.D., & Cherie Sohnen-Moe

the ETHICS *of* TOUCH

The Hands-on Practitioner's Guide
To Creating a Professional, Safe, and Enduring Practice

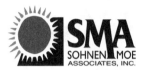

PO Boc 86913
Tucson, Arizona 85754-6913
520-743-3936
www.Sohnen-Moe.com

Publisher's Cataloging-in-Publication
(*Provided by Quality Books, Inc.*)

Benjamin, Ben E., 1944-
The ethics of touch : the hands-on practioner's guide to creating a professional, safe and enduring practice / by Ben E. Benjamin and Cherie Sohnen-Moe.
  p. cm.
Includes bibliographical references and index.
LCCN 2013918075
Print Edition-   ISBN-13: 978-1-882908-42-4 ISBN-10: 1-882908-42-2
Digital Edition- ISBN-13: 978-1-882908-43-1 ISBN-10: 1-882908-43-0
1. Touch—Theraputic use—Moral and ethical aspects.
2. Allied health personnel—Professional ethics.
I. Sohnen-Moe, Cherie. II. Title.
  RZ999.B465 2003   174'.29582
           QBI03-200040

Cover design: Tina Goins
Original artwork: Michaelangelo Buonarroti
Photograph ©iStock.com/estelle75
Editors: James Moe, Deanna Sylvester
Second Edition, 2014

Interior Design: Kathy Liddiard, James Moe
Illustrations: Paul Kraytman
www.TheEthicsOfTouch.com
Printed in the United States of America
Last digit is the print number: 9 8 7 6 5 4 3 2

Preface

Introduction

Ethics is an exciting, vital field of study for all professionals. Life is more fulfilling and satisfying if we live with honor and integrity in all our relationships and business dealings. Yet much confusion exists about what is and what is not ethical behavior. This confusion can be even more complex for somatic practitioners. This book helps to clarify an often vague, amorphous topic, easing the application of a professional code of ethics to practical behavior. It is our desire to assist practitioners in developing an ethical foundation beyond reproach.

We originally created this ethics book because of the lack of resource materials written specifically for somatic practitioners. Even though several books have been published since our first edition, we are committed to providing a breadth and depth of information not found elsewhere. Most massage therapists, bodyworkers, somatic practitioners, chiropractors, acupuncturists, physical therapists, personal trainers, and other somatic practitioners don't receive adequate ethics training. It is our mission to support hands-on professionals in expanding their knowledge about the field of ethics, enhancing their boundary management, and running ethical practices. We want to reach students as well as seasoned practitioners.

Those practitioners with a clear understanding of ethical behavior and professional communication skills are the ones who create and build successful practices. In the more than 10 years since the first edition of *The Ethics of Touch* was published, we have heard from employers and practitioners alike that there is still an increasing need, inside the treatment room and out, for these essential tools. As the wellness professions continue to evolve, we have collected more and more relevant information to share with beginners and seasoned practitioners. This second edition is the product of those collections.

The Ethics of Touch was also written to facilitate exploration. Throughout this book you'll find thought-provoking examples, models, points to ponder, practical applications, and activities that make this information personally relevant. We have also created a free downloadable workbook that contains chapter highlights, the activities from the book, and a few bonus activities.

We begin by developing a theoretical foundation and defining key terms. We, then, present methods for resolving ethical dilemmas and provide information on critical topics. We also incorporate specific methods and techniques for maintaining healthy boundaries, enhancing communication, fostering a sense of safety, working with other professionals, and managing your practice.

We encourage you to read each chapter and evaluate how to put these behaviors and skills in place. Some of these issues may not be critical at your current setting, nevertheless we have found that most practitioners are faced with these issues at some point in their careers. If you seriously think about these issues ahead of time, you're prepared when they arise. The information, models, and suggestions are meant as a starting point for you to customize and apply to the unique aspects of your practice.

▇ Terminology

What's In a Name?

The book is directed at healthcare professionals who touch the body as a primary method of delivering care. For consistency and when speaking of all providers we have most often chosen to use the words practitioner, healthcare provider, somatic practitioner, hands-on practitioner, and manual practitioner instead of specific titles such as massage therapist, bodyworker, acupuncturist, yoga instructor, chiropractor, Feldenkrais practitioner, physical therapist, Rolf© practitioner, polarity therapist, Shiatsu practitioner, or Alexander teacher. Some of the scenarios do refer to specific professions yet are relevant to almost every field. Also, the terms bodywork, body therapy, touch therapy, somatic therapy, manual therapies, treatment, and session are all interchangeable. It is our hope that all professionals in the healthcare field use the information in this book, as the same concepts and basic information applies equally to all these professions.

Patient or Client?

Depending on the context, a person who is receiving a session may be called either a patient or a client. In this book, we use whichever term seems most fitting for the situation. For instance, we use the word client when discussing a private massage therapy practice; we use the word patient when referring to a chiropractic or acupuncture treatment, or to massage that is performed in a hospital setting.

Him or Her?

Throughout most of history the male gender has been used exclusively to denote the generic pronoun when referring to women as well as men. As our culture and language has evolved, we have struggled to find the appropriate way to refer to all persons equally. Unfortunately, in English at least, a gender neutral pronoun doesn't exist and thus there's no simple way to accomplish this except by using clumsy terms like s/he, his/her, or himself/herself. We chose to alternate the use of the female and male pronouns throughout the book, but we intend for the principles illustrated by the examples to apply to both genders.

▇ How to Use this Book

The Ethics of Touch is intended for use both by hands-on healthcare practitioners in training and by professionals in the field. To fully assimilate the material in this book, it's best to read and study one chapter or even one section at a time. Although each chapter is self-contained, we suggest reading chapters One and Two first, to gain an understanding of the core concepts that are carried throughout the book.

Many of the chapters include useful activities and thought-provoking Points to Ponder for personal exploration. While you can do these on your own, they're much more valuable when you discuss them with peers and colleagues.

Special Features of the Digital Edition

The digital edition is interactive. On each chapter title page, the headings are hyperlinked to the corresponding section, and the key terms are hyperlinked to the appropriate glossary page. Throughout the chapters, the margin guides take you to the referenced chapter and page number, and the web addresses take you directly to the referenced website. Each endnote superscript takes you to the appropriate endnotes page, so you can research the reference materials yourself. Click away and have fun!

Online Workbook

Get the most out of *The Ethics of Touch* book by doing the exercises and regularly referring to them. We've made it easier by creating *The Ethics of Touch Workbook*, which includes chapter highlights and all of the written exercises from this book (plus more). We also recommend that you make this a journal to track your thought processes throughout this book (and throughout your career). In the workbook/journal you can keep your responses to the activities, your thoughts on the Points to Ponder, and your plans for using the Practical Applications. To download your free copy, go to http://www.TheEthicsOfTouch.com/workbook.php.

Pictograph Glossary

The following icons signal tips, resources, related information, and activities.

	Activities	Most of the exercises involve writing. This is your cue to get out your journal or go to your computer.
	Idea	Quick tips or suggestions for other ways to utilize the information.
	Publication Resources	Books, magazines, and other publications with more information on specific topics.
	Internet Resources	Links to related websites, articles, and other resources.
	Inspirational Quotes	Quotes from historical figures and thought-leaders.
	Point Forward	Lets you know where you can find related information in a subsequent section.
	Point Back	Reminds you to refer to an earlier section.

Continuing Education Credits

You can obtain Continuing Education Credits (CEs) for each chapter. Our courses are recognized by many organizations, and we are approved providers for the National Certification Board for Therapeutic Massage and Bodywork (NCBTMB Provider No. 031932-00), Florida State Department of Health (Provider No. MCE477-05), and many other healthcare practitioners' national and state boards.

If you're interested in using this material for CEs, please see page 389 for *The Ethics of Touch* Continuing Education Series, call 800-786-4774, or visit our web site, http://www.TheEthicsOfTouch.com. If you have any questions regarding CEs, please contact your professional organization or your state licensing board.

Teacher Resources

We offer a multitude of free teaching resources to schools requiring *The Ethics of Touch*: a 64-page guide on *The Art of Teaching*; Lesson Plan Builders for each chapter; PowerPoint® slides; a test bank; and more. Please visit http://www.TheEthicsOfTouch.com for more information.

About the Authors

BEN BENJAMIN holds a PH.D. in Sports Medicine. He was the founder of the Muscular Therapy Institute, in Cambridge, Massachusetts, and has been in private practice since 1963. As an educator and author, he has conducted seminars and workshops across the country, served as an instructor and trainer in a variety of settings, and written several books and countless articles. His books include *Listen to Your Pain, Are You Tense?* and *Exercise Without Injury.* He is the co-author of *Conversation Transformation: Recognize and Overcome the 6 Most Difficult Communication Patterns.*

Dr. Benjamin was the initiator and chairperson of the AMTA Council of Schools Professional and Sexual Ethics Task Force for four years and is considered an authority on ethics and boundaries in the body therapy field. He was one of the first to write extensively about boundaries, ethical issues, and sexual abuse in alternative health care, and since the early 1990s has published many articles on these topics in professional journals. Among the workshops he teaches throughout North America are Creating Healthy Boundaries in Health Care Settings, Working with Survivors of Trauma and Abuse, Assertiveness and Effective Communication, and Sexuality and Dual Relationships.

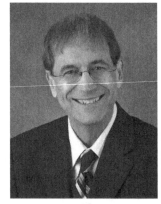

Long recognized for his contributions to the field, Dr. Benjamin's honors include the American Massage Therapy Association (AMTA) President's Award for the year 2000, the highest honorary recognition given by the organization; and the Distinguished Service to the Profession award, given in recognition of leadership and commitment to the massage profession and the AMTA. He has received awards naming him as one of the most influential people in the field by the AMTA, ABMP, and massage journals.

He trains teachers to be the best they can be, and coaches individuals toward success in both their personal and professional lives.

CHERIE SOHNEN-MOE is an author, business coach, international workshop leader, and successful business owner since 1978. Before shifting her focus to education and coaching, she was in private practice for many years as a massage and holistic health practitioner. Her background is diverse, having worked with individual therapists, small wellness centers, day spas that have multiple locations, and business in retail and the hospitality industry. Cherie holds a degree in psychology from UCLA and has extensive experience in the areas of business management, training, and creative problem solving.

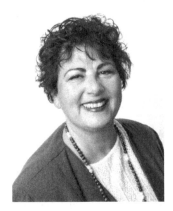

Cherie has served as a faculty member at the Desert Institute of Healing Arts, the Arizona School of Acupuncture and Oriental Medicine, and Clayton College of Natural Health. She has written more than 100 articles and is the author of the books *Business Mastery, Present Yourself Powerfully,* and *The Art of Teaching.* She is also a contributing author of *Teaching Massage,* and was interviewed for a chapter of *SAND TO SKY: Conversations with Teachers of Asian Medicine.* Her most popular workshops are Marketing from Your Heart, The Four Keys to Publicity, The Ethics of Touch, Therapeutic Communications, Present Yourself Powerfully, Profit with Products, and Creative Teaching Techniques.

Cherie is active in many professional and community organizations. Among her honors she has received the Distinguished Service Award and the Professional Achievement Award from the American Society for Training and Development (ASTD), and the Outstanding Instructor Award at the Desert Institute of the Healing Arts, and the MO AMTA President's Award.

Cherie is a firm believer in education. She serves on the exam committee of the Federation of State Massage Therapy Boards (FSMTB) and is a founding member and sits on the board of directors of the Alliance for Massage Therapy Education (AFMTE).

Contributing Authors

This book has been a work in progress for two decades. The first edition took us more than five years to write and it's been more than ten years since that first edition was published. The combination of our backgrounds, education, and experience created a dynamic, useful resource.

In the process of researching, writing, and updating this book, we sought the assistance of experts in a variety of fields to give breadth and depth to this book. Many people contributed ideas and stories, and several wrote major sections. Along with our original writing, we blended the contributed materials to fit the style, tone, and focus of this book. We are grateful for all the support from our colleagues and their permission to adapt and expand their writings. We are true believers in collaboration, and this book is the synergistic result of many creative minds. This list includes the people who contributed to the first edition, as well as those that contributed to the second edition.

JODI ALT, M.S., M.B.A., R.N., L.M.T., has worked in case management since 1992. She worked as a consultant with many hospitals nationwide in implementing case management programs. She co-authored "Nursing Case Management and Quality" in the *Handbook of Nursing Case Management*. Ms. Alt and Dr. Kathleen Stephens co-wrote the original Case Management section for the first edition of this book.

STEPHANIE BECK, owner of SRB Solutions, is an online marketing expert working with health and wellness practitioners for 15 years. Stephanie has served as a published columnist since 2003 for several magazines and is the author of *Social Trigger Points: Massage Therapist Guide to Marketing Online*. Connect with Stephanie at http://www.socialtriggerpoints.com/profiles today. She contributed the Ethical Social Media section in the Business Ethics chapter.

DOUGLAS BOLTON is a clinical psychologist and certified school psychologist. He received his PH.D. from the University of Vermont. Robert and Douglas Bolton were the primary authors of the Dynamics of Effective Communication chapter in the first edition of this book.

DR. ROBERT BOLTON is the co-founder of Ridge Associates, Inc., a consulting firm that serves Fortune 500 companies. He has designed training programs for the New York State Department of Mental Hygiene and co-founded a psychiatric outpatient clinic. He is the author of *People Skills: How to Assert Yourself, Listen to Others and Resolve Conflicts*; and *People Styles at Work...and Beyond*.

NANCY A. BRIDGES, L.I.C.S.W., is Faculty at the Cambridge Health Alliance, Harvard Medical School, and Massachusetts Institute for Psychoanalysis. She practices psychoanalysis, psychotherapy, and consultation in Belmont, MA. She was a primary contributor to the supervision section in the first edition.

DAPHNE CHELLOS, M.A., LPC has been moving between psyche and soma for over 35 years. As a massage therapist, she was named a pioneer in the field of sexual ethics by the Bodywork Entrepreneur in 1991 and taught and consulted nationally with bodywork schools and organizations. She has a private practice in psychotherapy, spiritual direction, and Authentic Movement. She is an adjunct professor in the Graduate School of Psychology at Naropa University in Boulder, CO. Ms. Chellos is the primary author of the chapter on Sex, Touch, and Intimacy.

NAOMI HEITZ, B.A., L.M.B.T., is a massage therapist, early childhood teacher, and artist. In her bodywork practice, Naomi specializes in teaching parents massage techniques for their children. She also researches ethics in the healing arts and has created the website http://www.healingethics.com. She contributed the Impacts of Ethical Breaches Chart in the Ethical Principles chapter and wrote information on boundaries, dual relationships, and trauma.

FRED N. LERNER, D.C., PH.D., F.A.C.O., has been in practice for over thirty years. He is a chiropractic orthopedist at Cedars-Sinai Medical Center—The Pain Center. He also serves as Chairman of the National Board of Acupuncture Orthopedics. Dr. Lerner wrote the section on the Health Insurance Portability and Accountability Act (HIPAA) in the Practice Management chapter.

LINDA MABUS JORGENSON, M.A., J.D., has considerable legal experience in the area of sexual exploitation by professionals. She has handled 400+ cases of therapist-patient sexual abuse allegations, as well as cases involving non-sexual boundary violations. Ms. Jorgenson has published extensively in this area in numerous law reviews and mental health journals. She contributed the Legal Issues information for the Business Ethics chapter.

CLIFFORD P. MARTIN, M.D., is an infectious diseases physician in private practice in Tucson, AZ and Assistant Clinical Professor of Medicine at The University of Arizona. He has a Master of Science degree in Healthcare Administration from the University of Texas at Dallas and is the Chairman of the Board of Massamio.com, an online directory, website, and booking service for independent massage therapists. He wrote the Care Coordination and Case Management section in The Team Approach chapter, plus general information throughout that chapter.

STEPHANIE MINES, PH.D., is the author of *We Are All in Shock: How Overwhelming Experience Shatters You and What You Can Do about It*, *New Frontiers in Sensory Integration*, and *Sexual Abuse/Sacred Wound: Transforming Deep Trauma*. Dr. Mines is the founder of the TARA Approach for the Resolution of Shock and Trauma. She trains therapists internationally in her synthesis of Western neuroscience and Eastern energy medicine. Stephanie contributed to the update of the Working with Trauma Survivors chapter.

SHAYE MOORE is a nationally certified bodyworker and registered yoga teacher whose practice is devoted to seniors, children, and adults with special needs. She was the recipient of a grant from the Community Health Program Fund of Boston Children's Hospital to bring infant massage instruction to disadvantaged young parents. Ms. Moore contributed to the first edition by writing sections on dual relationships, working with minors, boundaries, and definitions. She wrote the office ethics and working with others in the Team Approach chapter for the second edition.

LAUREN MUSER CATES, CMT, is founding director of the Society for Oncology Massage. She served as the Clinical Supervisor for Hospital/Oncology Massage at Virginia Hospital Center in Arlington, VA, and founded Healwell, a non-profit organization focused on hospital-based massage therapy education, service, and research. She has worked with hospice in home and clinical settings since 2003. Ms. Cates wrote the section on working in hospitals and hospices in The Team Approach chapter.

JULIE ONOFRIO is a massage therapist in Seattle, WA for over 25 years. She is the creator of many websites for the massage profession and the author of numerous books. She is an avid supporter of supervision and offers online supervision groups. You can visit http://www.facebook.com/MassagePracticeBuilder for many daily tips and tricks for building your massage business. She contributed to the expansion and revamping of the Support Systems chapter.

DIANNE POLSENO, L.M.T., passed away in May of 2012, and will be missed for much more than her contributions to this text. Dianne continuously advocated for ethical massage practice, and as the President of Cortiva Institute-Boston worked tirelessly toward thorough and professional massage education. She was a former chair of the AMTA National Ethics Subcommittee, and the 2006 AMTA Jerome Perlinski Teacher of the Year Award recipient, among many other accolades. She led ethics workshops and authored numerous articles on ethics. Ms. Polseno contributed information on Sexual Misconduct, Informed Consent, and Scope of Practice for the first edition of this book.

STUART N. SIMON, L.I.C.S.W., has over 35 years of experience as a Gestalt therapist, coach and organizational consultant. He has taught in the US, Canada, Europe, the Middle East, and Africa. He is member of the senior faculty of the Gestalt International Study Center (Wellfleet, Cape Cod), and a contributing author to numerous books and articles on psychotherapy and coaching from a Gestalt perspective. A graduate of the Gestalt Institute of Cleveland, he is also on the faculty of Boston University Corporate Education Group. Mr. Simon was a major author of the Boundaries Chapter.

KATHLEEN N. STEPHENS, D.C., L.M.T., has been involved in the Alternative Health field since 1977. She is the author of *The Stephens Method of Manual Therapy* and teaches her recognized technique nationally. Dr. Stephens also serves as a consultant in Case Management in private practices. She and Ms. Alt co-wrote the original Case Management section for the first edition of this book.

DEANNA SYLVESTER, L.M.T., is a massage therapist, shiatsu practitioner, and teacher. Ms. Sylvester is currently the Regional Director for the Arizona Schools of Integrative Studies, and formerly the President of Cortiva Institute-Tucson where she developed and provided comprehensive ethical massage curriculum for beginning therapists. Ms. Sylvester contributed to the second edition of this book as an editor, with content additions throughout.

DIANA THOMPSON, L.M.P., author of *Hands Heal: Communication, Documentation and Insurance Billing for Manual Therapists*, contributed the section on Insurance Issues for the Business Ethics chapter.

RUTH WERNER is a retired massage therapist and a working writer and educator for the profession. She is the author of *A Massage Therapist's Guide to Pathology, Disease Handbook for Massage Therapists*, and she contributes material to many other publications. Ms. Werner contributed to the Touch section in the Sex, Touch, and Intimacy chapter.

AMY YEAGER is a communication coach, trainer, and consultant. She is a co-author, with Ben Benjamin and Anita Simon, of *Conversation Transformation: Recognize and Overcome the 6 Most Destructive Communication Problems*. Ms. Yeager helped revamp the book, rewrote the Ethical Principles chapter, and updated the Communication chapters.

▮ Acknowledgments

We acknowledge all those individuals whose work and thoughts contributed to creating this book. First our thanks to those who graciously let us use information that they developed: Mark Annett; Lu Bauer; Joan Calgano, J.D.; Estelle Disch, PH.D., C.C.S; C Diane Ealy, PH.D.; Clyde Ford, D.C.; Steven Hassan, L.M.H.C.; Naomi Heitz; Judy Herman, M.D.; Krishnabai; Stephanie Mines; Shaye Moore; Angelica Redleaf, D.C.; Melissa Sault; Helene Sorkin, L.AC.; Charles Whitfield, M.D.; Janet Yassen, L.I.S.W.; and Amy Yeager.

We express our appreciation to the following people who shared their stories, gave us ideas, provided resources and information, and critiqued our material: Caroline Abreu; Virginia Anthony; Cindy Banker; Monque Barazone; Elaine Calenda; James Clay; Mary Ann DiRoberts, M.S.W., L.M.T.; Dave Epley, PH.D, L.AC.; Dian Fitzpatrick; Robert Flammia; Jackie Galloway; Susan Gottlieb; Susie Hale; Debbie Jedlicka; Helene Jewell; Paula Jilanis; Janet King, J.D.; Jennifer Kuhn; Karen Manning; Sue Mapel, L.I.C.S.W.; T.C. Merrill; Daz Moran; Bill Mueller, L.AC.; Doug Newman, J.D.; Betty Norris; Pamela Polley; Ken Pope, PH.D.; Julia Riley, R.N.; Mary Ringenberger; Daniel Schmidt; Gary Schoener, PH.D.; Rebecca Stephenson, P.T.; Sandi Straub; Nancy Tam, B.S.W; Stella Tarnay; Tracy Walton, M.S.W., L.M.T.; Christi Warner; Rebecca Wilcox; Tracy Williams, M.S.; and Gary Wolf, J.D.

Our deepest thanks go to the peer reviewers. The first edition reviewers were: Mark Annett; Elaine Calenda; Dave Epley, PH.D, L.AC; Judy Herman, M.D.; Shaye Moore; Bill Mueller, L.AC; Angelica Redleaf, D.C.; Julia Riley, R.N.; Mary Ringenberger; Rebecca Stephenson, P.T.; Christi Warner; and Tracy Williams, M.S. The second edition reviewers were: Tonya Aiossa; Daphne Chellos; Naomi Heitz; Shaye Moore; Zachary Potchinsky; Deanna Sylvester; and Amy Yaeger.

We are grateful for the following people who gave their time and expertise editing various drafts and giving input to make this book as accurate and useful as possible. The first edition: Joelle Andre; Mary Ann DiRoberts, M.S.W., L.M.T.; Ginevra Fay; Helene Jewell; Fran Knott; James Moe; Shaye Moore; Melissa Mower; and Tracy Williams, M.S. The second edition editors were: Tonya Aiossa; Stan Dawson, D.C.; James Moe; Sally Niemand; Terri Osborne; Deanna Sylvester; and Amy Yaeger.

We thank Tina Goins for her beautiful cover design, Kathy Liddiard and James Moe for the interior book layout, and Paul Kraytman for his drawings in the Boundaries Chapter.

Thank you to all of our students, clients, teachers, and colleagues.

The Ethics of Touch

Table of Contents

11. Working with Trauma Survivors

1

Ethical Foundations

"It is always the right time to do the right thing."
—Martin Luther King, Jr.

The Therapeutic Relationship
- Client-Centeredness
- Impacts from Ethical Breaches
- Safety
- Privacy
- Clear Structure
- Power Differential

Complications of Power Differentials
- Misuse of Power and Disempowerment of Clients

Transference and Countertransference
- Transference
- Countertransference
- Managing Transference and Countertransference
- The Body as a Storehouse for Emotions and Past Experiences

Universal Ethical Principles
- Justice
- Honesty
- Reverence for Life
- Adherence to Law

Sources of Ethical Guidance
- Official Codes and Regulations
- Personal Ethics and Self-Accountability

Resolving Ethical Dilemmas
- The Six-Step Resolution Model

Key Terms

Autonomy
Beneficence
Client-Centeredness
Code of Ethics
Countertransference
Duties
Ethical Congruence

Ethical Dilemma
Ethics
Fiduciary
Informed Consent
Morals
Nonmaleficence
Power Differential

Principles
Rights
Scope of Practice
Self-Accountability
Self-Determination
Transference
Values

For all of us who work as wellness practitioners, ethics is a topic that we simply can't afford to ignore. Whether you realize it or not, you confront ethical issues on a regular basis, some of which may be fairly serious:

- A client to whom you're attracted asks you out on a date, and you're not sure what to say.
- During a session, a client confides that he sometimes lashes out physically at his girlfriend, and you must decide how to respond.
- A regular client refers her father to you and then probes for details about his treatment, and you feel pressured to divulge confidential information.
- You suspect that a colleague is involved in an inappropriate relationship with a client, and you must decide whether and how to intervene.
- You think some of your clients would heal much more quickly with a treatment you don't provide, but you're reluctant to make referrals because of the income you'd lose.

Or the issues might be somewhat less serious but still concerning:
- Although you don't normally offer a sliding scale, one of your favorite clients asks for a lowered rate, and you feel tempted to make an exception.
- You realize that your new ad is potentially misleading (though technically accurate), but you'd prefer not to change it because it brings so much business.
- You have an opportunity to co-teach with a well-known practitioner in your field, and you'd love the exposure but are worried about appearing to endorse some of her techniques, which you believe are ineffective.

How do you decide which actions to take and which to avoid, or when to speak up and when to remain silent? Where do you turn for guidance when you're not sure how to proceed?

The purpose of this book is to help you build the knowledge, skills, and self-awareness to approach a wide range of ethical questions with clarity and confidence. Whether you're a massage therapist, acupuncturist, physical therapist, chiropractor, yoga instructor, personal trainer, movement teacher, nutritional consultant, esthetician, or bodyworker—professional or student—this material can equip you to run an ethical practice, prevent many ethical violations from occurring, and resolve ethical dilemmas when they arise. We begin in this chapter by discussing the unique combination of ethical issues that arise in therapeutic relationships, universal ethical principles that are relevant to healthcare practitioners, sources of guidance for ethical behavior, and a systematic process you can use to help resolve any ethical dilemma.

The Therapeutic Relationship

The study of ethics is the study of right and wrong conduct, of how we should and should not behave. Guidelines for ethical behavior depend on the context. What is ethically acceptable in one role or setting may be unethical in another. For instance, certain ways you interact with a close friend or family member may be unethical in the context of your business practice, such as the way you joke around, the type and amount of self-disclosure, and the kinds of physical contact.

Therapeutic relationships involve several key elements that differentiate them from other human relationships: client-centeredness; safety; privacy; a clear structure; and a power differential. Each of these elements directly affects both your duties (your obligations as a practitioner) and your clients' rights (what they're entitled to receive). Gaining an understanding of these issues will deepen your awareness of how your behavior affects your clients, and thereby help protect you from inadvertent ethical violations and from behaving unethically, even in difficult situations.

Client-Centeredness

Therapeutic relationships are often referred to as client-centered. The practitioner is in the role of fiduciary, a professional in whom the client places his trust. The client is asking for help and placing himself in a vulnerable position by becoming a client. As a result, there's an implicit contract that the practitioner puts the client's interests above and before her own. Trouble often begins when the practitioner takes an action just because she feels like it and not because it's therapeutically necessary. For example, a therapist has just learned a new technique that she wants to practice, and she tries it on a client who hasn't asked for it and doesn't really need that type of work.

In client-centered relationships, clients have the right to expect that the practitioner always act in their best interest. Practitioners have two related duties:

1. Do no harm (nonmaleficence) and
2. Do positive good (beneficence).

Many practitioners consider "do no harm" to be the more compelling obligation in situations where these two duties conflict. For instance, if a client has a suspected sprained ankle and asks you to help, your duty to work on the ankle (which might help the injury) is outweighed by your duty to refer the client to a physician for an x-ray to see if the ankle is broken (to ensure that your work does no harm).

Another implication of client-centeredness is that the client is viewed as a partner who shares decision-making power with the practitioner. The client has a voice in the therapeutic process and must agree to a course of treatment for it to proceed. In other words, clients have the right to direct what happens to their bodies, and practitioners have a duty to obtain their clients' informed consent. This means, for example, that a practitioner should never treat a client's injury without permission.

Impacts from Ethical Breaches

To determine what is ethical or unethical, many professions have created guidelines based on what generally harms clients. The impacts from ethical breaches are diverse. Figure 1.1 depicts possible damage created for the client by a practitioner's intentional or unintentional breach of ethics. On one end of the spectrum could be short-lived confusion and unease in a client when a practitioner fails to clearly communicate her fees in advance of a session. A more serious instance is a practitioner's request of a client to invest in a business venture that could create more complex impacts for a client, including feeling pressured, anxiety, confusion, and a derailed healing process. The most egregious breaches involve sexualization of sessions and working outside the scope of practice for the profession. In these cases, it can be many years before clients fully heal from severe emotional or physical damage such as depression, PTSD, physical pain, and touch avoidance. By crossing boundaries outlined by generally accepted codes of ethics, practitioners risk the wellbeing of clients.[1, 2]

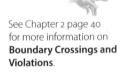

See Chapter 2 page 40 for more information on **Boundary Crossings and Violations**.

Safety

The client has the right to expect that the therapeutic environment is safe, both physically and emotionally. The practitioner is responsible for ensuring that safety by keeping strong boundaries (for instance, not making inappropriate personal comments or sexual advances). At times, the obligation to protect the client's health means not providing a treatment. This is the case when the therapist is sick and infectious, or when the client shows signs of a condition that precludes physical contact, such as an undiagnosed rash.

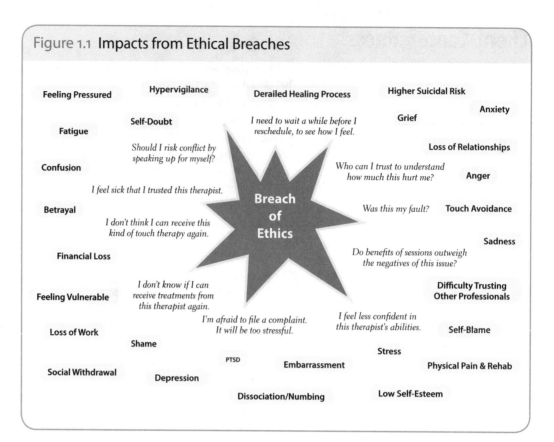

Figure 1.1 Impacts from Ethical Breaches

Do you have a personal story of how a breach of ethics impacted you as a client or as the practitioner? Participate in ethics research.

http://www.healingethics.com/

See Chapter 7 page 188 for in-depth information on **HIPAA** and other aspects of **confidentiality**.

Privacy

As healthcare providers, we have access to very personal information about our clients. It is our duty to keep that information confidential, respecting every client's right to privacy. In addition to being bound by ethical considerations, our privacy practices are also governed by stringent laws—most notably the Health Insurance Portability and Accountability Act, or HIPAA.

Clear Structure

Within a therapeutic relationship, contact between the practitioner and client is limited and structured. Structured aspects of the relationship include:

- **TIME:** The client comes for a session once a week, or at some other time interval, with each session lasting for a prescribed time frame.
- **ACTIVITY:** During each session, the client receives specific, agreed-upon types of treatment, which are within the practitioner's scope of practice.
- **ROLES:** Each person has a clearly defined role. The client comes for help, and the practitioner directs her energy toward providing that help (a focus referred to as being service-oriented).

It's the practitioner's duty to establish and maintain a clear structure in each of these ways.

Power Differential

It is difficult to understand the therapeutic relationship without comprehending the power differential that it entails. In our society, power differentials arise from differences in age, economic status, gender, education, and many other factors. In addition to these societal power differentials, several factors specific to professions that involve touch or movement create even greater differences in power within the therapeutic relationship: the practitioner's role as professional; the practitioner's base of knowledge; the client's state of awareness; and the physical aspects of the practice.

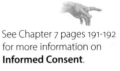

See Chapter 7 pages 191-192 for more information on **Informed Consent**.

Power differentials exist in many different types of relationships: between parent and child; between teacher and student; between employer and employee; and of course between practitioner and client. The practitioner, as the authority figure whose actions directly affect the wellbeing of the client, automatically has more power. In theory and in ethical practice, the power differential exists for the purpose of bringing benefit to the more vulnerable individual (the child, student, employee, or client).

The power differential is also enhanced by differences in knowledge bases. A practitioner's training and experience in working with bodies typically far exceeds that of the client. The client trusts that the practitioner will provide beneficial care by drawing on the practitioner's knowledge of techniques, therapeutic relationships, and ethical conduct. Out of respect for this component of the power differential, the practitioner educates the client about techniques before using them and gets informed consent from the client for any changes to the therapeutic plan.

Differences in states of awareness and consciousness augment the power differential.[3] For instance, during a bodywork session, the client may become inwardly focused, entering a deep state of relaxation which heightens her vulnerability. Rather than keeping normal levels of vigilance and awareness of her surroundings and the actions of the practitioner, the client may enter meditative states, sleep states, or states of awareness of memories and past traumas. The practitioner's tracking skills of the client's nonverbal cues become even more important when the client is not in a normal state of alertness, as the client may be less likely to give prompt feedback.

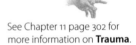

See Chapter 11 page 302 for more information on **Trauma**.

In the healthcare field, the power differential is amplified by the physical aspects of the practice. The client takes a position—usually lying or sitting—in which he allows the practitioner access to his body. The practitioner positions herself within the client's physical space, often leaning over the client. Furthermore, in many instances the client is partially or fully unclothed. Although draping is used for privacy, the psychological effect of the unclothed client and the clothed practitioner increases the imbalance of power. Finally, as the practitioner's hands make physical contact with the client's body, the client's physical safety is literally in the practitioner's hands.

Because healthcare professionals are in positions of power relative to their clients, they're held to a higher standard of behavior than professionals in business relationships with smaller power differentials. Maintaining professional boundaries is the responsibility of the practitioner, even if the client requests or instructs the practitioner to behave otherwise. Therefore, if a client makes an inappropriate request—for instance, asking for a type of work that's outside the practitioner's scope of practice, or asking to be treated without draping—it's up to the practitioner to decline. The practitioner also has a duty to stay aware of how the power differential may affect the client's ability to raise concerns. To avoid unintentionally misusing their power, practitioners should always keep in mind their clients' essential right to self-determination (freedom from interference with their personal life and autonomy).

In the following section, we explore several different types of ethical complications related to power imbalances.

Figure 1.2 Duties and Rights in the Therapeutic Relationship

The fundamental elements of the therapeutic relationship each carry with them certain duties for the practitioner and rights for the client.

	Practitioner Duties	**Client Rights**
Client-Centeredness	• Place the client's interests first • Do no harm (nonmaleficence) • Do positive good (beneficence) • Obtain informed consent	• Have one's own interests placed above and before the therapist's interests • Have an active role in directing the course of treatment
Safety	• Protect the client's physical and emotional safety	• Receive treatment within a safe environment
Privacy	• Keep confidential all information shared by the client during the session • Protect the privacy of all health records and other personal client information	• Be assured that one's health history and any other personal information remain private
Structure	• Maintain clear time boundaries • Provide agreed-upon treatments, within the appropriate scope of practice • Remain service-oriented	• Receive treatment within a context of structured time, activity, and roles
Power Differential	• Take responsibility for maintaining professional boundaries • Use own authority to enhance, and never endanger, the client's wellbeing • Stay aware of how the power differential is affecting the client • Respect the client's autonomy	• Benefit, rather than suffer, from the professional's authority • Remain free from interference with autonomy/self-determination

Complications of Power Differentials

The power differential between practitioner and client raises two crucial questions: How is the person with more power (the practitioner) using that power? How is the person with less power (the client) responding? Problems on either end of the relationship may lead to ethical complications.

Misuse of Power and Disempowerment of Clients

When practitioners misuse their power (either intentionally or unintentionally) or when clients feel disempowered to actively participate in their care, the clients' safety and wellbeing are at risk.

Misuse of Power in Attempts to Help

A common ethical error occurs when a practitioner tries to override a client's autonomy because the practitioner is worried about the client's behavior. For instance, a chiropractor insists that a client change her diet because he "knows" it will help her heal more quickly from her injury. In this example, the client's right to self-determination clashes with the practitioner's perceived duty to do positive good. In truth, simply mentioning something once fulfills the duty to do good.

The client's right to self-determination always overrides the practitioner's duty to do positive good unless the anticipated negative consequences are extreme. For instance, if your assessment indicates that the client has a serious, possibly life-threatening medical condition, and needs to see a medical doctor, you would more strongly encourage the client to see a specialist even if she is hesitant to do so.

Misuse of Power for Personal Gain

Practitioners may also misuse their power for their own personal benefit, taking advantage of their clients either physically, sexually, emotionally, financially, or professionally. Consider the following examples:

- A practitioner is treating a client who happens to be a lawyer. In the middle of the session, she asks, "Since I have you here, could you just answer this quick little question I have about my divorce?"
- A practitioner who is running in a charity race solicits sponsorship during a session.
- During a session a client mentions an executive whom the practitioner has wanted to meet, and the practitioner asks for a personal introduction.

Clients frequently test boundaries by offering things that may be inappropriate. For instance, a client may suggest that he tell you about some exciting new stock options while receiving a treatment, or volunteers to take your computer home to repair it because he sees you're having trouble with it.

To maintain an ethical practice, the person in power must choose to regularly say no to something she could easily get, and instead pay special attention to the needs of the person with less power. The practitioner must consciously decide to maintain the integrity of the client's boundaries in a situation where the client has significantly relaxed those boundaries.

> But the relationship of morality and power is a very subtle one. Because ultimately power without morality is no longer power.
>
> —James Baldwin

Disempowerment of Clients

The power differential in a hands-on session puts the client in a highly vulnerable position. It may be difficult for her to raise concerns, make requests, say no, or question the practitioner's behavior, even if she feels uncomfortable or mistreated. She may refrain from communicating anything that could possibly be construed as negative for fear of reprisal or loss. Consider this scenario:

An active businesswoman has received massage twice monthly from the same massage therapist for more than two years. She recently began having sharp pains in the big toe of her right foot. On one occasion, she mentioned the pain to the practitioner at the beginning of the session in hopes that the therapist would spend some time vigorously working the area. As the massage proceeded, the practitioner moved through the foot area rather quickly.

Disappointed, the client debated about asking the therapist to go back to the toe area. She couldn't understand why it was so difficult to ask. After some thought she realized she felt vulnerable lying naked on the table having someone standing over her, touching her body (even though she was covered by a sheet). And asking someone to do something to her (especially on a big toe) might seem silly. She might be imposing, or maybe the practitioner would become upset since it was close to the end of the session. She didn't want to appear needy or self-centered. Plus, if the request were to aggravate the therapist, she'd have to risk feeling the therapist's irritation conveyed through the therapist's hands for the remainder of the session.

Finally, the client muttered in a very unsure, child-like tone, "Um, ah, do you think, I mean, would it be OK, could you, um, work on that toe that hurts?"

The practitioner responds, "Sure!"

Points to Ponder

Does the power differential ever diminish over time, as a therapeutic relationship continues and the client and practitioner get to know each other better?

In this case, even though the client and practitioner had worked together for a couple of years, the client became hesitant to make a request out of a sense of vulnerability, a fear of appearing foolish, and concerns over possibly upsetting the practitioner. The client was unaware of the psychological effects of the power differential until a need arose that required her to make a request. And even after recognizing the effects, she still asked as a child who was feeling very unsure of herself around an adult.

Realize that the power differential always exists in any therapeutic relationship, even though you may be doing your best to foster an atmosphere of equality. The power differential makes it particularly difficult for clients to take an active role in making decisions about their health care. To counter the effect of the power differential, the practitioner must regularly ask clients for permission to examine, to treat, or to reschedule. Consistently asking clients what they want puts the clients back in power and minimizes the effect of the power differential. It doesn't matter how powerful clients are in their jobs or in life in general, the practitioner must remember that in the role of client, even a normally powerful person feels diminished. Also, the power differential can change over time, such as when: a teenage client becomes an adult; a client increases his ability to communicate; a client feels more comfortable receiving sessions.

 Evaluating Power Differentials

- What types of relationships do not inherently have power differentials?
- Why is a power differential inherent in any therapeutic relationship?
- What are the conditions that make for a greater or lesser power differential?
- What are the conditions that might contribute to an inappropriate power differential?
- Describe positive and negative experiences you have had in relationships where there is a power differential.

▏▎ Transference and Countertransference

To behave responsibly and ethically, every practitioner must understand the core psychological concepts of transference and countertransference. Often discussed in the context of psychotherapy, these phenomena also have a powerful influence on hands-on therapeutic relationships.

Transference

Whenever there is a power differential in a relationship, there is a strong tendency for the more vulnerable person to respond to the more powerful person in the same way he responds to other authority figures. In doing so, he may recreate, within that relationship, complex elements of similar relationships he has had in the past. This is known as transference.

Transference is a normal, unconscious psychological phenomenon characterized by unconscious redirection of feelings from one person to another. This often occurs during the therapeutic process and typically doesn't cause serious problems for wellness practitioners. Professional helping relationships usually have a strong transference element in which the parent-child relationship is unconsciously re-established. The client's unresolved needs, feelings, and issues from childhood are transferred onto the helper.

Although the power of touch in stimulating transference has not been formally studied, anecdotal evidence suggests that touch—especially when it's intentional and done with care—can quickly create transferential or regressive experiences. When someone in a vulnerable position is touched in a caring way by a person of greater perceived power and authority, the touch often evokes a vulnerable, childlike state. One consequence is that clients often expect practitioners to help them emotionally, or to help in other areas that are outside their scope of practice. Somatic practitioners hear comments on a daily basis that confirm this reality. Clients frequently disclose very personal information in a first or second session, tell the practitioner about their emotional problems, or forcefully demand special treatment.

Emotionally mature adult clients are more likely to recognize transference-related feelings and not let them control their behavior. In individuals who are unaware of or unable to handle

Figure 1.3 Signs of Transference

- The client frequently asks you very personal questions.
- The client calls you at home even though your policies state that calls should be placed to your office.
- After only one or two treatments, the client is overly complimentary of your work and effuses about what a wonderful person you are.
- The client keeps trying to bargain with you for a reduced rate even after you have clearly stated your policy.
- The client regularly requests that you accommodate his schedule by changing your own schedule to work at a time when you don't normally see clients.
- The client develops a "crush" on you.
- The client seems overly attached.
- Every time you see the client, she brings you a gift.
- The client repeatedly invites you to social engagements and feels rejected when you explain your policy of not socializing with clients.
- At the end of most treatment sessions the client asks you to do just a little bit more, and expresses disapproval if you don't comply.
- The client often asks you to help him solve personal problems.
- The client frequently asks you questions in areas that you have previously explained aren't in your scope of practice.
- The client often mentions that you remind her of someone.
- The client has difficulty maintaining a physical boundary and attempts to inappropriately hug or touch you at the end of each treatment session.
- The client has great difficulty leaving after the session and tries to engage you in conversation.
- The client gives you details of his personal life, which feel too intimate and make you uncomfortable.

these feelings, transference may become the dominant reality, leading them to experience frequent disappointment and rejection, often followed by anger and withdrawal. To ensure that transference reactions don't negatively impact the therapeutic relationship, somatic practitioners must respond in a gentle, appropriate manner and maintain clear boundaries at all times.

Countertransference

Countertransference is simply transference occurring in the opposite direction, from practitioner to client. When a practitioner unconsciously transfers his unresolved needs, feelings, and issues onto a client, he begins to feel toward the client the same way he felt toward someone in his past.

Countertransference is a strong force that can adversely affect the therapeutic relationship, resulting in less effective therapy, loss of clients, or psychological harm to clients. Practitioners who are aware of the phenomenon of countertransference are more likely to recognize it when it occurs. This awareness can help make their responses more appropriate and help them to refocus on the client's actual needs. If you notice any of these phenomena in your behavior or experience, take this as a signal of something happening on an unconscious level and get help from a supervisor, counselor, or psychotherapist.

Figure 1.4 Signs of Countertransference

- Feeling a strong emotional charge, either positive or negative, toward a client.
- Feeling irritable or angry with a client for not changing, not improving, or not cooperating with the treatment plan.
- Distorted thinking about a client: having an idealized view or feeling very negatively toward the person.
- Distorted thinking about your work in relation to a client: believing that your work is much better for the person than most practitioners' work, or that your work is totally ineffective and worthless for the person.
- A pattern of feeling exhausted, exhilarated, depressed, or uneasy when seeing a particular client.
- Recurring themes such as frequent sexual attraction to clients or the recurrent desire to make friends with clients.
- The expectation of praise and resulting disappointment when clients don't praise your work.
- Feeling guilty when a client experiences a painful reaction that lasts for an extended period after the treatment.
- Frequent experiences of anger when a client crosses minor boundaries, questions your competence, or otherwise "pushes your buttons."
- Undergoing secondary trauma upon hearing painful stories about a client's past.
- Frequently helping a client in matters outside the sessions, such as offering rides or introducing the client to social contacts.

Managing Transference and Countertransference

Transference and countertransference affect the answers to the questions we mentioned earlier: how is the person who holds the power using that power, how is the person with less power responding? When both individuals in the relationship are psychologically mature, there is a greater likelihood that they'll use power or handle the other's use of power in a healthful way. Nevertheless, maturity doesn't ensure that transference and countertransference won't occur.

The practitioner working with a less psychologically savvy client has an especially serious responsibility, for such a client may be unaware of the transference he brings to the therapeutic relationship. Individuals who are more prone to transference include children and adolescents, clients who behave in a needy manner, and clients who have been referred by a mental health professional for bodywork to assist in the processing of psychological issues.

Wellness practitioners have a responsibility to cultivate their own awareness of both transference and countertransference and consciously guard against their effects. This can be challenging. Getting supervision on a regular basis provides a valuable opportunity to explore these issues, gain clarity, and learn methods for behaving ethically and effectively.

The Impact of Transference and Countertransference

- Describe one example of transference that you have experienced.
- Describe one example of countertransference that you have experienced.
- What are the positive and negative effects of transference and countertransference?

The Body as a Storehouse for Emotions and Past Experiences

While some behaviors and emotional responses within the therapeutic relationship can be classified as transference or countertransference, others are a result of a phenomenon that many practitioners and recipients of bodywork have experienced: the human body seems to hold patterns, not just of physical tension, but also of related emotions, thoughts, past experiences, or beliefs.

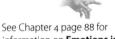
See Chapter 4 page 88 for information on **Emotions in the Treatment Room**.

As is frequently stated among bodywork practitioners, "our issues are in our tissues." Bringing awareness to an area of the body, especially through a practitioner's touch, can allow emotional or mental energies to emerge and then be expressed, acknowledged, witnessed, or processed internally by the client. Past experiences, especially those with unresolved traumatic impacts, are sometimes at the root of body-related emotional releases. The process of healing body, mind, and soul can be a delicate, emotional journey that puts the client into places of great vulnerability. Respecting this process, or even the potential for this process, is a core reason why ethical intentions and conduct are vital for protecting clients.

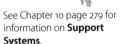
See Chapter 10 page 279 for information on **Support Systems**.

▊ Universal Ethical Principles

Beyond the duties and rights specific to therapeutic relationships, practitioners should also keep in mind basic principles of ethical behavior that apply to all human interactions. Behaviors that are unethical outside the therapeutic context are likely to be unethical within it as well. Four principles of great relevance to healthcare practitioners are justice, honesty, reverence for life, and adherence to law.

Justice

To touch the surface is to stir the depths.

—Deane Juhan

PROVIDE EQUAL TREATMENT TO ALL INDIVIDUALS. To be an ethical practitioner, you must consider what it takes to provide equal treatment to all individuals who seek your care. The following would be considered ethical violations under the Justice Principle:

- Refusing to adapt your office (or make some reasonable accommodation) for those with physical challenges.
- Refusing to work on someone due to race, religion, size, or sexual orientation.

Honesty

BE UP-FRONT AND TRUTHFUL IN YOUR COMMUNICATIONS. Practitioners need to remain factual with their communications, without exaggeration or false claims. You should always be direct and forthcoming when presenting boundaries, goals, and expectations. The following would be considered ethical violations under the Honesty Principle:

- Misrepresenting your educational status (for instance, calling yourself a craniosacral therapist after taking a three-hour workshop).
- Making misleading claims of your curative abilities (for instance, telling a client you guarantee her pain will be gone in two sessions).

Reverence for Life

RESPECT CLIENTS BY NOT HARMING THEM EMOTIONALLY, MENTALLY, PHYSICALLY, OR SPIRITUALLY. This principle encompasses the "do no harm and do good" principles of non-maleficence and beneficence, discussed earlier in this chapter.[4] The following are examples of relevant ethical violations:

- Providing care to a client with a medical condition for which you don't know the indications or contraindications.
- Behaving in a seductive manner toward a client.

Adherence to Law

ABIDE BY ALL OF THE LEGAL REQUIREMENTS THAT APPLY TO YOU AND YOUR PRACTICE. Studying and knowing the laws regulating your profession helps you maintain compliance. The following would be considered ethical violations, in addition to legal violations:

- Charging a cash-paying client a different fee than an insurance-paying client.
- Practicing out of your home when it isn't permitted by law.

▌ Sources of Ethical Guidance

In attempting to behave ethically, we can turn to a variety of guides, from federal laws and professional codes of ethics to our own internal sense of right and wrong. The following sections discuss a variety of valuable sources of guidance.

Official Codes and Regulations

Ethical conduct is of concern not just to individual practitioners and clients, but also to provider organizations, to our industry as a whole, and to the local, state, and national governments that regulate our practices. When you're faced with a major ethical decision, it's often worthwhile to consult the laws, codes of ethics, and other policies that apply to you.

Laws

Laws are codified rules of conduct set forth by a society and are generally based on shared ethical or moral principles. Laws often set the minimum standard necessary to protect the public's welfare and are enforceable by the courts—which means that violations may be punished by fines, imprisonment, or other penalties (such as a revoked license). Specific laws relating to scope of practice may vary by locale. For example, in some locations massage practitioners aren't permitted to give clients exercises, while in other places no such restrictions exist. Other ethics-related issues addressed by legal statutes include:

- requirements for obtaining and renewing a license to practice
- sanitation and safety precautions in the treatment location (e.g., a nearby sink for therapists to wash their hands and a smoke detector and fire extinguisher)
- draping of clients during treatment
- prohibition of sexual activity in the therapeutic context
- mandatory hours of continuing education

For information about the laws and regulations that apply in your state, consult the state board for your profession (if there is one) or any of the major professional organizations for your type of work.

Professional Codes of Ethics

All major professional organizations have established guidelines for practitioner behavior, known as Codes of Ethics. Their major functions are to:

- inform practitioners of appropriate ethical norms and behavior
- supply direction for challenging situations
- encourage practitioners to provide excellent service
- protect clients
- provide a means for enforcing desired professional behavior

Penalties for violating a professional code of ethics are generally less severe than those for breaking the law; an act deemed unethical but not illegal won't carry a jail term. However, depending on the situation, a practitioner may be barred from membership in the professional organization, have her license revoked, or face other types of disciplinary measures.

Codes of ethics also tend to be much broader and vaguer than laws. There are certain instances where they clearly dictate the desired behavior. For instance, the American Chiropractic Association Code of Ethics states, "It is unethical for a doctor of chiropractic to receive a fee, rebate, rental payment, or any other form of remuneration for the referral of a patient to a clinic, laboratory, or other health service entity." The American Physical Therapy Association Code of Ethics states, "A physical therapist shall not engage in any sexual relationship or activity, whether consensual or nonconsensual, with any patient while a physical therapist/patient relationship exists."

In most cases, however, further research, consultation, and self-exploration are required to determine what is appropriate and ethical. For example, the National Certification Board for Therapeutic Massage and Bodywork (NCBTMB) Code of Ethics states, "Provide treatment only where there is reasonable expectation that it will be advantageous to the client." Some somatic practitioners may interpret the word *advantageous* somewhat narrowly, as referring to an enduring, measurable physical change in the client's body. Others may have a looser interpretation, viewing relaxation as an "advantageous" goal in and of itself, whether or not it's accompanied by lasting physical changes.

As another example, the National Certification Commission for Acupuncture and Oriental Medicine (NCCAOM) Code of Ethics states, "I will continue to work to raise the standards of the profession." This leaves room for wide interpretation; one practitioner might think this means affecting public policy or giving public talks, while another practitioner simply takes it to mean conducting an ethical practice.

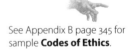

See Appendix B page 345 for sample **Codes of Ethics**.

Organizational Policies and Procedures

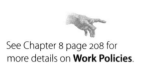

See Chapter 8 page 208 for more details on **Work Policies**.

In addition to laws and professional codes, practitioners who work in a spa, clinic, group practice, or other business are also bound by the policies or procedures of that organization. Many organizations that employ somatic therapists have detailed guidelines on issues such as tipping, relationships with clients, product sales, and the type of hands-on work a practitioner performs. If you encounter an ethical challenge in one of those contexts, their policy statements should provide you with helpful answers.

Personal Ethics and Self-Accountability

No matter what laws, codes, policies, and other external guidelines we follow, we all are powerfully influenced by internal factors as well. These include our personal morals, values, and principles, as well as our sense of self-accountability.

Figure 1.5 Comparing Ethics, Morals, Values, and Principles

Ethics	• System of moral principles and appropriate conduct • Uphold the dignity of the profession • Be client-centered • Adhere to prevailing laws • Stay committed to quality • Respect each client • Remain service-oriented • Work within appropriate scope of practice
Morals	• Standards of right or wrong • Shared assessment, undertaken by a group of people • Usually based on cultural or religious standards • Actions can be judged as moral in one culture and immoral in another
Values	• Beliefs about what is intrinsically worthwhile or desirable • Based upon beliefs and attitudes • Desirable rather than right and correct • People don't necessarily agree on what is worthy • Value structure may change many times over the course of life
Principles	• Individual's rules of behavior • Principled people modify behavior so that each action arises from a deeply held sense of self • Based at least in part upon one's values and morals • May differ widely from one individual to another

---

Morals, Values, and Principles

The concepts of morals, values, and principles are related but not interchangeable. **Morals** are standards by which we judge behaviors and character traits as right or wrong. It's your moral judgment that tells you it's wrong to continue treating a client just because you need the income, when you believe a client would benefit more by seeing a practitioner in a different field. Typically people's morals are shaped by their cultural or religious backgrounds; an action can be judged as moral in one culture and immoral in another. For instance, in the religion of Islam, a woman is forbidden to be unclothed in a room with a man who isn't her husband.

Values are beliefs about what is intrinsically worthwhile or desirable, rather than what is right and correct. For example, if you have a strong value of making your services accessible to everyone, regardless of their economic means, you may be motivated to incorporate a sliding scale into your fee structure. This doesn't mean that you feel a moral obligation to have a sliding scale, to avoid acting unethically; you just view this as a better, more worthwhile arrangement. Individuals don't necessarily agree on what is important as a value, and may even change their own value structures many times over the course of their lives.

An individual's **principles** are the rules or laws of behavior that enable her to behave with integrity. They are based in large part upon personal values and morals. For example, someone who acts upon the principle "Communicate clearly and directly" may be reflecting her value of openness, as well as a moral conviction that it's wrong to be dishonest or mislead people. Like morals and values, principles may differ widely from one individual to another.

Ethical Behavior Evaluation

- Make a list of behaviors you deem unethical.
- What are some behaviors, while unethical in your profession, might be fine in others?
- What unethical behaviors by your colleagues would you feel compelled to report?

Core Values

Your values, and the principles that spring from them, are major conscious and unconscious influences on the decisions you make throughout your life. Many professional and personal conflicts arise because there is a clash of values either within oneself or with others. By investing the time to explore your values, you can help ensure that these values are in synchrony with the way you lead your life and run your business.

The exercise below is designed to help you clarify your core values. Ask yourself the following questions and write down your responses, taking time to carefully consider each one. We have listed sample responses to stimulate your thinking (if needed). When you finish this exercise, we recommend you discuss it with a fellow student, friend, or colleague. Engaging in a dialogue with others is another way to more fully explore your own values.

Core Values Assessment

- What values are most important to me?
- What are the character traits I deem essential?
- Who and what have been major influences in my values development?
- What are my attitudes and beliefs about wellness?
- What are my attitudes and beliefs about my profession?
- What are the most important personal characteristics for someone in my field?
- What are the most important professional characteristics for someone in my field?
- What are the crucial characteristics for a practitioner in my field to be effective?
- How do my values affect my work with clients?
- Which of my personal values could conflict with professional rules of conduct?
- Which of my personal values could conflict with laws or regulations?
- How do my values enhance my professionalism?

Practical Application: Core Values Assessment

Here are some sample responses to the questions asked in the previous activity:

- **WHAT VALUES ARE MOST IMPORTANT TO ME?**
  Being honest; treating myself and others with respect and kindness; trusting my intuition; appreciating nature; acknowledging people for their support.
- **WHAT ARE THE CHARACTER TRAITS I DEEM ESSENTIAL?**
  The ability to communicate; patience; a sense of humor; the ability to listen without giving advice; honesty; integrity.
- **WHO AND WHAT HAVE BEEN MAJOR INFLUENCES IN MY VALUES DEVELOPMENT?**
  My mother; my father; my third grade teacher; my mentor; Martin Luther King, Jr.; psychotherapy; my decision to pursue this profession; Outward Bound experiences.
- **WHAT ARE MY ATTITUDES AND BELIEFS ABOUT WELLNESS?**
  If people exercise regularly they live long and healthy lives; good health involves a balanced body, mind, and spirit; it takes a lot of work to be healthy; just because you have a disability doesn't mean you're sick; the best path to wellness is through acupuncture/massage/chiropractic/yoga.
- **WHAT ARE MY ATTITUDES AND BELIEFS ABOUT MY PROFESSION?**
  It is really the best path to getting and staying healthy; it complements other types of health care; it feels like a good vehicle for me to make a difference in other people's lives; this profession has a proven track record for effectiveness.
- **WHAT ARE THE MOST IMPORTANT PERSONAL CHARACTERISTICS FOR SOMEONE IN MY FIELD?**
  Intuition; empathy; a sincere desire to help others; patience; humor; good boundaries.
- **WHAT ARE THE MOST IMPORTANT PROFESSIONAL CHARACTERISTICS FOR SOMEONE IN MY FIELD?**
  Hard work; punctuality; skillful touch; professional proficiency; dedication; excellent communication skills; integrity; good professional boundaries.
- **WHAT ARE THE CRUCIAL CHARACTERISTICS FOR A PRACTITIONER IN MY FIELD TO BE EFFECTIVE?**
  The ability to connect with people and create a safe environment; the ability to admit mistakes; the ability to recognize conditions in individuals beyond my professional expertise capabilities; investing in continuing education; using high-quality products and equipment.
- **HOW DO MY VALUES AFFECT MY WORK WITH CLIENTS?**
  I believe everyone should behave responsibly, therefore I charge when people cancel without giving 24 hours notice; one of my values is giving back to the community, so I hold a free clinic one day a month; I believe people should participate in their care, therefore I discuss my overall treatment plan and give self-care exercises for clients to do on their own.
- **WHICH OF MY PERSONAL VALUES COULD CONFLICT WITH PROFESSIONAL RULES OF CONDUCT?**
  I believe I should be allowed to mention the names of my celebrity clients to my friends and family but the confidentiality code of my profession prohibits it; I like to reward people when they help me in my business with referrals, but my professional code of ethics doesn't allow me to do that.
- **WHICH OF MY PERSONAL VALUES COULD CONFLICT WITH LAWS OR REGULATIONS?**
  I believe in limited government regulation, but my profession requires a license; I believe I should be allowed to work out of my home, but the zoning laws in my area don't permit home offices.
- **HOW DO MY VALUES ENHANCE MY PROFESSIONALISM?**
  My commitment to open communication with my clients makes me a more effective practitioner; my good boundaries create a safe environment for my clients; my honesty with my clients instills trust in me as a professional and in my profession as a whole.

Points to Ponder

Which of the above questions were hardest for you to answer? What kind of purposeful study and consideration can you give those subjects as you build your ethical practice? Which of your answers motivate you to change your attitude or behavior?

Self-Accountability

Self-accountability is the cornerstone of ethics. It is about who you are and what you do when no one's watching you. When you have a well-developed sense of self-accountability, you're honest with yourself, and you're answerable and fully responsible for what you say and do at all times. Part of self-accountability is to refrain from blaming others for your behavior. You have the ability to look beyond the immediate moment to consider all the consequences and know if you're willing to accept them. You have personal ethics. As individuals, it's our capacity for self-accountability that keeps us functioning ethically and responsibly.

Personal ethics are the precursor to professional ethics: you're not likely to be more ethical in your professional life than you are in your personal life. As the saying goes, "No matter where you go, there you are." If you're dishonest in your personal life, you're most likely dishonest in your business affairs as well. Likewise, if you can't keep the secret of a friend, your client's confidentiality is at risk.

Dan Ariely, in his book, *The (Honest) Truth About Dishonesty*,[5] makes the following statement:

> Most people think of themselves as honest, but, in fact, we all cheat. From Washington to Wall Street, the classroom to the workplace, unethical behavior is everywhere. None of us is immune, whether it's the white lie to head off trouble or padding our expense reports. Generally, we assume that cheating, like most other decisions, is based on a rational cost-benefit analysis. But it's actually the irrational forces that we don't take into account that often determine whether we behave ethically or not.

According to Mark Annett in his book *The Scruples Methodology*,[6] whenever you decide to take an action that some might construe as unethical, or neglect to act when it's ethically required, you should be aware that you're taking a risk at three different levels:

> The first level of risk is personal. People are always observing other people's behavior. If you act unethically in one situation then people will assume you might act that way in others. Consequently, people may begin to distrust you and your judgment, even under unrelated circumstances. For instance, if a co-worker hears you convincingly lie to a customer then your co-worker might think, "Wow, she is really good at lying. I wonder if I could tell I was being lied to or not." From that moment on, mistrust begins to build.
>
> The second level of risk is to your company. People learn by example. If top management is doing things that are unethical then people might get the message that it's okay for them to do the same. For instance, if the company just cheated another company out of $50,000, then my stealing $50 in office supplies doesn't seem so bad.
>
> Finally, being unethical also places your industry at risk. For instance, take telemarketers. I will absolutely not give out my credit card information, even to charities. Now, not all telemarketers are unethical. But, the ones that are have so badly damaged their reputation that the whole industry is tainted.

Ethical Congruence Checklist

In practicing self-accountability, we strive for *ethical congruence*: making decisions that are congruent—consistent or in alignment—with the ethical values that apply to each situation. Whenever you're contemplating an action (or inaction) that you find questionable, you can use the following questions to test for ethical congruence. Ask yourself:

- ❏ What does your gut say?
- ❏ Do you get butterflies just thinking about the issue?
- ❏ Do you have doubts?
- ❏ Do you need to sacrifice any of your personal or professional values?
- ❏ Is it against the law, policies, or a professional code of ethics?
- ❏ Is this fair to all concerned parties in the short term as well as the long run?
- ❏ How would it hold up to scrutiny if all the details were made public?

Why Cheaters And Liars Think They're Honest, Wonderful People (video)

http://www.upworthy.com/why-cheaters-and-liars-think-theyre-honest-wonderful-people

" Whenever you do a thing, act as if all the world were watching.

—Thomas Jefferson

□ How would you feel if the people you hold in high esteem knew your decision?

□ How would you feel if your decision was emblazoned on the headline of your local newspaper?

□ How would you feel about yourself when all is done?

If any of your answers suggest that you're facing an ethical conflict, use this information as a cue to step back and re-evaluate your options. You might find it helpful to proceed to the next section on resolving ethical dilemmas.

Practical Application: Ethical Congruence in an Academic Setting

The situation: The instructor in one of my classes has given us a take-home exam. Although I got the impression that she expected everyone to complete it independently, she never explicitly stated that or prohibited collaboration. Two of my friends in the class are planning to work on the exam together and they invited me to join them. I'm considering whether I should.

1. **WHAT DOES YOUR GUT SAY?**
   I'm excited at the idea of getting help with the exam, but also feel a bit uneasy about it. I feel as though I'm being sneaky and trying to get away with something.

2. **DO YOU GET BUTTERFLIES JUST THINKING ABOUT THE ISSUE?**
   Yes, a little bit.

3. **DO YOU HAVE DOUBTS?**
   Yes. I'm not entirely sure what to do.

4. **ARE YOU NEEDING TO SACRIFICE ANY OF YOUR PERSONAL OR PROFESSIONAL VALUES?**
   Possibly. One of my values is to be very clear, direct, and honest in my communication. If I did decide to collaborate with my friends, I wouldn't want to talk openly about it with my instructor or with other students, in case they thought it was wrong. I might even be tempted to lie. To stay true to my values, I would need to ask the instructor up-front whether collaborating on the exam was okay.

5. **IS IT AGAINST THE LAW, POLICIES, OR A PROFESSIONAL CODE OF ETHICS?**
   No, not directly.

6. **IS THIS FAIR TO ALL CONCERNED PARTIES IN THE SHORT TERM AS WELL AS THE LONG RUN?**
   Possibly not. If other students assumed they needed to work independently, this collaboration could give me and my friends an unfair advantage.

7. **HOW WOULD IT HOLD UP TO SCRUTINY IF ALL THE DETAILS WERE MADE PUBLIC?**
   Even though I wouldn't be breaking any explicit rule, other people might still think of this collaboration as unethical.

8. **HOW WOULD YOU FEEL IF THE PEOPLE YOU HOLD IN HIGH ESTEEM KNEW YOUR DECISION?**
   I'd be nervous about how they might judge me, and worried they might lose trust in me.

9. **HOW WOULD YOU FEEL IF YOUR DECISION WAS EMBLAZONED ON THE HEADLINE OF YOUR LOCAL NEWSPAPER?**
   Nervous and embarrassed.

10. **HOW WOULD YOU FEEL ABOUT YOURSELF WHEN ALL IS DONE?**
    I think I'd regret the decision and feel badly about myself.

Using the Ethical Congruence Checklist helped this student to identify the uneasy feelings she was having and why she was having them. In this case, the student probably needs to ask her teacher directly if collaboration is allowed or do the assignment by herself.

Points to Ponder

Have you ever found yourself in a similar situation? Did you ignore your own feelings, or did you reach out for assistance with the situation?

Exploring how any situation matches up with your own personal ethics is the first step in self-accountability. Taking responsibility for your personal and professional ethics, and honestly evaluating tricky situations, is crucial to resolving ethical dilemmas.

Resolving Ethical Dilemmas

Earlier in this chapter we talked about the concepts of duties and rights. In some situations, two or more duties, rights, or a combination of duties and rights are in conflict. As a result, regardless of what action you take, something of value will be compromised. These situations are referred to as ethical dilemmas.

Consider two examples:

1. A minor comes to see you for an evaluation. He is in pain from a soft tissue injury and you feel confident that you can relieve his pain after several weeks of treatment. You tell him you need parental permission before you can work on him. He informs you that his parents refuse to let him see you for treatment and he has come to see you without their knowledge. He pleads with you to work on him without getting parental consent. In this case your duty to do good (beneficence) conflicts with your duty to obtain informed consent (which, for a minor, must come from the parents).

2. A client, in discussing her stress, reveals that she is excessive in her corporeal punishment of her child. You feel torn between your client's right to confidentiality and your duty to protect the welfare of the child, which would lead you to report her to the child welfare authorities. (In many places the law requires that you report suspected child abuse.)

Points to Ponder

How does it feel when you're faced with an ethical dilemma? How can you be sure to consider all the options and consequences before making a decision?

"How to resolve ethical dilemmas"

http://www.ehow.com/ how_5904872_resolve-ethical-dilemmas.html

Ethical dilemmas are by their nature complex, troubling, and difficult to resolve. In addition to ethical codes, laws, organizational policies, and the community's expectations, you must also examine your personal values and practical considerations.

Many ethical dilemmas involve a strong emotional component. From a purely logical, detached standpoint, the "right" decision may be relatively clear, and yet in practice we feel conflicted about what to do. For instance, you may have a policy of never socializing with clients, but have trouble saying no when a client you really like offers an extra ticket to a sold-out concert you've been longing to attend. Or suppose a close colleague gives you a treatment that you don't particularly enjoy, and then asks for a testimonial; you may worry that saying anything negative will hurt her feelings or damage your relationship.

The Six-Step Resolution Model

When you're facing an ethical dilemma, the following model can help you to think through the problem and make an informed decision. It is adapted from the problem-solving process outlined by Corey, Corey, and Callahan in their book *Issues and Ethics in the Helping Professions*.[7] Keep in mind that this processing model is just a starting point. In the words of Frank Navran, a leading consultant on organizational ethics, "The process alone doesn't guarantee an ethical outcome. Unfortunately, only the decision maker can do that."

1. **IDENTIFY THE PROBLEM**
   - Gather as much relevant information as possible.
   - Talk to the parties involved.
   - Clarify the nature of the problem: legal, values, moral, ethical, or a combination.

2. **IDENTIFY THE POTENTIAL ISSUES INVOLVED**
   - List and describe the critical issues.
   - Evaluate the rights, responsibilities, and welfare of those affected by the decision.
   - Consider the basic moral principles of autonomy, beneficence, nonmaleficence, and justice.
   - Ascertain the potential dangers to the practitioner, client, and the profession. (Refer to the Impacts from Ethical Breaches chart on page 4.)

3. **REVIEW YOUR PROFESSION'S CODE OF ETHICS AND RELEVANT LAWS**
   - Determine if this issue violates either the letter or the spirit of applicable laws, regulations, or professional codes (on a national, state, or local level).
   - Check if your policies or procedures address this issue.

4. **EVALUATE POTENTIAL COURSES OF ACTION**
   - Brainstorm lots of ideas. Usually the first few options are based upon your personal values or an emotional response to the issue. Delve deeply for potential courses of action that aren't necessarily apparent at first.
   - Enumerate the benefits, drawbacks, and possible outcomes of various decisions.
   - Consider the consequences of inaction.
   - Contemplate how you'll feel about yourself when all is done.

5. **OBTAIN CONSULTATION**
   - Engage in self-reflection. Identify which of your personal and professional values could be impacted by the various actions. Walk through the Ethical Congruence Checklist.
   - Consider how members of your community and the larger society might view these actions.
   - Determine the impact these actions could have on your profession. (Colleagues or a supervisor can add an outside perspective.)
   - Ask colleagues or supervisors for their reflections on the dilemma and what they might decide if they were in your position. Use the Ethical Congruence Checklist as a guide for your discussions.
   - Justify a course of action based on sound reasoning which you can test in a consultation. (It is a serious warning sign if you don't want to talk to another person about actions you're contemplating.)

6. **DETERMINE THE BEST COURSE OF ACTION**
   - Map out the best way to resolve the problem: If multiple parties are involved, who should be contacted first? Do you need outside support? Do you need to talk to a supervisor?
   - Consider who, if anyone, should know about the problem (such as a work supervisor, friend, client, doctor, police, professional association, school, or colleague).

> You'll never have all the information you need to make a decision. If you did, it would be a foregone conclusion, not a decision.
>
> —David Mahoney

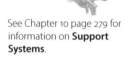

See Chapter 10 page 279 for information on **Support Systems**.

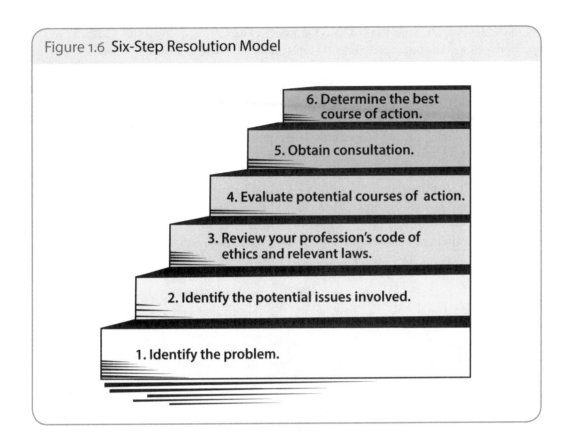

Figure 1.6 Six-Step Resolution Model

6. Determine the best course of action.

5. Obtain consultation.

4. Evaluate potential courses of action.

3. Review your profession's code of ethics and relevant laws.

2. Identify the potential issues involved.

1. Identify the problem.

Practical Application: Ethical Dilemma Resolution

A chiropractor offers you financial remuneration for every client you refer to her. You like the chiropractor's work and you refer clients to her even without financial incentive. You're fairly confident you won't yield to temptation and send additional clients for financial motives. You need to decide whether you should accept the offer. You're under financial pressure and every dollar helps.

1. **IDENTIFY THE PROBLEM**
An opportunity exists to make more money. You feel reasonably sure that the financial incentive won't influence your referral decisions. You lean toward saying yes, but want to make sure you have thoroughly examined the issue and are acting ethically.

2. **IDENTIFY THE POTENTIAL ISSUES INVOLVED**
You think the critical issue is: Can this action and my desire to earn more money conflict in any way with my duty to do no harm and to benefit the client? Also, would it in any way harm my profession?

You consider the possible dangers of taking this action. First, you acknowledge there is a risk that you'll be influenced to refer some clients who only have a borderline potential for benefitting from chiropractic work. You also realize that a client might suffer emotional harm if he later found out that you were given a financial kickback for the referral. You imagine it would create a general sense of mistrust toward you; the client couldn't be sure that you did not refer at least partially for your own financial gain. Depending on the nature of the treatment relationship, this realization could create a small or very large negative impact on the client. It seems quite unlikely that any clients will find out, but the fact you don't want them to know about the arrangement raises a red flag for you.

Additionally, you identify a possible risk for your profession. If someone found out that you accept financial incentives, they might conclude that your discipline is a less than legitimate profession, because many healthcare professions prohibit this type of arrangement.

3. **REVIEW YOUR PROFESSION'S CODE OF ETHICS AND RELEVANT LAWS**

You review your professional organization's code of ethics and read, "Refuse any gifts or benefits which are intended to influence a referral, decision, or treatment that are purely for personal gain and not the good of others." You review the chiropractic code and nothing in this code explicitly states that a chiropractor can't *offer* a "reward." After reading the various codes you aren't entirely sure whether the action you're considering is prohibited. You don't intend to refer purely for personal gain. But you can imagine that the action you're considering could be seen as a failure to act with honesty and integrity.

You review the laws governing your discipline and find no relevant statutes prohibiting the giving or receiving of financial incentives. By talking to friends and colleagues, you find out that this behavior is generally viewed as an unacceptable practice in health care.

4. **EVALUATE POTENTIAL COURSES OF ACTION**

The possible courses of action are: a) accept the offer; b) propose a change to the offer; and c) refuse the offer.

   a. **Accept the offer**

   The obvious benefit associated with this option is the financial gain. However, given all the risks you identified in step 2, you decide that if you accept the chiropractor's offer, you'll disclose the arrangement to your clients.

   b. **Propose a change to the offer**

   Instead of receiving direct financial rewards, you could set up an alternative type of incentive system. For instance, for each referral, the chiropractor could give you a $10 gift certificate for chiropractic services, redeemable by you or anyone you designate. A variation on this would be a special reward after certain levels of referral (e.g., a certificate for a full treatment after the third referral). This option feels better to you, particularly since you plan to mainly offer the certificates to clients in financial need who could benefit from those services. This arrangement raises many of the same concerns that you identified with the original proposal. You determine that if you decide to go with this option, you'll disclose the arrangement to your clients.

   c. **Refuse the offer**

   A straight refusal would allow you to avoid the risks associated with accepting or changing the offer. As you contemplate this option you feel some sense of relief, knowing you don't need to have those lingering concerns hanging over your head. The only drawback that occurs to you—apart from the lost potential for financial gain—is the possibility of straining your relationship with the chiropractor.

5. **OBTAIN CONSULTATION**

Talking to colleagues, you get a mixed reaction. Some think the arrangement is okay, and others don't. Although no consensus exists, you're surprised by how strongly several colleagues express their sense that the action you're contemplating is wrong.

6. **DETERMINE THE BEST COURSE OF ACTION**

You choose to refuse the offer. As an alternative, you suggest to the chiropractor that you and she show appreciation for each other's support through the professional courtesy of working on each other when needed. You also suggest negotiating a strategic partnership in which you offer mutual clients discounted fees.

Points to Ponder

Is this resolution model complete? Are there other questions you can ask yourself or other steps you can take when you find yourself in an ethical dilemma? Would you have taken the same action as the practitioner in this example? Why or why not?

Sometimes working through these six steps can be done quickly. Other times it can take many hours to do the research, contemplate, and get feedback. It can be tempting to skip some of the steps or only look for one or two potential solutions. We encourage you to invest the requisite time so that you make better informed decisions when you encounter ethical dilemmas.

▌ Conclusion

After reading this chapter, you have all the background knowledge you need to start exploring the specific ethical challenges we discuss in the remainder of the book. You've learned about the unique combination of factors involved in therapeutic relationships, together with the duties and rights they entail, as well as several universal ethical principles that apply to all human interactions. You've also learned about various sources of guidance on ethical issues, from laws and ethical codes to your own personal ethics and self-accountability.

In addition, you now have a set of tools to reference whenever you encounter a tough ethical issue. Your completed Core Values Assessment serves as a lasting record of the personal and professional values you strive to embody. The Ethical Congruence Checklist gives you a relatively quick way to test whether the action you're contemplating might be ethically questionable. And the Six-Step Resolution Model provides a comprehensive framework for thinking through all the relevant ethical factors, to ensure that the decision you make is a truly informed and responsible choice.

2
Boundaries

"Good fences make good neighbors."
—Robert Frost

Key Terms

Attitude	Interactive Boundary	Privacy
Boundary	Permeable Boundary	Rigid Boundary
Boundary Crossing	Personal Boundary	Self-Disclosure
Boundary Violation	Power Differential	Semi-Permeable Boundary

S ome types of boundaries are very simple and clear cut. For instance, any competent surveyors can clearly draw the boundary that separates the property of two neighbors. Unfortunately, that kind of simplicity and clarity doesn't exist in the relationships between people, especially in practitioner/client relationships. In relationships, a boundary is a limit that separates one person from another. It protects the integrity of each person. A boundary can be as tangible as the skin that surrounds our body or as intangible as an attitude. The primary problem in defining boundaries is that in most instances they're intangible.

Understanding boundaries is crucial to creating an ethical practice and building professional relationships. By increasing your awareness of your clients' boundaries (as well as your own), you improve the therapeutic relationship and avoid many inadvertent slips into unethical behavior. To begin this process it would be good to clarify the knowledge you already possess. If the following activity doesn't seem clear to you, don't worry—it takes time to understand the breadth of this material. And it's an ongoing learning experience.

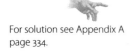

For solution see Appendix A page 334.

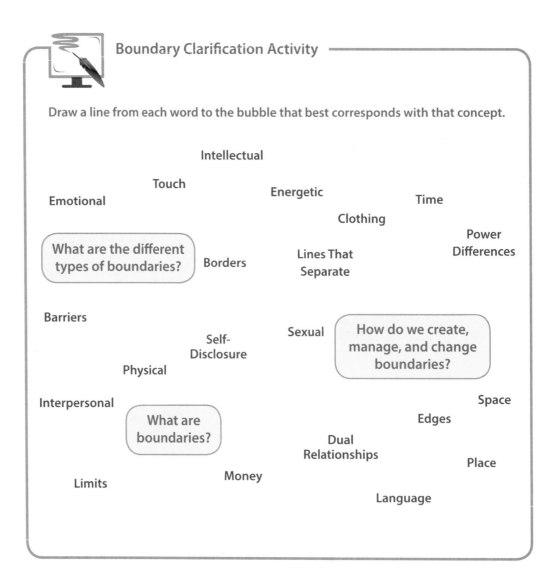

Boundary Clarification Activity

Draw a line from each word to the bubble that best corresponds with that concept.

Intellectual

Touch

Emotional

Energetic

Time

Clothing

Power Differences

What are the different types of boundaries?

Borders

Lines That Separate

Barriers

Sexual

How do we create, manage, and change boundaries?

Self-Disclosure

Physical

Interpersonal

Space

Edges

What are boundaries?

Dual Relationships

Place

Limits

Money

Language

▌ What Are Boundaries?

Boundaries separate people from their environment and from other people. They are elusive, yet personally discernible, lines that distinguish you from everything and everyone around you. They define your personal space—the area you occupy which you appropriately feel is under your control.

Most likely, you have had the experience of someone standing too close to you or touching you without your permission. What that person has done, knowingly or not, is invaded your space and crossed your physical boundary. Boundaries are not only physical though. They also protect emotions and thoughts. Boundaries provide a sense of safety. They help you to sense how close or far away you want people, both physically and emotionally. Often you're unaware of your boundaries unless they're threatened or crossed.

Each person faces innumerable boundary decisions each day. Whom do you greet with a smile, with a handshake, with a hug, or with a kiss? What information about yourself do you disclose to which people? With whom do you cry when you're sad, or vent when you're angry? To make things even more confusing, the boundaries may fluctuate because they're both idiosyncratic and contextual. Boundaries are idiosyncratic because they reflect each person's likes, dislikes, cultural background, temperament, and history. They are contextual because they can change depending on the situation. Behavior that is deemed appropriate at one time may be highly offensive in another setting. For instance you don't touch a client in the same way off the treatment table as you do when he is receiving a treatment because the context is different. Even involving the same person, the context can influence boundaries becoming more fluid or rigid. For example, some people who like to be affectionate in private are very uncomfortable with public displays of affection. Although some interpersonal boundaries are fairly stable, others require ongoing sensitivity to changes in time, place, and emotional state.

See Chapter 4 page 81 and Chapter 5 page 109 for **Communication Skills** and for specific **Communication Techniques**.

Most people find it stressful to discuss boundary issues. Their upbringing seldom prepares them to do this effectively. In her book, *Parents, Teens and Boundaries*, Dr. Jane Bluestein notes that for most people there has been a severe shortage of healthy role models in this important aspect of family relationships. Furthermore, knowledge of how to set and maintain boundaries "isn't typically a part of a child's education. If anything, most of us have been conditioned not to set boundaries as a way to avoid the negative reactions of others."[1] Thus, most clients and many, if not most, practitioners are ill-equipped to freely discuss boundaries.

Negative reactions can occur as part of any personal boundary discussions. People like to think well of themselves. So if you suggest that their behavior is causing you discomfort because they're encroaching on your space, they're apt to feel hurt or angry—or both. Then you must communicate about their feelings and your boundary needs. Unless you're a very skilled communicator, you may decide it isn't even worth the effort to raise the issue.

Boundary issues between a practitioner and a client are especially sensitive. Helping relationships often require the client to make unusual boundary adjustments. For example, in very few settings other than health care are people expected to undress shortly after meeting practitioners, then permit the practitioners to touch them or insert needles into their bodies. In this vulnerable state, they may be expected to tell the practitioners aspects of their life history that they have told no one else, or allow practitioners to manipulate their muscles and bones in ways that are uncomfortable. The healthcare practitioner is accustomed to these types of boundary adjustments. They are part of his daily work life, year in and year out. For the client, though, these adjustments may be an unusual and stressful experience. In this uncharted territory, clients may not even be aware of their own needs, options, or of what constitutes appropriate boundaries and behavior.

Types of Boundaries

The five major types of interpersonal boundaries are physical, emotional, intellectual, sexual, and energetic.

> ### Figure 2.1 The Five Major Boundary Types
>
> ## Physical • Emotional • Intellectual
> ## Sexual • Energetic

The Physical Boundary

In day-to-day human interactions, people regularly monitor their physical boundary—usually without being aware of it. For example, when standing in line at the bank or milling around with strangers on a public transportation platform, with little effort, they all find the appropriate "comfortable" distance to keep—their physical boundary. In the American culture, the majority of people prefer a space in front and back that extends about an arm's length from the body (approximately two to three feet). The space deemed comfortable at the sides of the body seems narrower for most people, about a foot or so.

In nearly all human interactions the physical space contained within this invisible line may expand or shrink depending on the individual's level of comfort and safety. People generally allow someone they like and know well to move closer to them than someone they don't know. However, if they're upset about something or angry with another person, the limit of the boundary changes dramatically. If you feel fear toward someone, you may create more distance from that particular person. If you feel safe with someone and you feel sad, your boundary may change to allow that person to be very close. When there is a perceived threat to the boundary, monitoring becomes more heightened. Being on an elevator with only one other person who has an unkempt appearance and a menacing look may cause uneasiness. Most often, people purposely attempt to create some small measure of personal space in an effort to minimize the discomfort of having their physical boundary crossed. These changes in the physical boundary may occur instantaneously. For instance, when you get really annoyed at your spouse, you don't want him to touch you at that moment.

Physical boundaries also vary in a professional setting. When a somatic practitioner is in an actual session, it's appropriate to be in physical contact, yet during the pre- and post-session, that same physical contact is inappropriate. As another example, clothing which often serves as a protective boundary may be removed to some extent in the treatment setting. The physical boundaries also shift depending on the part of the body being treated and the intensity of the treatment. For instance, working in the mouth may elicit thoughts such as, "Get out of my mouth!" whereas working on the hand or shoulders is usually less threatening. The setting modifies the boundary. While a physical boundary may be more tangible than other types, it must always be carefully considered.

> It is what we think we know already that often prevents us from learning.
>
> —Claude Bernard

The Emotional Boundary

In many ways people are defined by their emotions and how they feel in the moment. The people we love, the things that make us afraid, the sadness and losses in our lives, and the situations that bring us joy, are major components of our personal identity. To reveal our feelings means that we have decided to trust another with an important part of ourselves, and thereby create a kind of intimacy with that person. The emotional boundary may change with each situation; and it influences whether a person expresses his feelings and how he chooses to do that with others.

Consequently, it's important to be conscious of your own and your clients' emotional boundaries. If not, and boundaries are crossed, it can be as painful and as difficult to heal (or even more so) as a violation of our physical boundaries. For example, everyone knows the anger, anguish, and shame that occur when someone reveals a personal confidence to others. The actual content of what is revealed is often less significant than the sense of violation that occurs from the betrayal of trust.

Respect for emotional boundaries is essential to any healthy relationship.

The Intellectual Boundary

Like emotions, a person's thoughts, beliefs, and opinions form a significant part of her identity. They help to create a world view and define an individual as different and separate from others. If our belief system is accepted, encouraged, or even respectfully challenged, we feel respected and validated. If our ideas and beliefs are ridiculed, criticized, ignored, dismissed, or punished, our sense of self may be shaken, and we may become hesitant to speak openly about our ideas. For instance, it might be challenging to remain open with a fellow practitioner if, after you share some of your deeply-held beliefs about wellness, he responds, "You don't really believe that, do you?!"

The Sexual Boundary

The sexual boundary can be thought of as a subset of the physical or the physical and emotional boundaries. Sexual boundaries are created by determining with whom, when, where, and how we wish to express our sexuality. Any of these boundaries can be treated respectfully or violated.

See Chapter 6 page 129 for more information on **Sex, Touch, and Intimacy**.

The sexual boundary is also determined by the context of the relationship. Healthcare professionals should not have sexual relationships with their clients. Period. Issues of crossing sexual boundaries in the healthcare professions are of such significance and concern that they have led to numerous regulations and professional ethics statements regarding inappropriate sexual behavior with clients and in the workplace. Violation of the sexual boundary can also be a violation of the law. Know the requirements of your state or regulatory board. Ignorance of the law is not a defense.

Violating the sexual boundary with a client can violate all the other boundaries as well. Respecting it isn't only the ethical choice, it's the therapeutic choice as well.

The Energetic Boundary

For thousands of years, various cultures throughout the world have shared a belief in the existence of an energy flow within the body. Whether we call it chi (Chinese), prana (Sanskrit), mana (Polynesian), lung (Tibetan), or élan vital (French), the basic idea is the same: the energy that runs through us is an essential part of who we are, influencing both our physical and mental wellbeing. Even from a purely scientific perspective, there is no doubt that we are energetic, as well as material, beings. Human bodies are composed of substances that conduct electrical currents, and the body actually generates an electromagnetic field.

The energetic boundary can be considered to encompass the other four types of boundaries, reflecting our overall way of being in the world. Consciously or unconsciously, we all shift this boundary depending on the context we're in. When we're enjoying time with our family or close friends, we tend to open up; we express ourselves more freely, in a variety of ways, and are generally receptive to what's happening around us. When we're in a situation that's not safe or comfortable—emotionally, physically, intellectually, or sexually—we tend to shut down and close our energetic boundaries. Imagine getting lost in a foreign city and ending up in a potentially dangerous area. The natural response is to energetically withdraw, staying quiet and avoiding eye contact or any other interactions with the people around you.

Somatic therapists need to strike a fine balance energetically. It's important to stay sufficiently open and receptive to connect with the client and track their responses through the course of a session. At the same time, practitioners must maintain a clear boundary, both to protect themselves from being excessively influenced by the client's energy and to prevent their own energy from crossing the client's boundary inappropriately. Consider the following two scenarios:

1. A massage therapist was having some business difficulties that caused him a great deal of worry. During one of his sessions with a female survivor of abuse who was extremely sensitive to the quality of his touch, his thoughts wandered back to those issues. He performed all the same techniques as he usually did, but his mind was elsewhere. At the end of the session, the client told him she didn't feel good about the treatment. "You weren't really there," she said. "I could feel it in your hands." The therapist realized she was right, offered a sincere apology, and waived his fee for the session.

2. A chiropractor seeking healing from an early trauma has started visiting a psychotherapist on her day off. The therapy leaves her feeling open and vulnerable, in a way she hasn't experienced since childhood. One week, due to a change in the therapist's schedule, she has her session during a lunch break. Immediately after her return to the office, she treats a patient who is going through a messy divorce and experiencing severe back pain. While she's working, he tells her a long story about the latest crisis in his battle to get custody of his children. By the end of the session, he says he's feeling much better. The chiropractor, on the other hand, feels nauseated and exhausted. She cancels the rest of the day's appointments, drives home, and breaks down in tears.

Points to Ponder

The scenarios above illustrate two ways in which a practitioner may fail to manage their energy effectively—not being energetically present, and not having a clear energetic boundary. If these problems were to continue over time, what effects might that have on the practitioners' therapeutic relationships? How might these problems contribute to other types of boundary crossings?

The idea of managing your energy can seem vague and mysterious until you experience the effects of not doing it well, as the practitioners in these two scenarios did. If you find yourself feeling drained or sick after working with certain people, or if you start to develop some of the same symptoms as your clients, make an effort to strengthen your energetic boundaries. Your own health and safety, as well as that of your clients, may depend on it.[2]

Touch and the Energetic Boundary

Ask a friend to join you in this exercise. While you're seated, ask your friend to stand behind you, with her hands resting on your shoulders. Have your friend think of an angry or peaceful experience from her past, and ask her not to tell you which experience she has chosen. Her hands remain on your shoulders for a minute while she remembers the experience. Notice how you feel. Does the contact feel pleasant or unpleasant? Does it trigger any emotions, thoughts, sensations, or urges within you? Can you guess which type of experience she recalled? Switch places and do the exercise again.

Put one hand on your friend's arm and really focus on making contact with her arm. At some point, allow your mind to wander off to an unrelated topic, and then later bring your attention back. Her job is to see whether she can tell each time your attention shifts, and if so, notice how she knows it has shifted. Then switch roles and repeat the activity.

How Boundaries Develop

Boundaries are innate, developmental, and learned. By innate we mean that there seems to be a genetic quality to the types of boundaries humans develop. Many characteristics of personality and boundaries are discernible in children at very young ages. For example, traits of reticence or of openness are often observable very early in life, and appear to have little to do with learned behavior or environmental influence. Research studies of twins separated early in life and tested as adults, suggests that the quality of their boundaries are quite similar.[3]

However, many boundaries (socially appropriate as well as self-defeating ones) are learned early in life. Boundary development is influenced by experiences with the environment, family, teachers, neighbors, culture, and the world as a whole.

The environmental influences include both the culture at large and the culture within the family. However, the family's influence on boundaries is always influenced by cultural ethnicity, societal mores, social class, laws, and educational experiences. In this section we look at the effect of family and culture on boundary development.

Figure 2.2 **How Boundaries Develop**

The Family	The Culture at Large
• Privacy • Physical Contact • Emotional Connection and Expression • Sexual Attitudes • Sensitivity • Intellectual Expression	• Schools • Media • Religion and Religious Groups • Voluntary Social Groups

The Family

Boundaries emerge and become shaped through relationships with a close circle of caretakers such as parents or other significant individuals who help raise the child. This occurs gradually and primarily unconsciously. All families are guided by both spoken and unspoken rules—sometimes in conflict. Among the factors in family life that shape early boundary development are privacy, physical contact, emotional expression, intellectual freedom, and sexual attitudes.

A family's attitudes about each of these areas are themselves influenced by culture and family history. Clearly there are different ethnic norms about each. For example, in some cultures emotions are expressed loudly and passionately, while in others such explosiveness would be inappropriate and frightening. Similarly, there are different ethnic/cultural expectations about issues such as privacy and physical contact. Therefore, it's important to consider each of the following areas within the context of ethnic or cultural expectations.

"
Our first line of defense in raising children with values is modeling good behavior ourselves. This is critical. How will our kids learn tolerance for others if our hearts are filled with hate? Learn compassion if we are indifferent? Perceive academics as important if soccer practice is a higher priority than homework?

—Fred G. Gosman

Privacy

In some family environments, a right to privacy is clear and guides behavior about dressing and undressing, bathroom privacy, and the right to personal space. In other family settings, the code of accepted behavior may be entirely different; doors may always remain opened, or even if closed, a family member may enter a room at any time without requesting permission. If the family style is one that provides for privacy, a person's boundaries may move easily from permeable to rigid within the whole range of boundary interaction. However, if there is limited privacy, a person may develop rigid or distancing boundaries as a way of creating privacy. Or he might have mostly permeable boundaries, having lost a sense of privacy.

Physical Contact

Demonstrating physical affection in some families is a significant part of family relationships. Physical contact, if present, occurs in varying degrees and may be expressed through hugging, physical playfulness, kissing, and holding hands. In some families open and warm contact is expected and children are included without inquiring whether touch is wanted; in others children are asked if they want physical touch. Some families experience little physical contact among family members; hugging may be very rare and children rarely witness physical affection expressed between their parents. These behaviors influence how the child responds to her body's physical boundary and what characterizes her degree of comfort with physical contact as she grows into an adult.

Emotional Connection and Expression

Emotional connection is the process by which a person is known emotionally within the family. Emotional expression refers to how emotions are dealt with in the family. Is it common for emotions to be expressed, or is this rare? Are certain emotions acceptable and others not? Do emotions explode or modulate according to the situation? Is emotional expression acknowledged and attended, or avoided? Is there emotional warmth or coolness in the family? Some families maintain a wide range of emotional connection and expression, while in others it's rather narrow. These factors influence how humans set emotional boundaries as they grow and mature.

Intellectual Expression

Some families support intellectual development while others suppress this natural expression of human curiosity and exploration. In one family, a child's independent thoughts and ideas are encouraged and engaged with attention and care. In another family no forum or space is provided for this self-expression to occur. In the extreme circumstance, a young person may be berated and their ideas ridiculed.

Sexual Attitudes

Parents transmit their feelings about sexuality in both overt and subtle ways. Children have many questions about the sexual parts of their bodies: they may engage in sex play, touch themselves, and later may begin to masturbate. How parents respond to these situations gives the child early cues to parental sexual attitudes. Sexual attitudes are cemented into the child's belief system through the parents' attitudes and beliefs about premarital sex, sex education, how comfortable they are talking about sexuality, religious influences, and whether they feel sexuality is something to feel guilty about or to enjoy.

Sensitivity

Hypersensitivity in childhood may be a sign that the child's energetic boundaries are weak or underdeveloped. Sometimes this can be from the child's natural temperament. Other times the child's boundaries may have been damaged by abuse or other trauma. A hypersensitive child can be a challenge for any family. Some sensitive children quickly learn to hide, deny or repress their sensitivity because the family shames, ridicules, or ignores it. On the other hand, the child whose sensitivity is acknowledged and nurtured can learn how to connect with that sensitivity without being overwhelmed by it. These skills form the basis for successful management of energetic boundaries in adulthood.

When understood and directed, a high degree of sensitivity can be an advantage for practitioners. Highly sensitive practitioners often sense when energy is stuck in a particular tissue and are receptive to what the body is communicating. However, they must take great care to establish clear energetic boundaries to protect themselves from becoming overwhelmed or flooded by all the information they pick up on from their clients.

> If the elders have no values, their children and grandchildren will turn out badly.
>
> —Chinese proverb

The Culture at Large

While we could identify any number of cultural institutions and influences, the most significant impact on boundaries comes from schools, the media, religion and religious groups, and voluntary social organizations.

Schools

As children enter the primary grades, their daily lives typically become more structured. Children are required to gain greater control over their bodies. For example, the expectations that groups of children move through hallways in an orderly fashion, or maintain an organized classroom, require increased physical boundary maintenance by the child, and an increasing awareness of other's boundaries.

As the child begins to explore and learn in a structured environment, performance expectations increase. At this early age, and in a new environment, a child's thoughts and intellectual boundaries are particularly vulnerable.

Consequently, depending on the philosophy and competence of the teacher, the school, and often the school system, the development of a child's intellectual boundary is supported or inhibited. For example, a second-grader had raised her hand to answer a question, and was told that she wouldn't be called on because "she always had the right answer." In a similar situation, a third grade child was told that he wouldn't be acknowledged because, "You're only raising your hand to get attention!" In these two situations the adults relaying their childhood stories recalled that it was months in the first case and years in the second before each child felt comfortable contributing ideas in class.

Media

Everyone is susceptible to both overt and subliminal messages that print and broadcast media convey. Sexuality is often used as a tool to deliver an advertiser's message and is a predominant theme in the television and motion picture industry. Teenagers in particular are regularly influenced by sexual images, complicating their own boundary development pertaining to when and how they want to be sexual. Ultimately, this can make it difficult for them to develop their own or respect anyone's sexual boundaries.

At the same time media images have supported a highly polarized view of men and women. Women are often imbued with the ability to understand and manage a range of emotions, with diminished intellectual competence. Men are typically portrayed with intellectual and physical prowess, but with a narrow range of emotions.

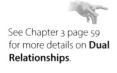

See Chapter 3 page 59 for more details on **Dual Relationships**.

Of particular concern for healthcare practitioners is the number of television and motion picture scenarios in which inappropriate dual relationships are presented in a positive light. These include lawyers, doctors, and psychotherapists having sexual or other types of intimate, dual relationships with their clients. Presenting these unethical relationships with humor makes them more damaging. When responsibly and purposefully developed, the media can also teach the importance of healthy boundaries.

Religion and Religious Groups

Most religious organizations have some sort of adjunct school or social group that focuses on child development. Whether overt or covert, there are often specific messages regarding human sexuality, the role of free thinking and emotional expression. Key to children's emotional or intellectual boundary development is how they're taught to deal with strong feelings (sadness, anxiety, fear, anger, excitement, and love), or thoughts that may not be congruent with the organization's teachings.

This is also true when considering how children are taught to think about their bodies. Is the body simply a vessel for the spiritual self, or is a child taught to value the body in its own right? How are questions about the body handled? Religious organizations play a pivotal role in many people's boundary development.

Voluntary Social Groups

Social groups such as Scouts, camps, after-school programs, and sports often become an integral aspect of children's lives and social education, and consequently their boundary development. The leaders serve as strong role models and are often unaware of the influence of seemingly insignificant comments and actions. For instance, if an adult leader makes statements about sexuality, it can impact the children who look up to the leader. This of course has an effect on the child's sense of a sexual boundary. One individual recalled his experiences in the Scouts as the first clear communication from an adult about homophobia:

> At the age of twelve I had already begun to feel that I was different—you know, odd. Then I heard my scout leader making jokes about 'boys that like boys,' and it was the first real proof from an adult that I knew and liked that I was strange. It was horrible. From then on, I knew that I would have to keep this secret to myself.

Youth sports are extremely popular. Boys and girls of school age through college are offered year-round opportunities to play sports such as soccer, basketball, baseball, softball, and football. How coaches deal with these young athletes impacts their physical and emotional boundary development. When coaches encourage children to ignore injuries, or to push beyond their bodies' appropriate limits, they're teaching children to ignore their physical boundaries. One man who had played football in his youth remembered injuring his knee. The coach told him to get up and keep playing since there was "no time for injuries on this team." From that day forward, he tried to numb his body—thickening his physical boundary—so that injuries wouldn't interfere with his athletic success. Similarly, if coaches convey the message that certain feelings are "weak" (e.g., sadness, apprehension, or fear), this encourages children to devalue their emotional boundaries.

Through awareness, sensitivity, and modeling, coaches and other organizational leaders can empower children to develop appropriate boundaries.

Influences on Your Boundary Development

Describe the experiences in your culture, environment, or family that have influenced the development of your boundaries. What are some boundaries that are idiosyncratic to your cultural background (e.g., touch, disclosure)?

Students:
   Describe how your school experiences have influenced your boundaries.

Practitioners:
   Describe the cultural diversity of your practice. What are your clients' cultural considerations?

Boundary Models

Understanding interpersonal boundaries can be complicated because while some boundaries remain rigid and consistent through a person's lifetime, others fluctuate by context or condition. It is helpful to take a look at several boundary models when identifying the boundaries of ourselves and others, and in determining how best to react to boundary crossings or violations.

In this section we draw from the work of family therapist Salvador Minuchin, M.D.[4] and Gestalt Theory[5] to help make the often amorphous concept of boundaries more concrete. We look at how boundaries function under different circumstances in human interactions and how that awareness is useful in the somatic practitioner's work. With fuller awareness you can consciously make adjustments in your own boundaries and behavior, thus preventing an automatic response.

Context determines which boundaries are the most appropriate. For instance, if you feel compassion for a client, it may be appropriate for your boundary to be thinner and more "permeable" to allow you to feel more empathy. If you feel threatened in a therapeutic situation, it may be more useful for your boundary to thicken and become more "rigid" to protect you. These models also give a conceptual picture of what happens when a boundary is crossed or when you feel you're doing just the right thing for a client.

Personal Boundaries

Minuchin describes the nature of boundaries as a continuum of permeable to rigid. The degree of permeability also represents vulnerability. The following series of diagrams illustrate selected points along that continuum.

Permeable

A permeable boundary allows information and feelings to flow easily in and out without barriers. Figure 2.3 illustrates a permeable boundary by a series of dots surrounding the drawing of the person. In this state, a practitioner working with a seriously ill client may feel empathy and the boundary might become more permeable while she gently and compassionately works with the client. If the practitioner becomes identified with her own feelings of loss or sadness and is overwhelmed by the client's pain, a permeable boundary may interfere with the practitioner's effec-

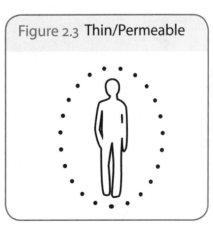

Figure 2.3 **Thin/Permeable**

tiveness. In a different situation, a practitioner might encounter a client who is very strong and dominant. In this case, the practitioner with a permeable boundary may lose a sense of identity, subordinating her opinions and beliefs to the client.

Semi-permeable

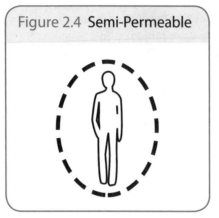

Figure 2.4 **Semi-Permeable**

In the middle range of the continuum is the semi-permeable (also referred to as flexible) boundary represented by a series of dashes around the person (Figure 2.4). This boundary indicates a flexible relationship with the outside world. Allowing closeness if appropriate and keeping someone at a distance when necessary characterizes this boundary.

A flexible boundary is useful when scheduling appointments with a client whose work limitations, illness, or children's needs are involved. On the other hand, inappropriate flexibility can interfere with the therapeutic relationship. For instance, excessive flexibility in scheduling which interferes with your personal time may lead to resentment and models a lack of self-care. Usually a limit is set for the length of a session but flexibility in the boundary would be called for if the client had an extreme physical reaction to part of the treatment and more time was needed.

Rigid

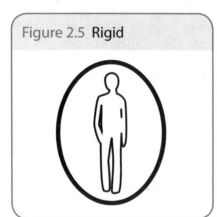

Figure 2.5 **Rigid**

At the far end of the continuum is what could be described as a rigid or thick boundary[6] which is very firm and distinct (Figure 2.5). A rigid boundary severely limits the flow of information and feelings moving in or out. This is illustrated by a solid line that encircles the person. In this case, the person is well protected from external harm or stimuli but may feel isolated. This boundary is often valuable when someone is berating or attacking you.

A firm boundary is necessary when a client attempts to engage a practitioner in constant conversation or attempts to elicit too much personal information. If a practitioner is treating a terminally ill client, a thicker boundary may be needed to maintain objectivity. However, if the practitioner's boundary becomes too rigid and he becomes distant, the therapeutic relationship is negatively affected.

Doing your best work is difficult if your history and belief systems contain certain prejudices about people (e.g., race, size, sexual orientation, eating habits, smoking, drinking, and philosophy) because prejudice makes for a rigid boundary.

 Personal Boundaries Assessment

Describe examples of permeable, semi-permeable, and rigid boundaries you have with people in your life. How do those boundaries change depending on the context and condition?

Interactive Boundaries

The Gestalt theory views boundaries from an interactive perspective. They are described as existing in relationships between individuals. The three interactive situations useful in understanding the client/practitioner relationship are: meeting at the boundary; crossing the boundary; and being distant from the boundary.

Meeting at the Boundary

In Figure 2.6 one person is meeting another at the boundary. This is illustrated by two people whose boundaries touch each other. In regards to client and practitioner, the point of contact (where they touch) occurs when the practitioner communicates in a way that the client can easily receive and understand. For example, using the appropriate amount of pressure during a treatment meets the client at his boundary. Sometimes the interaction pushes at the boundary, moving it slightly but never crossing it.

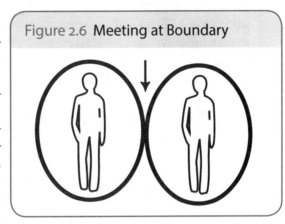

Figure 2.6 **Meeting at Boundary**

Boundary Crossing or Violation

When the boundary is crossed or violated, as in Figure 2.7, the boundaries overlap. The arrow illustrates that the boundary of one person (A) is crossing the boundary of the other (B). The boundary is considered crossed or violated when the person (B) experiences discomfort or perceives being attacked. Examples of this situation are asking inappropriate or invasive questions, or hurting the client by applying too much physical pressure.

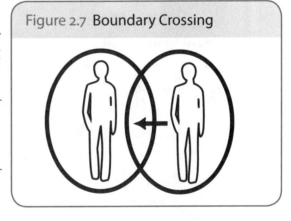

Figure 2.7 **Boundary Crossing**

Distance from the Boundary

In Figure 2.8 the people are separated by a considerable space indicating no meaningful contact. The individuals have difficulty communicating and there is hesitation and coolness in the interaction. Attempts to communicate are incomplete and unsuccessful. The practitioner's comments and questions may seem out of context or irrelevant to the client which contributes to a sense of isolation and separation between them.

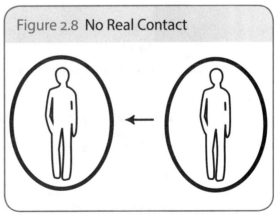

Figure 2.8 **No Real Contact**

Boundary Indicator Activity

As you consider these various models you may be assessing where your characteristic boundary lies along this continuum and how your boundaries function in interactions with others. This exercise, adapted from the work of Charles Whitfield, M.D.[7] helps you understand how your boundaries function. Circle the answer which most accurately represents how you react in these situations. Answer as honestly as you can; don't choose the answer you think is "correct" as there is no right answer.

1. **It is difficult for me to say no to people I am close to.**

    Usually   Often   Occasionally   Seldom   Never

2. **I feel my happiness depends on other people.**

    Usually   Often   Occasionally   Seldom   Never

3. **I am overly sensitive to other people's feelings.**

    Usually   Often   Occasionally   Seldom   Never

4. **I would rather attend to others than to myself.**

    Usually   Often   Occasionally   Seldom   Never

5. **It is hard for me to make decisions.**

    Usually   Often   Occasionally   Seldom   Never

6. **I trust others easily.**

    Usually   Often   Occasionally   Seldom   Never

7. **I feel anxious, scared, or afraid.**

    Usually   Often   Occasionally   Seldom   Never

8. **I put more into relationships than I get out of them.**

    Usually   Often   Occasionally   Seldom   Never

9. **I spend my time and energy helping others so much that I neglect my own needs and wants.**

    Usually   Often   Occasionally   Seldom   Never

10. **I tend to take on the moods of people close to me.**

    Usually   Often   Occasionally   Seldom   Never

11. **When I awake, it takes me a while to realize I am awake.**

    Usually   Often   Occasionally   Seldom   Never

Add up your responses in each of these categories to determine where your tendencies lie. The statements where you circled **USUALLY** or **OFTEN** are the areas of your boundaries which are on the permeable side. Where your response was **SELDOM** or **NEVER** indicates aspects of your personality that tend toward the rigid side. Statements where you circled **OCCASIONALLY** indicate a semi-permeable boundary. If you answered most or all questions with **NEVER** you may not be aware of your boundaries. Underline or circle the key words or phrases to which you answered **NEVER**, **USUALLY**, and **OFTEN**. These are indicators of potential boundary issues.

The various models described are useful in learning about boundaries. But models, by their very nature, are guides and have their limitations. In reality, our boundaries are in constant flux. They can quickly change from rigid to permeable, depending on the situation and context (see the Practical Application below). Moreover, our boundaries may combine qualities. For example, a person can simultaneously have a permeable boundary and a partially rigid boundary.

Once again, it's essential to remember that one type of boundary is no better than another. Each person needs all of these types of boundaries according to the situation and context. Boundaries need to be contextually appropriate. People experience difficulty with boundaries when they become stuck in a single mode or when the boundary doesn't match the context.

Practical Application: A Day in the Life of a Practitioner

The following example illustrates how dramatically boundaries can fluctuate, although it's very unlikely that all of these occurrences would happen on the same day (or even in the same month). This imaginary massage therapist and her partner have an infant son and in-home childcare. The practitioner works in her home office.

1. PERMEABLE
   The practitioner sits with her baby and nurses him. Her boundaries are wide open and she merges with the baby.

2. LESS PERMEABLE
   She and her partner are very close. Her partner awakes with a back pain and she lovingly offers to work on her partner's back. They feel very close and in love—almost merged but not quite.

3. PART FLEXIBLE—PART RIGID
   The practitioner greets a new client in her home office and as the treatment session begins the client asks very intrusive and personal questions about her life and her family. She wants to remain open to the client but feels herself pulling away and closing down at times during the session.

4. PERMEABLE, FLEXIBLE, AND RIGID
   The next client is a war veteran. As she begins to work on his head and neck, he has a flashback. This has never happened to the practitioner and while she feels great empathy for the client, she is also apprehensive and afraid she may not handle the situation well.

5. SEMI-PERMEABLE AND PERMEABLE
   In her afternoon break a close friend drops by to visit. Her friend's father suddenly died in an accident and the friend begins to cry uncontrollably. This reminds the practitioner of her own father's death two years ago and she quietly begins to cry as well.

6. MORE PERMEABLE
   Her fourth session is with a twelve year old girl who has headaches. This girl was referred by a physician. While taking the history from the girl and her father, it emerges that the mother has been physically abusive to the child. As the practitioner begins to work with the girl, she feels focused but tender and sad.

7. LESS FLEXIBLE
   The next client arrives late for the third time and the practitioner becomes annoyed. Lateness isn't something she tolerates well.

8. **RIGID**

   This same client makes a sexual comment during the treatment. They talk about it and clear the air, but the practitioner continues to feel wary of this client.

9. **MORE RIGID**

   The practitioner receives a call from someone wanting sexual services. She attempts to educate the caller about her professional services, and the caller becomes irate and obscene. The practitioner gets filled with anger during this interaction and her boundary becomes rigid and thicker.

10. **FLEXIBLE AND PERMEABLE**

    As she closes her office, her partner returns home and they embrace. They sit together processing what happened during her difficult day ending with the disturbing telephone call. The practitioner becomes calm, they laugh together and begin to enjoy the evening with their child.

As is evident in this example, boundaries can dramatically shift many times throughout a day depending on the situation.

Remember that these models are designed to assist you in better understanding your own responses and behaviors in relation to boundaries. Boundaries aren't as clear-cut and simple as the theories suggest. It is more realistic to think of boundaries as multifaceted and multidimensional.

 Boundary Management

What are some areas of boundary management that may be difficult for you? How can you identify and address these areas?

After answering the questions above, spend several days noticing your thoughts and how they affect your mood. At the end of each day, take at least five minutes to record how your thoughts have affected your mood. Next, reflect on whether you can influence your boundaries by separating your mood from your thoughts.

▌ Boundary Crossings and Violations

A *boundary crossing* is a transgression that may or may not be experienced as harmful. Often the difference in degree is minute that makes an action shift from being considered a boundary crossing to a violation. It is also relative: what is a mere boundary crossing to one client may be a major violation to another. A *boundary violation* is a harmful transgression of a boundary. Differentiating a boundary crossing from a violation needs to be done on a case by case basis taking into account the context and facts of the situation. "The difference between a harmful and a non-harmful boundary crossing may lie in whether it is discussed or discussable; clinical exploration of a violation often defuses its potential for harm."[8]

No boundaries are inherently right or wrong, yet when confronted with someone whose boundaries are different from ours, we may become uncomfortable and consequently judgmental. At these times, identifying our own discomfort helps us avoid creating value judgments about other people's boundaries. For instance, some cultures use very personal questions in an attempt to create safety. Such behavior is normal in that culture.

Most healthcare practitioners would agree that the boundaries between the client and practitioner must be respected. There is also agreement about the nature of gross boundary invasions such as sexual exploitation of any kind. However, while sexual abuse is egregious, there are far subtler kinds of intrusions which are harmful both to the client and to the treatment relationship. Unlike sexual abuse, these intrusions may occur without such clarity, leaving the client or the practitioner unable to recognize or articulate them.

These kinds of subtle intrusions aren't usually the result of intentionally invasive behavior. More often they occur because the practitioners don't completely understand personal boundaries. Practitioners may also lack awareness of how boundaries are affected by the power dynamics in the professional helping relationship.

The foundation of any therapeutic relationship is an implicit contract between the client and the practitioner which defines appropriate behavior. To act inappropriately is to break the contract. To avoid violating a client's boundaries a practitioner must only do what is included in the professional contract. Several distinct areas hold the potential for boundary violations on the part of the practitioner including: the kind of physical touch permitted by the client; probing for personal or private information about the client's past; the use of intimate words; and value judgments about the client's body or lifestyle. Each of these behaviors is a way of crossing a client's boundary physically or verbally. To do so without permission is at best an intrusion, at worst a violation.

See Chapter 1 page 5 for more information on the **Power Differential**.

These same actions, if done with co-equals (friends, peers, and colleagues), don't usually have quite the same impact. Co-equals by definition have equal power and don't have an implicit contract about certain kinds of boundaries.

Everyone commits minor violations and allows others to do the same. Consider the following examples: someone may put his arm around you when you don't expect it or want it; you might interrupt someone who is having an important telephone conversation; and a loved one may call you sweetheart when you're angry and don't want any closeness. Though these "violations" may be annoying and intrusive, and even feel hurtful, they typically don't do serious damage. This is because as co-equals, no implicit power dynamic keeps us from defending ourselves. You can tell the loved one not to call you sweetheart right now; the person on the telephone can ask you to not interrupt; and you can find a kind way to remove the person's arm from your shoulder.

Limitations of Terminology

Words sometimes create distance from truer meanings. This can be the case for the word boundary, especially in regards to boundary crossings and violations. When a practitioner chooses to follow through with an unethical intention or behavior, she isn't truly violating an abstract boundary. She is violating a human being. The term boundary can seem to imply that just the person's outer edges are impacted when in actuality the damage can be core-deep. Keep this in mind when discussing breaches of ethics. Terms that mean something to psychologists and other healthcare practitioners can sound less meaningful to others.

What Constitutes Boundary Crossings

The following scenarios serve to clarify what constitutes crossing a boundary. As you review this section, ask yourself these questions for each scenario:
- Has a boundary been crossed?
- If so, what was the boundary that was crossed?
- If so, was the crossing intentional or unintentional?
- What could have been done differently to avoid the boundary crossing?
- What should be done after the boundary crossing occurs?

Inappropriate Touch

The following scenario illustrates inappropriate touch:

> For several months, Steve has been giving weekly chiropractic treatments to his client Gail for chronic pain. The treatments have been going extremely well. Since Gail had unsuccessfully tried several other approaches, both client and practitioner have been excited about the progress being made. As they're saying good-bye after a particularly good session Steve spontaneously gives his client a hug. Touch to this point has been limited to the treatment. Not wanting the hug, Gail tenses but says nothing. Gail goes home feeling unsettled rather than relaxed. She wonders if he would be offended or embarrassed if she were to ask him not to hug her again. She feels ashamed for being sensitive and uncomfortable with his hug. She delays her next appointment for a couple weeks and doesn't say anything to Steve about hugs.

Points to Ponder

Is it possible for Steve to offer a hug in this circumstance without crossing a boundary? How would this scenario be different if Gail had spontaneously given Steve a hug? Would this still be a boundary crossing?

Although Steve's hug was a sincere and warm gesture towards Gail, it was also a boundary crossing. Steve may have decided that a hug was fine in the moment, and that a hug wouldn't have felt invasive to him. Boundaries are idiosyncratic so he can't be sure what the experience is like for his client. Gail didn't want a hug. Possibly the hug made her uncomfortable, confused, and even afraid. Although Gail has invited touch in the form of therapeutic manipulations, she hasn't invited any other kind of touch. Since Gail didn't want a hug, Steve crossed Gail's boundary without her permission.

For whatever reasons, Gail didn't express her discomfort. She may not have wanted to offend Steve, feeling concerned that future treatments could be jeopardized. She may even have felt that a hug was somehow expected of her.

The point here is not that practitioners should never hug their clients, rather that it would be difficult for most clients to refuse if a practitioner initiated a hug. Non-violating crossings could go like this: After the session, Gail might have asked for a hug. If Steve was comfortable with the idea, he might have appropriately responded by giving one. In this case, he would be crossing Gail's physical boundary only in response to a clear invitation. In other words, Steve would be certain that it was wanted. Whenever a practitioner hugs a client, many decisions about the hug need to be made in an instant: how close; how long; is there full body contact; and is there movement or stroking while hugging. There are no easy solutions for this. The practitioner needs to determine how to make sure the hug stays in the friendly, professional hug category.

> He who has never made a mistake is one who never does anything.
>
> —Theodore Roosevelt

Careless or Uninvited Words

The following scenario illustrates careless or uninvited words:

> Joan is working for the first time with her new client Sarah who has come for physical therapy to build strength. During the course of the treatment, Joan notices that Sarah has a dark mole on her back. Without asking for permission to give her opinion, Joan says to Sarah, "Are you aware that you have a huge, hairy mole on your back?" and proceeds to inform her of the potential dangers of moles and suggests several methods of treatment for the problem.
>
> ### Points to Ponder
>
> How might Joan have approached the subject without crossing a boundary? Is it ethical for a practitioner to remain silent about potential physical issues?

It is easy to imagine that Joan thought she was being helpful to Sarah by pointing out the mole of which Sarah might not even have been aware. However, it's neither feedback nor professional judgment that Sarah has invited. It is quite possible that Sarah would feel injured and insulted, as anyone might if told something uncomplimentary about her body without her asking. Because Joan didn't have explicit permission to offer feedback about Sarah's body, Joan committed a boundary crossing.

This example demonstrates how words that convey any type of judgment are an intrusion. A fine line exists between increasing a client's awareness of a potential physical problem and overstepping your role. Joan could have said, "Is it okay with you if I point out things I notice such as bruises, bites, rashes, or moles—particularly those in areas that might be difficult for you to see?" If Sarah were to agree, Joan could be much more diplomatic in describing the mole. Then instead of immediately proceeding to tell Sarah about the implications and steps to take regarding the mole, Joan should wait for Sarah's response. Sarah might say, "Oh, yes, I've had that since I was a child. I had my doctor check it out and she says it's fine." If Sarah doesn't respond, then a simple statement such as, "You might want to have a dermatologist check this out" would suffice. Joan could also ask Sarah if she is interested in learning more about moles or if she would like recommendations (such as a referral to a dermatologist).

In some circumstances a boundary crossing is necessary. A practitioner has a responsibility to inform the client if certain things are noticed. For example, when a practitioner notices facial bruises or a pattern of multiple bruises, the issue of domestic violence must be considered. The practitioner must use her judgment in determining if the bruises seem like a normal occurrence or something for concern. The client may think the concern is silly, but it's better to be safe. A practitioner might say, "I noticed you have several bruises. As healthcare practitioners we're obligated to inquire if you're in a situation where someone is hurting you. If this is the case, I want you to know that there are many resources to help you out of this situation, and I can provide you with referrals."

Without invitation, even compliments or words of affection may put a person in an awkward position. To be called by intimate names (e.g., sweetheart, honey), or to be told you're attractive or appealing by someone you know and trust, generally makes you feel good. However, without trust, safety, and the appropriate context, words like these feel invasive. And in the treatment relationship where power is so unbalanced, they almost always serve to confuse the professional boundary.

We know stories about every type of practitioner who unintentionally offended a client by making uninvited comments (positive or negative) about the client's body. Significantly, when this type of boundary crossing occurred in one of the first few sessions, none of these clients went back to the practitioner (we assume because they were too upset or angry).

> If you think you're too small to make a difference, you haven't been in bed with a mosquito.
> —Anita Roddick

Sexual Misconduct

The following scenario illustrates sexual misconduct:

> After several months of treatment, Tracy's client Chris expresses a personal interest in Tracy by making subtle, sexual comments. Tracy finds the client attractive and begins to fantasize about a social relationship. Chris invites Tracy to go out for coffee and they meet after the next session. They decide to see each other socially and become friends. After several dinners the friendship develops into a casual sexual relationship. The professional relationship continues for a few more months, sometimes becoming sexual during the treatment sessions. The treatment relationship slowly ends in several months but the two enjoy each other for six more months until the relationship ends suddenly when Chris realizes that Tracy is also dating someone else. Chris feels betrayed and angry, seeks psychotherapy, and ends up suing Tracy for sexual misconduct.

Points to Ponder

How many boundary violations were committed? What were Tracy's options for acting ethically without violating boundaries? Is it possible for an ethical and appropriate transition from professional relationship to social relationship to occur in this or any case?

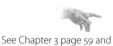

See Chapter 3 page 59 and Chapter 6 page 153 for more details on **Sexual Misconduct**.

This is a clear case of sexual misconduct. It also demonstrates the rapid move along the continuum from a client/practitioner relationship to friendship to a sexual relationship. There were several strong indicators of boundary violations along the way that could have signaled Tracy to seek help or to stop the process: when Chris began to make subtle, sexual comments; when Tracy noticed an attraction to Chris and began to fantasize a social relationship; when the invitation to coffee and then dinner was made. By the time they decided to become friends, the slide to sexual misconduct was almost complete.

When Chris began to make sexual comments, Tracy could have stopped it and opened a conversation by saying, "I notice that you're making some personal comments to me with sexual innuendos. This makes me a little uncomfortable and I am wondering if there's something else behind it?" If Chris then says, "I think that I would like to be friends with you," Tracy could have responded by saying, "I feel flattered but in my professional life I avoid mixing my personal and professional relationships. This feels more professional, protects my clients and makes life simpler."

Some disciplines have strict guidelines about the length of time between a therapeutic relationship ending and a social relationship beginning. It is highly recommended to reviewing Chapter 10 page 281 before acting on this impulse.

A red flag to immediately seek professional or peer supervision should have been signaled when Tracy noticed an attraction to Chris and began to fantasize about a social relationship. Most practitioners have occasionally felt attracted to a client but when it progresses into fantasizing this indicates that a boundary has been crossed in the practitioner's mind. If Tracy had sought help at this time, the following would have become clear: strong boundaries needed to be put in place or the client/practitioner relationship terminated.

Two other choice points came when Chris invited Tracy to coffee and when Tracy accepted. Both of these occurrences indicated that the relationship was about to change in a manner that wasn't strictly professional. Going out to coffee with a client that the practitioner has been having fantasies about and who has made sexual comments is a clear recipe for trouble and eventual disaster. At this moment Tracy could have said, "Thank you for the invitation but my policy is to refrain from developing social relationships with my clients." Or Tracy could have said, "I find myself also interested in developing a personal relationship with you, but if this were to occur, I could no longer work with you in a therapeutic role. If you want to develop a social relationship with me, we need to end our professional relationship first. We need to consider this decision very carefully and perhaps get some outside help."

Excessively Permeable Boundaries

The following scenario illustrates excessively permeable boundaries:

Arianne was a young somatic therapy student who was generally regarded as highly intuitive and naturally gifted. When she practiced with other students in class, she always seemed to know just where to put her hands, sensing which part of the person's body needed the most attention. She was also a very attentive listener, someone with whom both personal and professional acquaintances tended to share their troubles.

After Arianne graduated, her peers and instructors expected her to go on to have a very successful career. But as she started to build her private practice, she began feeling fatigued and overwhelmed—particularly after seeing clients who were experiencing high levels of stress or strong negative emotions and who talked extensively to her about their problems. Working with a client who expressed grief or anxiety left her feeling sad or anxious. Working with someone who suffered from tension headaches left her own head and neck feeling tense and achy. It got to the point where she was having trouble sleeping and spent most of her non-working time resting and recuperating.

After a particularly challenging week, Arianne made an appointment with a body-based psychotherapist. Over the course of several sessions, this therapist helped her develop strategies for centering and grounding herself and strengthening her emotional and energetic boundaries. Arianne started to use these techniques at the start of each workday and after every client session. She also got some supervision from one of her former instructors on how to set appropriate limits on client self-disclosure. Gradually, as her boundaries grew clearer, Arianne's level of stress and fatigue decreased significantly, and her head and neck pain disappeared.

Points to Ponder

Whose boundaries were crossed in this scenario? Whose responsibility is it to set boundaries in this type of situation? What other issues could have resulted if Arianne had not worked on strengthening her emotional and energetic boundaries?

Practitioners like Arianne who have overly permeable boundaries frequently suffer from fatigue, overwhelm, burnout, and other complications. Treating even one individual who's experiencing deep physical or emotional pain can leave them feeling drained and physically ill. Clients are rarely aware of this reaction unless the practitioner mentions it. (If they do find out, they usually feel uncomfortable for any number of reasons, including guilt for "causing" the problem and uncertainty about the practitioner's ability.) However, the influence can also work in the other direction, with a practitioner unintentionally passing on her own distress of discomfort to those she treats.[9] Practitioners who encounter any of these difficulties have a responsibility to learn ways to get more grounded, contain their energy, and maintain clearer boundaries throughout their practice to protect both themselves and their clients.

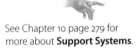

See Chapter 10 page 279 for more about **Support Systems**.

Client Reluctance to Personal Disclosure

The following scenario illustrates a client's reluctance to personal disclosure:

Before working on her new client, Jim, Susan hands him a history form to fill out. Jim becomes somewhat annoyed and suggests that they skip the history and proceed with the massage therapy session. Susan explains that to do her work well a history must be taken. Jim remains truculent but agrees.

Points to Ponder

How could Susan determine that Jim's boundaries have been crossed? What other approaches could Susan have used to elicit the information she needs to provide an appropriate treatment?

It seems obvious that taking a history helps a practitioner in working with clients. However, in this example, taking the client's history makes him feel upset and invaded in some way. Although the reasons aren't yet obvious, it's apparent that Jim isn't comfortable with the history. Perhaps he generally feels uncomfortable disclosing information about himself. Maybe he feels unsafe revealing particular pieces of his personal history. He might even have difficulties reading. Whatever the cause, it's reasonable to interpret his resistance as an attempt to establish a boundary. The practitioner's insistence may serve as a threat to the boundary he is trying to establish.

Jim's agreement may be the result of feeling intimidated. Perhaps he believes that the therapist knows best, or fears that without acquiescing he won't get his treatment. A boundary crossing has occurred because Jim wasn't offered a real choice about giving a history. Susan could have chosen other options: do the history and intake verbally; pare down the intake form—checking off the questions that are vital to providing an appropriate, safe treatment; and ask Jim if he wants to discuss his reluctance to filling out the history.

Remember that because boundaries are unique to each person, what constitutes crossing a line is different for different people. What feels like decent respectful behavior to one client (taking a medical history) may feel like a violation to another client like Jim. Therefore, even the most careful and respectful practitioner must be willing to learn about and assess each client individually.

Inappropriate Self-Disclosure

The following scenario illustrates inappropriate self-disclosure:

During a chiropractic treatment with new patient Mary, Dr. Bill discloses that his wife is pregnant with their first child. Dr. Bill was unaware that just last year at this time Mary had lost a baby. Although Mary was happy for Bill and his wife, her vulnerable position on the adjustment table allowed her to be instantly overwhelmed by grief. Mary tried her best to conceal her sadness, but could only mutter, "I'm so happy for you." Bill noticed Mary's subtle mood change, but didn't inquire and he continued the treatment.

Points to Ponder

How would this situation be different if Mary had been Bill's client for years, and knew Bill and his wife personally? Might Bill have chosen a different time to share this information had he known Mary's history?

It is quite common for people to share joyful events with friends and acquaintances, even clients. But somatic practitioners must be mindful of how and when personal information is shared. When a client is on the treatment table, she is in an open and vulnerable position, where the safety of her physical body and emotions is in the hands of the practitioner. It is in this position that the practitioner must only communicate information that is related to the treatment and in the best interest of the client. In this case, Bill was sharing information that in no way related to the treatment, in fact he was more focused on himself than he was on his patient.

This type of boundary crossing may seem minor and is unintentional, of course, but can be avoided by remaining client-centered during the treatment. There is no way for practitioners to always avoid every subject that might upset a client. But they can feel confident in the appropriateness of what they're sharing, as long as it relates to the session. This is a case where the information wasn't necessarily inappropriate, but how and when the information was shared was inappropriate.

Tardiness

The following scenario illustrates tardiness:

> Sam has been a regular client of Denise's since she began her private practice. He is habitually 15-20 minutes late for his appointments, usually due to his unpredictable schedule. In the beginning, Denise would accommodate him and give him his full treatment, but now Denise's schedule is filling up. She doesn't want to lose a reliable client, but she is frustrated that his tardiness may begin affecting others on her schedule. She knows she has created this issue by always accommodating his schedule.
>
> ### Points to Ponder
>
> How can Denise set new time management boundaries? How can she discuss this with Sam and elicit his consent?

Frequently, new practitioners make special accommodations for clients, in an effort to build their practices and create long-term relationships, even at the expense of their own boundaries. Time management is an important boundary that needs to be created and maintained from the start. Denise feels that she just has to figure out how to continue accommodating Sam, since she allowed this situation to continue for so long.

As her business grows, Denise will likely have to create and update office policies and procedures to accommodate that growth. Boundaries around tardiness and missed appointments can be stated in an office policies statement. In this particular case, Denise should sit down with Sam and explain that it has been her pleasure to accommodate his varying schedule in the past, but her schedule is now less flexible. Denise could ask Sam to schedule his appointments on his days off, or when his schedule is more predictable, so that he can make it to his appointments on time. Denise also needs to let Sam know that in the future, she will be adhering strictly to her time slots, so when he is late, she will do her best to provide a treatment within the time remaining. In this way, Denise has stated her new boundaries as well as the consequences for any future lateness.

See Appendix A page 338 for **Sample Policies**.

Inappropriate Use of Social Media

The following scenario illustrates inappropriate use of social media:

> Jan is very active on Facebook and invites all of her clients to be Facebook friends with her. She often uses Facebook to promote her personal training business. John is one of Jan's clients, and becomes friends with her on Facebook. Jan's birthday was last week, and she posted several photos from her birthday party. She and her friends in the photos were dressed in sexually provocative clothing and appeared to be drinking alcohol. John saw the photos and became very uncomfortable about his next appointment with Jan. He felt sure that if his wife saw these photos, she wouldn't feel comfortable about him continuing to work with Jan as his personal trainer.

> ### Points to Ponder
>
> Were boundaries crossed here? If so, how could Jan avoid potential boundary crossings like this one in the future?

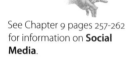

See Chapter 9 pages 257-262 for information on **Social Media**.

Jan dresses and acts appropriately in her training business. She doesn't think that what she does on her personal time should matter, as long as she is performing professionally while training her clients. Jan has many friends who are also clients, and so she believes that sharing both personal and professional information on her Facebook page is just fine.

When considering our actions, both personally and professionally, we need to consider our audience. Clearly, drinking and letting loose isn't offensive to Jan and her friends, but could be offensive to others that have joined her on Facebook. It is a fairly new, yet increasingly controversial issue, that of Facebook disclosure. We discuss this concept more in Chapter 9, but in Jan's case, if she wants to have her business clients join her on Facebook, she should only disclose information on her Facebook page that is appropriate in the business setting as well. Many businesses and private practitioners create a separate Business Page on Facebook for their businesses, keeping their personal pages separate.

Identifying Boundaries

- How do you know when a client's boundaries have been crossed?
- Identify behaviors that might indicate that a client's boundaries have been crossed.
- Make a list of questions that would help a client identify when boundaries have been crossed or violated.

Why Boundary Crossings Occur

Most practitioners genuinely intend to maintain clear boundaries and act ethically. Subtle boundary crossings generally occur for several reasons: a lack of understanding of boundaries in general; the practitioner isn't aware of her own boundaries; the practitioner may not comprehend or pay attention to a particular client's boundaries; the practitioner may make incorrect assumptions about a client's ability to communicate when a boundary has been crossed; and the practitioner may choose to ignore certain therapeutic boundaries. This section explores how each of these may have been involved in the boundary transgressions described in the previous scenarios.

Without a good understanding of the nature of boundaries, and their own boundaries in particular, practitioners might assume that clients feel the same way they do. Consequently practitioners may do things such as move too close physically or emotionally, or offer unwanted advice. It is unlikely that the practitioner who offered unwanted feedback about the mole in the second scenario did so callously (although flippantly). More likely, she was trying to offer good advice or inspire confidence by demonstrating her expertise. However, without understanding that unwanted advice may feel invasive, she obliviously crossed a boundary.

Similarly, in the first scenario, it's likely that Steve's initiation of a hug was based in his belief that what felt appropriate for him would also apply to Gail. Steve lacks a conceptual understanding of boundaries: a hug might have a different meaning to a client than to a practitioner. He didn't realize that while his own boundaries allow for an easy expression of affection, Gail's may not. And in the self-disclosure scenario, Bill assumed that anyone would be just as excited as he was about he and his wife expecting a child. This confusion was also true for Susan in the fifth scenario. Had she been in touch with her own boundaries, she might easily have realized that the client, Jim, was trying to establish a boundary.

Sometimes practitioners choose not to explore their boundary issues before going into practice. Luckily, Arianne's bodywork delivered no known detrimental effects to her clients during the time before she established her energy boundary. Arianne overestimated her abilities and beliefs, and underestimated the power of the energy connection that happens between practitioner and client. She found out that she needed to take another look at her boundary issues altogether and was willing to do so.

See Chapter 3 page 59 for more information on **Dual Relationships**.

Not exploring and setting boundaries before going into practice became problematic for Denise with her tardy client, Sam. Issues may have been avoided if Denise was aware of the need to set boundaries, and she could have set time management expectations with Sam right away.

In the third scenario, Tracy's desire for a social relationship with Chris turned into a gross violation of therapeutic boundaries. Sometimes practitioners ignore the precepts of ethical client/practitioner interactions, attempt to bend the rules, or simply believe the rules don't apply to them. This manifests most often when in dual relationships (having more than one type of relationship with the same person). Jan's Facebook post was much less serious than Tracy's sexual misconduct, but still an example of how dual relationships can lead to problems. While dual relationships aren't necessarily harmful, they're often difficult and effective management requires attention and careful consideration.

As demonstrated in all the scenarios, practitioners need to get more information about a particular client's boundaries and learn more about their own. Getting this information is important work that can also be difficult. Patience and good communication between client and practitioner are required to discuss issues which may feel very personal and private to the client. Those issues might also appear threatening for the practitioner.

Figure 2.9 Boundary Crossing Signals

- Client pulls away when certain areas are touched.
- Client changes communication style (gets overly quiet or overly talkative).
- Client avoids eye contact.
- Client breathing changes: halts, becomes shallow, or increases.
- Client or client's significant other makes comments to the staff.
- Client doesn't reschedule.
- Client brings another person to stay in the treatment room.
- Client serves you with a complaint.

Difficulties in Identifying Boundary Crossings

A practitioner may mistakenly assume clients know how to identify when their boundaries are being crossed. In reality, some clients may not initially be aware of this type of discomfort. Their personal history with emotional distress, physical pain, or abuse may have taught them to deny these feelings. Therefore, in another version of the first scenario, it's possible that a different client might not want a hug, and not be aware of it. In this case, the client would feel uncomfortable afterwards but not know why.

The practitioner may also mistakenly assume that when clients are aware that their boundaries have been intruded, they're then willing to talk about it. In some cases past experiences have taught people to avoid conflict by remaining quiet, particularly when they're uncomfortable. Others may simply feel it isn't worth the effort. For example, neither Gail (the huggee in the first scenario), nor Sarah (who had the mole in the second scenario), nor Mary (who lost the baby) told the practitioner how she felt.

In addition to personal histories, the power dynamics of the treatment relationship often make it difficult for clients to talk about their discomfort to a practitioner. The point here is that practitioners shouldn't rely on clients speaking up to ensure that boundary crossings and violations don't occur.

Boundary Crossings Evaluation

- Identify behaviors that might indicate that a client's boundaries have been crossed.
- List actions you can take when a client's boundaries have been crossed.
- What are the areas in which you might be in danger of disregarding these boundary signals?
- What professional or personal situations make you uncomfortable because your boundaries have been crossed?

Steps to Avoid Boundary Crossings and Violations

Practitioners make mistakes. Given the power that is accorded to healthcare professionals, they often feel enormous pressure to know everything that a client needs. This pressure may lead practitioners to avoid acknowledging mistakes to themselves or to others. Yet if the practitioner wants to learn about boundaries and identify when crossings or violations occur, it's useful to remember that even the most skilled and careful practitioners make these errors. In fact, by noticing mistakes when they occur and speaking about them with clients, practitioners are demonstrating awareness and respect for their clients' boundaries.

With this in mind, you can take several steps to avoid boundary crossings or violations and identify and correct them when they occur.

Increase Empathy

Increasing empathic awareness of clients' experiences means that the practitioner regularly works on expanding awareness of what the client may be experiencing. In the first scenario, Steve gave Gail a hug because he wanted to, not because he was attending to her needs. If Steve increases his empathetic awareness, he will be more considerate of how Gail might experience touch that is separate from the treatment. He will also pay attention to what Gail is and is not requesting.

> Nothing is more important to the future of an idea than the first step you take to try it out.
>
> —O. A. Battista

Figure 2.10 Avoiding Boundary Crossings

- Increase Empathy
- Manage Energy
- Identify Clients' Behavioral Cues
- Ask Questions
- Teach Boundary Identification and Establishment
- Encourage Clients to Speak Up

Manage Energetic Boundaries

Practitioners can avoid the problems experienced by Arianne, whose overly permeable boundaries began to compromise her physical and mental wellbeing, by consciously managing their energetic boundaries. There are a variety of ways of doing this, ranging from visualizations and meditations to more physically-oriented centering methods. Some practitioners choose to use specific rituals or focusing techniques before and after each client session. Such precautionary steps are particularly important for individuals whose boundaries have been damaged by past traumas or who have a heightened level of sensitivity for any other reason.

Identify Clients' Behavioral Cues

Enhance skills for identifying clients' behaviors that indicate crossed boundaries. Because clients can't always articulate the fear and discomfort that accompany unwanted boundary crossings, practitioners must become better at identifying behavior that indicates an intrusion. If the client can't easily set a boundary, or tell the practitioner when they feel crossed, their indirect verbal or nonverbal behavior may provide clues. For example, if Jim (the client who resisted giving his history) had felt comfortable enough to set a boundary, his response to the request for a history might have been to calmly say, "I'd really prefer to skip the history. I don't feel comfortable right now saying a whole lot about myself. Perhaps we could do it another time." However, without such emotional clarity and verbal skill, clients may set the boundary indirectly. If the practitioner had understood that Jim's stubborn behavior was his best attempt at setting a boundary, she could've helped him set the boundary more easily and directly. An alternative interaction might look like the following practical application:

> "
> Everything we do seeds the future. No action is an empty one.
>
> —Joan Chittister

Jim:

I really don't see why I have to give you all this information. I just came here to get a massage.

Susan:

I'm hearing that this seems like more information than I'd need to give you a treatment. Is that right?

Jim:

Yeah. I've had massages before and I didn't have to tell my whole life story.

Susan:

That makes total sense. After having that experience in the past, I can see why this detailed history would seem unnecessary. There are actually very specific reasons behind each question—with the main goal of making sure that my treatment will be as helpful as possible to you, without aggravating any injuries or other existing conditions you may have. Is there a particular reason why you'd rather not do a history?

Jim:

Yes.

Susan:

Do you feel comfortable telling me that reason?

Jim:

Not really.

Susan:

No problem. I have a suggestion then. There is some basic information I need to know before we begin. Why don't we just go over those few questions and skip the rest for now? Then, if you like the treatment and decide you want future sessions, we can talk about the best way to move forward. How does that sound?

At this point Jim may accede. Either way, Susan's message to him is that while a history is important, she is willing to respect his boundary. Further, she has communicated that she is open to learning more about his reluctance when Jim feels comfortable. This also communicates respect for his boundary.

Points to Ponder

What other approaches could Susan take to demonstrate her respect for Jim's boundaries? How else could she get the information she needs to develop a treatment plan?

Ask Questions

Ask questions that identify when clients' boundaries may have been violated. Practitioners must learn to ask questions when they feel they may have violated a client's boundary.

I just realized that for the past several minutes I've been asking you some very personal questions that aren't actually an integral part of the medical history. Have any of them made you uncomfortable?

Of course this type of intervention only works if the client identifies her discomfort. If the practitioner suspects that the client might avoid conflict by not acknowledging the problem, the practitioner may simply have to make a statement.

I just realized that for the past several minutes I've been asking you some very personal questions. Let me apologize if any of them made you uncomfortable.

Teach Boundary Identification and Establishment

Teach clients how to identify and establish their own boundaries. Practitioners can prevent boundary crossings and violations by teaching clients to identify and establish their boundaries.

This encourages clients to be aware of what feels right and wrong for them in all aspects of the professional relationship. This training begins from the first moment of contact with the client: the practitioner establishes an environment of choice, which teaches clients to identify their boundaries. You could say:

> Regarding disrobing, people feel comfortable getting a massage in a variety of ways. Some people remove all their clothes before getting under the sheet. Others choose to leave their underwear on or wear a gown. Still others feel most comfortable leaving their clothes on. Do what's right for you. I'm going to leave the room for a few minutes, and while I'm out please choose what feels best for you.

Asking specific questions is often effective in helping the client identify their boundaries:

> I'm going to show you a diagram of a back. Are there parts of your back you would prefer I focus on or avoid?

-or-

> Occasionally pain is experienced in the process of relaxing the muscles. I want to work with you to limit discomfort. How do you typically respond to pain? If it becomes too painful, do you say nothing and hope it eases, or would you tell me so I would know to reduce pressure or stop?

Encourage Clients to Speak Up

Establishing an atmosphere of choice encourages clients to pay attention to their boundaries and articulate their experience. Depending on the client's answers, the practitioner might inquire further. This allows for more refined understanding of the client's boundaries and encourages the client to notice any feelings of violation.

Practical Application: Encourage Clients to Speak Up

PRACTITIONER:

Would you say nothing or would you tell me so I would know to stop or change my technique somehow?

CLIENT:

Come to think of it, I probably wouldn't say anything. I've had treatments from other people and I guess I sort of hang on during the real painful parts. I've always assumed that good work would most likely elicit some pain. Is that true?

PRACTITIONER:

Not always. If you're in so much pain that you're tensing against it, it may be counterproductive.

CLIENT:

Well, the truth is I guess I do sometimes put up with more pain than I really want to. It just never occurred to me to ask anyone to go easier.

PRACTITIONER:

Now that we've established it's okay, will you tell me when I'm working too hard?

CLIENT:

I'm not sure.

PRACTITIONER:

How about if I check in with you regularly and I ask you if you're comfortable with the intensity? Would that make it easier?

CLIENT:

Maybe. Let's try.

Points to Ponder

Have you had direct conversations such as these with your clients? How do these types of questions help you learn about your clients' boundaries, and understand your clients' style of communicating those boundaries?

These types of questions teach the practitioner about clients' boundaries. Note: these questions also teach clients to pay attention to, and learn about, their own boundaries. It is clear from the above scenario that when this type of interaction goes well, both the practitioner and the client benefit.

 Discovering Your Boundary Issues

Oftentimes, as a healthcare practitioner, you may be unaware of when you're overstepping boundaries with clients. You may feel uneasy about your relationship with a particular client, yet the reason eludes you. This checklist (adapted from the work of Estelle Disch[10]) helps you illuminate boundary issues with one or more of your clients. To do this exercise, imagine a problematic relationship that you're having or have had with one of your clients. Place a check mark next to the statements that apply to you in this situation.

1. _____This client feels more like a friend than a client.
2. _____I often tell my personal problems to this client.
3. _____I want to be friends with this client when treatment ends.
4. _____I think the good-bye hugs last too long with this client.
5. _____Sessions often run over the scheduled time with this client.
6. _____I accept gifts or favors from this client without examining why the gift was given.
7. _____I have a barter arrangement with this client that is sometimes a source of tension for me.
8. _____I sometimes choose my clothing with this particular client in mind.
9. _____I have attended small professional or social events where I knew this client would be present, without discussing it ahead of time.
10. _____This client often invites me to social events and I don't feel comfortable saying either yes or no.
11. _____Sometimes when I'm touching this client during our regular sessions, I feel like the contact is sexual for either or both of us.
12. _____This client is very seductive, and I often don't know how to handle it.
13. _____This client owes me a lot of money and I don't know what to do about it.
14. _____I have invited this client to public or social events.
15. _____I am often late for sessions with this particular client.
16. _____I cajole, tease, and joke a lot with this client.
17. _____I am in a heavy emotional crisis myself, and I identify so much with this client's pain that I can hardly attend to the client.
18. _____I allow this client to comfort me.
19. _____I feel like this client and I are very much alike.
20. _____This client scares me.
21. _____This client's pain is so deep I can hardly tolerate it.
22. _____I enjoy feeling more powerful than this client.
23. _____Sometimes I feel like I'm over my head with this client.
24. _____I feel that I am the only person who can really help this client.

25. ____I often feel hooked or lost with this client, and advice from colleagues and former teachers hasn't helped.

26. ____I often feel invaded or pushed by this client and have difficulty standing my ground.

27. ____I feel overly protective of this client.

28. ____I do things for this client that I don't usually do with other clients.

29. ____I sometimes drink alcohol or use recreational drugs with this client.

30. ____I do so much on this client's behalf I feel exhausted.

31. ____I am reluctant to discuss certain client/practitioner interactions in my peer supervision group.

32. ____I accommodate this client's schedule and then feel angry/manipulated.

33. ____This client has invested money in an enterprise of mine or vice versa.

34. ____I have hired this client to work for me.

35. ____I find it difficult to keep from talking about this client with my close friends and colleagues.

36. ____I engage in a lot of self-disclosure with this client—telling stories and carrying on peer-like conversation.

37. ____I feel emotionally drained after working with this client.

38. ____My body, especially my arms, feels heavy after working with this client.

39. ____I feel strong irritation and even anger toward this client.

If you check off any of these items, boundary issues may be interfering with your ability to work effectively and ethically and we highly recommend you seek professional supervision to assist you in developing stronger boundaries.

We suggest that you periodically do this exercise to give you insight into areas where you might want to further your knowledge or get support.

Establish, Maintain, and Change Boundaries

There are a variety of factors that influence the ways we establish, maintain, and change boundaries. Including these issues in a policy statement and addressing them at the beginning of the professional relationship, lessens the possibility of inappropriate, embarrassing, harmful, or legally damaging situations. The following eight major areas should be considered when establishing and maintaining boundaries, and again when boundaries need to be changed.

Figure 2.11 Boundary Change Agents

- Location of Service
- Interpersonal Space
- Money
- Appearance
- Self-Disclosure
- Language
- Touch
- Time

Location of Service

Treating a client in a professional office sets a different contextual boundary than treating the client in her home or in an office located in your home. Always create a professional environment regardless of your office location. If you're in your home or making a visit to the client's home, more attention must be given to establishing and maintaining appropriate boundaries. For example, it's helpful for home offices to have a separate entrance and separate bathroom facilities. If this isn't possible, eliminate as many personal items as possible from the "office areas."

Interpersonal Space

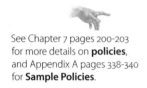

See Chapter 7 pages 200-203 for more details on **policies**, and Appendix A pages 338-340 for **Sample Policies**.

Note the distance you allot when talking with your clients before and after sessions. Be mindful of the height differential (e.g., do you stand while clients are seated or sit on a higher stool/table?). Being at the same height helps level the power differential. If crossing a physical boundary is necessary to perform your work, act with awareness and respect as you move through this zone. Create an appropriate space boundary by maintaining a physical distance that makes both you and the client comfortable—always defer to whoever requires the greater distance.

Money

Money also helps to establish professional boundaries. The exchange of money reinforces the business nature of relationships. Friends don't pay to help each other. Be clear about your financial interactions. Boundaries are altered if a client owes you money over a long period of time or if a client never pays for sessions.

Appearance

The way you dress establishes a certain tone and carries a message to those you meet. Your primary goal is that your clothing and appearance foster feelings of trust and safety in your clients. Care is needed to avoid overly informal, revealing, or sexually provocative clothing. Visible tattoos and multiple piercings can make certain clients uncomfortable, which has led to many employers and healthcare facilities imposing strict policies around these items. Professionalism involves dressing appropriately for your daily work, maintaining good hygiene, and modifying your appearance for the therapeutic relationship (e.g. tie back long hair, trim fingernails, cover tattoos when required). Requirements differ by the specific work environment and are likely to change as individual expression becomes more acceptable.

Self-Disclosure

Self-disclosure occurs when practitioners reveal professional or personal information about themselves. Decisions about this must be made carefully. Completely avoiding any disclosure may create an unnecessary distance from a client. Too much self-disclosure often institutes an inappropriate closeness.

Appropriate professional disclosure includes describing training and experience to instill confidence in a client. An example of appropriate personal disclosure is sharing a personal experience that communicates empathy and understanding regarding the client's present situation.

Self-disclosure creates a danger to the boundaries of the relationship when the practitioner reveals information which isn't pertinent to the healthcare relationship and which may result in the client feeling uncomfortable or inappropriately intimate with the practitioner. Self-disclosure is a powerful factor in regulating the emotional distance between practitioner and client. In all cases, self-disclosure must be guided by a belief that the information revealed is helpful to the client.

Language

Language is one of the most potent means for creating and maintaining healthy boundaries. The words you choose, your voice intonation, timbre, and overall skill as a communicator are vital aspects in creating effective boundaries. Clients are more likely to know what they can expect from you and understand your expectations of them if you're respectful, articulate, clear, and have a sincere and honest tone of voice. In this way, a clearly defined boundary is created. Conversely, if you're imprecise, unclear, hesitant, or insensitive, expectations of both parties are more likely to be cloudy and the boundaries unclear.

> It doesn't matter how strong your opinions are. If you don't use your power for positive change, you are, indeed, part of the problem.
>
> —Coretta Scott King

Touch

The type of touch either establishes a sense of safety and reassurance, or it makes the client feel uneasy, apprehensive, and uncomfortable. The practitioner needs to be very sensitive to the physical boundaries of touch both on and off the treatment table. A major touch boundary is the actual depth of touch. Working or probing too deeply or too lightly may be perceived as inappropriate. Another example of touch boundaries concerns greeting and saying good-bye to a client. In general, the more conservative approach of shaking hands is advised. Make certain it's appropriate (and beneficial) before hugging a client or putting a hand on the client's shoulder or back.

Time

How you deal with time delineates your boundaries. In personal relationships, the time spent in social interaction is usually very flexible; clear limits aren't often stressed. A distinguishing feature of professional relationships is the limit placed on the time spent with clients. Clients often test the seriousness of your boundaries by asking for more time at the end of a session, coming late and expecting a full session, or canceling without adequate notice. Your responses to these situations either build or weaken the client's trust.

▌ Conclusion

The foundation of an ethical practice is built upon establishing, maintaining, and respecting personal and professional boundaries. A large measure of your professional success will be determined by the clarity with which you communicate expectations, the integrity in how you manage the business aspects of your practice, and the delicacy and grace with which you acknowledge the pain and vulnerabilities of your clients. Honoring your own boundaries and the boundaries of your clients promotes understanding and healing.

3
Dual and Sequential Relationships

"It is not the great temptations that ruin us; it is the little ones."
—John W. De Forest

Key Terms

Accountability
Countertransference
Dual Relationships

Maturity
Non-Fraternization
Power Differential

Sequential Relationships
Supervision
Transference

Dual relationships commonly consist of many layers and encompass a number of professional and social components. Some dual relationships evolve easily and naturally, and initially seem relatively simple. Upon closer examination, their dynamics can be surprisingly complex with ramifications ranging from vital and stimulating to tragically harmful. Potential benefits enrich dual relationships when both parties are emotionally developed and able to handle the multiple roles without confusion. The major benefit is a fuller experience of each other, including shared talents and gifts.

Unfortunately, judging your ability to successfully juggle multiple roles is often very difficult and problematic. Failure to navigate the risks involved in a dual relationship can result in financial, educational, social, or personal loss. Conscious consideration and discernment are important prior to engaging in a relationship of this nature, and clinical supervision is strongly recommended.

In the healthcare setting it's the practitioner's responsibility to be educated and informed about the nature of dual relationships, and it's the practitioner who is accountable for informing the client about the parameters and possible impact of entering another dimension of the relationship. The power differential that exists in a helping relationship demands that the practitioner behave ethically by clearly defining and maintaining relationship boundaries. This concept appears fairly straightforward on the printed page. However, the work of a helping professional often occurs within complex sets of relationships where boundaries and matters of authority take on shades of gray. We examine the nature of this complexity in this chapter.

What Are Dual Relationships?

The term dual relationships describes the overlapping of professional and social roles and interactions between two people. Human beings naturally develop multiple relationships in various arenas—among family, friends, neighbors, employees, employers, professional peers, clients, students, and teachers. It is clear that people often fit into more than just one of those categories and that certain individuals play a mixture of roles. The classic depiction of a dual relationship is when two persons who interact professionally develop other roles of social interaction. For example, you and a working colleague discover a mutual interest in tennis and begin to play together, or you and your teacher develop a longstanding friendship. Dual relationships also develop in the other direction, from the social to the professional realm: you and your sister decide to go into business together; or a social acquaintance or a friend seeks your professional services.

There are 1,500 people in Browns Valley, and only one alternative health center. When one neighbor strains his back, or another develops hay fever, their only choice for massage or acupuncture is Lisa's clinic. Lisa grew up in Browns Valley and, after training as a massage therapist and then as an acupuncturist, returned home to open her clinic. Lisa markets her practice by talking to her church group, her kids' 4-H club, and her extended family. There are very few people she doesn't know in the valley, so most of her clients are also friends. Understanding the physical lives of the farmers in the community helps Lisa develop appropriate treatment plans. Because they have known Lisa all her life and they trust her, the people in the community aren't afraid to try complementary health care.

Points to Ponder

Does Lisa need to approach her social life differently than a therapist in a larger community since she is far more likely to run into clients in many situations? Does this make it more difficult for Lisa to maintain a separation of her personal and professional life, or does this situation eliminate the pressure to keep those aspects of her life separate in the first place?

Dual relationships are even more common in small towns or rural communities because of the limited numbers of people and choices for professional services.[1] Practitioners living in large cities can be more selective about dual relationships.

▌A Historical Perspective

Awareness of the risks involved in dual relationships in health care has evolved slowly over the past 40 years, beginning in the field of psychology. At the beginning of the 20th century, the situation was often handled in a fairly loose manner. Doctors had social relationships with their patients and very little clarity or agreement existed about whether dual relationships were a good or a bad idea. Awareness of the risks of dual relationships was limited to the idea that doctors shouldn't treat their own family members because their judgment might be clouded.

In the 1940s and '50s, there was much debate among different schools of psychology about the limits and propriety of dual relationships. Consensus gradually moved toward strict rules. Psychotherapists didn't treat members of the same family or even friends of their patients. It was generally felt that the temptations within dual relationships were too big and falling prey to them was too much of a risk—therefore all dual relationships were to be avoided.

In the early 1960s, with the advent of what is referred to as the Human Potential Movement, attitudes and cultural norms began to loosen, and some of the advantages of dual relationships emerged. For instance, if a couple were seen together there were advantages to the therapy, or if a sister and brother were seen by the same therapist, the therapist would have more knowledge about the dynamics of the family. In this period, it was commonplace for doctors to become friends with, or socialize with, their patients: university professors dated their students; and somatic practitioners treated all their friends and family members. As the helping field struggled to find a balanced approach with regard to multiple relationships, norms began to swing very far in the permissive direction.[2]

> The greatest homage we can pay to truth is to use it.
> — Ralph Waldo Emerson

The dangers became apparent when evidence of sexual impropriety and misconduct between psychotherapists and patients became more widely known in the 1970s and '80s. Victims of sexual exploitation, supported by the women's movement, began to speak out publicly, lawsuits were filed, insurance companies came under legal pressure to pay out large judgments, and advocacy groups demanded accountability and change.

In the field of psychiatry, Nanette Gartrell, Chair of Committee on Women for the American Psychiatric Association, along with Judith Herman (and many others), began researching the frequency of sexual inappropriateness within psychiatry.[3] Jean C. Holroyd and Annette M. Brodsky spearheaded research on sexual exploitation in the field of psychology.[4] These examinations of sexual misconduct cases prompted much thinking, research, and writing to clarify why and how dual relationships shift from simple to complex and eventually to damaging.

Until the late 1980s, very little thought was given to the importance of understanding multiple relationships and how they might interfere with the therapeutic relationship in the somatic therapy field. The massage therapy industry was one of the first to consistently demonstrate concern about dual relationships.[5]

Throughout the 1990s, a more balanced view of dual relationships emerged in many healthcare disciplines and educational institutions. Important wisdom will be gained when more healthcare and educational providers realize that they have the responsibility of dealing with the issues surrounding dual relationships.

As complementary healthcare disciplines evolve, so does the understanding that somatic practitioners develop strong therapeutic relationships with their clients. They need to behave with the responsibility that comes along with the power of that position. There are still many practitioners who don't take the risks and dangers of dual relationships seriously. We hope that after reading this chapter that they exercise careful judgment when considering or engaging in dual relationships with clients.

The Range of Dual Relationships

Dual relationships range from personal to financial. What follows are common circumstances where professional relationships, including those between clients and practitioners or students and school personnel, add new roles and thus become dual relationships.

Figure 3.1 Types of Relationships

- Socializing
- Group Affiliation
- Friendship
- Social Media
- Dating
- Sex
- Family
- Financial Arrangements
- Students

Socializing

Socializing is defined as an unplanned personal interaction occurring outside of the therapy time. Socializing implies that neither party would have sought this more personal experience of the other if the interaction hadn't transpired. It may occur when a client and practitioner find themselves at the same social event, such as a concert, movie, lecture, or party. In a school setting, socializing occurs at functions outside of classroom or office hours such as at workshops, retreats, or celebrations. Meeting in a social setting expands an otherwise limited professional relationship to include the experience of the event itself and more personal knowledge of each other.

Group Affiliation

Group affiliation refers to the special case where a practitioner invites a client (or a client invites a practitioner) to attend an activity focused on a group with which he is personally involved. Various kinds of groups include professional associations, educational classes or workshops, political organization meetings, product marketing programs, religious group meetings, therapy groups, PTA meetings, or recovery programs. In contrast to the more accidental meetings that take place in socializing, there is intention or purpose behind the invitation to the group. The motivation rests somewhere in the nature of the group itself and may not be clear to the person at the time the invitation is extended.

Unexpected consequences may arise if a practitioner accepts an invitation to a group or invites a client to a group in which he is personally involved. If the shared group experience turns negative, either party could feel awkward continuing the professional relationship. This can be particularly problematic when the motive behind the invitation, or the nature of the group itself, isn't made clear to the invitee at the time the invitation is extended. For example, if a client or practitioner accepts an invitation to a dinner meeting, only to find that it's a multi-level marketing recruitment meeting or religious group meeting, this could create unexpected conflict depending on the beliefs and values of the persons involved. Also, if extremely personal information is revealed in this context, it could damage the trust and safety of the professional relationship.

Friendship

Friendship implies that two people have an intimate interaction based on personal sharing, mutual liking, and loyalty. Friends actively seek out one another's company in settings that often include other acquaintances and friends. Any power differential in the professional relationship must, in a friendship, yield to a greater equality of connection. In a friendship both parties want and expect their needs to be met equally in a give-and-take manner. Maintaining both a friendship and a professional relationship is usually very difficult and puts both at risk.

Social Media

Connections on social media sites can vary from the simple unplanned personal interactions of socializing to the more intimate interactions of friendships. Social media presence usually involves more than a professional presence, where practitioner and client gain personal knowledge of each other. When either party shares personal information in the social media venue, the other party may feel more connected if they perceive similar interests, or they may feel alienated if they perceive differences. It may become difficult to maintain the professional relationship once personal knowledge is gained indicating major differences in beliefs or lifestyles.

See Chapter 9 pages 257-262 for tips on **Ethical Social Media Interactions**.

For instance, even if a practitioner has a business page on Facebook, that practitioner can be at risk for inappropriate self-disclosure if the public can see posts and photos on the practitioner's personal profile page. Another example of creating a dual relationship in social media is when a practitioner solicits donations for a charity on her business page.

Dating

It is generally inappropriate for a wellness practitioner to date a client. If a practitioner and a client are interested in dating each other, it's advisable to discontinue the professional relationship and wait for some time before starting to date. Dating involves a high level of interaction. When people date, their time together is more exclusive and generally is for the purpose of exploring each other as potential partners. As the couple's intimacy increases, the professional relationship takes a secondary role to the dating relationship, boundaries tend to blur, and the professional relationship becomes more difficult to manage.

See page 71 for more details on **Dating Clients**.

Sex

Sexual activity may occur as an isolated incident or may progress from socializing to friendship to dating. Even when sexual activity occurs only once, its impact on the professional relationship and, most importantly, on the client can be devastating and far-reaching.

Family

Dual relationships involving family members are among the most challenging to manage. Family members frequently expect to be treated differently than a usual client. They will "push" your boundaries. While this can happen at any stage of a practitioner's career, students are especially susceptible to this type of dual relationship. Family members may be the only folks you can find to practice on while in school. Students are essentially thrown into the deep end of the pool and forced to learn about dual relationships early in their careers because of the circumstances of the schooling process.

Financial Arrangements

Money adds an additional dimension to dual relationships. The three most common types of financial dual relationships are bartering, exchange of healthcare services, and employment.

BARTERING occurs when a practitioner and client exchange service for service rather than money for service. For example, a practitioner may offer sessions in exchange for laundry service, office cleaning, marketing assistance, or website design. This type of arrangement illustrates how dual relationships may consist of trading professional roles.

EXCHANGE OF HEALTHCARE services involves two healthcare practitioners who exchange services. For example, a chiropractor and an acupuncturist agree to exchange sessions. The effects on the professional relationship of this specialized type of barter center around the reversal of roles each practitioner makes, from client to practitioner and back again.

EMPLOYMENT refers to cases where a practitioner or school hires a client or student to work for financial remuneration. The types of jobs may vary widely, from secretarial work to designing brochures to building a cabinet. Work-study employment, for example, is one way students afford their training. The multiple professional roles involved have varying levels of impact on one another.

Students

In addition to the kinds of dualities described above, students may experience other permutations in the professional relationship. For example, a student who is a public relations specialist may have as a client one of his teachers or administrators; a student with an injury may undertake long-term therapy with a teacher. Any duality can significantly influence the core relationship between student and school personnel.

Identifying Dual Relationships

- Make a list of the current and past dual relationships in your life.
  Which dual relationships have been successful? Why?
- Identify any negative outcomes from your dual relationship. In retrospect, do you think the negative outcome could have been avoided? If so, how?

▌ The Benefits of Dual Relationships

Dual relationships are common occurrences, and not necessarily something to be avoided. Where practitioners get into trouble is in their lack of understanding of the complexities in multidimensional relationships. When practitioners learn how to work within these complexities, and maintain appropriate boundaries in the various roles, they can actually enjoy many benefits from their dual relationships.

People are often apprehensive about trying somatic therapies because it's hard to trust someone they don't know. That's where dual relationships become beneficial. For example, someone who needs bodywork but who otherwise wouldn't receive it may very well try it if the practitioner is a dear friend or family member. Consider the following scenarios:

1. Sue and Tracy had been in a drumming circle together for several years and considered each other dear friends. Sue recently experienced breast cancer resulting in a double mastectomy. Tracy, a massage therapist, knew that massage might help Sue with her healing process and offered to treat her. Sue was uncomfortable about being touched, but agreed because she loved and trusted Tracy. Tracy provided the needed safe space for Sue to feel comfortable in her own skin. Because of their previous relationship, they worked through the trauma, alleviating both physical and emotional pain. Without that dual relationship, Sue may not have reached out for the help she needed.

Points to Ponder

Should Tracy have offered her services to her friend? Are there any potential negative outcomes to Tracy having offered her services to Sue? Are there any other potential benefits to this particular type of dual relationship?

2. Joey is in massage school and plays basketball on Thursday nights with friends. This week, his friend Jim complained of some plantar fasciitis during their game. Joey had learned some techniques for plantar fasciitis just last week and asked Jim if he felt comfortable receiving a treatment. Joey had also just learned about dual relationships in school and told Jim about the risks. They mutually agreed that if the therapeutic relationship didn't work out, they wanted to continue their friendship on the basketball court. Joey helped Jim with his plantar fasciitis and other structural problems later on, as he had witnessed Jim's physical patterns in his basketball style.

Points to Ponder

Do the benefits of this dual relationship go both ways? While the benefits to Jim may be obvious, are there any benefits to Joey?

This last scenario illustrates how dual relationships can also enhance the therapeutic relationship. The better you know a person, the easier it is to navigate his idiosyncrasies. For instance, you might take the same communication skills class with a client and thereby gain increased compassion and understanding for each other. Also, you might discover the client's communication weaknesses and take different action in the treatment setting. If you were on the same volleyball team as a client, you might notice how the client uses her body and adjust your treatments to help her to avoid injuries.

The Risks of Dual Relationships

If dual relationships are common, why are they of such concern? This question generates a great deal of debate. When one of the interactions in a dual relationship is between a helping professional and a client, questions of concern include the following: To what extent does mutual and equal consent exist in making this relationship dual? Where does accountability lie? Will the therapeutic nature of the relationship be enhanced, hindered, or unaffected by the dual relationship?

For example, the person who becomes a client of her physical therapist friend, is surprised when the therapist charges her for a missed appointment, believing the "friend" part of the relationship would understand and excuse a last-minute schedule change. This belief is particularly understandable if the "professional" part of the relationship hadn't clearly communicated different expectations. Misunderstandings such as this often lead to an estrangement and the end of a friendship. Therefore, when communication is lacking or cues are misread in a dual relationship, feelings get hurt, one or both parties in the relationship suffers, and the relationship itself in all its manifestations is endangered.

Some experts contend that all dual relationships are harmful in the context of the helping professions. Others believe that dual relationships are often benign or even potentially beneficial. Mindful observation of the effects of a dual relationship is advisable. If problems develop, both parties can decide how to adapt to the issues.

Many elements are involved in dual relationships, and these elements often interact in subtle ways. All practitioners should receive special training in recognizing, evaluating, and communicating about dual relationship issues. In these ways, the risk in a dual relationship from a lack of understanding or poor communication is minimized. Furthermore, certain kinds of dual relationships are never ethical, when the risks are so high and the benefits so low that the relationship is unjustified.

If problems arise in a dual relationship, the relationship itself and the wellbeing of those involved suffer. What this means depends upon which human aspects are engaged (e.g., financial aspects, educational, social, romantic). Whatever issues are most prominent around the relationship are potentially vulnerable to harm if the relationship fails. Therefore, failed dual relationships can conceivably be related to failure in business, at school, or on a personal level.

Consider the following situations: In the first, a practitioner needs a website and knows that one of her clients has the experience to design it. In the second, a practitioner needs a shelf built in her office and knows that one of her clients is a carpenter. The wise practitioner uncovers any potential for harm in either case by asking many questions of herself, her client, and her supervisor or peer group. How much professional experience does the client have in web design or shelf building? How successful has his other work been, and how similar were those jobs to what the practitioner envisions for herself? How invested is the practitioner in the outcome of the work—in other words, how much does the practitioner stand to gain from a successful website or a sturdy shelf; and how much could she expect to lose from a job badly done? What is the potential impact of the outcome of the work on the client—will he gain significant exposure and referrals from a good job, or lose the goodwill of his therapist if his work isn't up to her expectations? If the outcome proves to be negative and the therapeutic relationship ends, how much of a loss is this to the client and the practitioner? Does the potential for emotional harm to the client outweigh the potential benefit? Would it be better to just hire a carpenter or web designer recommended by a friend or found in a directory?

The most important factor to remember about professional helping relationships is that they deal directly with people's wellbeing. Issues regarding mental, emotional, or physical health are near the core of the relationship and are therefore potentially vulnerable. For instance, a client with an injured shoulder invests his hopes for healing in a specific practitioner; or a client suffering from stress comes to rely on a hands-on session for relief. Will these clients lose therapeutic ground if a dual relationship with their practitioner goes awry?

Evaluating the Potential Risks

The potential for risk may be seen along a continuum. Sometimes a single element in the relationship signals a high risk potential. A strong need or an emotional component can signal that entering into a dual relationship with this client has a high risk factor. An illustration of this is a client who is in a great deal of pain and has come to rely on your expertise over many years. A number of factors work together to heighten or lessen the risk implied by any single factor. For instance, the risks are greatly multiplied if your client with chronic back pain is also the son of your friend, lives next door to you, and dates your daughter. In other cases, the risks are probably very low, such as if your neighbor sends his daughter for a one-time birthday session. In addition, risks must be evaluated not just between clients and practitioners but also between two practitioners who have a dual relationship. Consider the following example:

A mature person is one who does not think only in absolutes, who is able to be objective even when deeply stirred emotionally, who has learned that there is both good and bad in all people and all things, and who walks humbly and deals charitably with the circumstances of life, knowing that in this world no one is all-knowing and therefore all of us need both love and charity.

—Eleanor Roosevelt

An acupuncturist who had been in private practice for just a year referred a client to a massage therapist who was a close friend and a seasoned professional. The client was so impressed after visiting the massage therapist once that he decided to pursue massage for his pain problem and decided to terminate the acupuncture treatments because of the expense.

The acupuncturist was quite dismayed for several reasons. Foremost was his concern for his client's wellbeing because he felt this client needed more acupuncture treatments. He also felt a personal loss because he enjoyed working with this client, and because his income would be diminished. He wondered if he should refrain from referring more clients to this massage therapist until he felt more secure in his practice. He feared that if more referrals resulted in his loss of clients and income that it could create tension in the relationships between himself and the massage therapist, yet he knew his potential income loss was a bad reason to stop referrals and might not be in his clients' best interest. At this point, he realized he needed to get some supervision about this issue.

Points to Ponder

How would you handle a referral such as this? Was it appropriate for the massage therapist to continue to see the client, knowing that the client had decided to discontinue treatment with the referring acupuncturist?

The following questions help you evaluate the risk potential of a dual relationship you're either engaged in or considering:

> The truth of the matter is that you always know the right thing to do. The hard part is doing it.
>
> —Norman Schwarzkopf

Figure 3.2 **Evaluate Dual Relationship Risks**

- What is the intimacy level?
- What is the impact of the power differential?
- To what extent does mutual and equal consent exist?
- Who is accountable for what in the relationship?
- What is the relative maturity level?
- Will the therapeutic nature of the relationship be enhanced, hindered, or unaffected?
- What are the consequences of non-participation?

What is the Intimacy Level?

As the level of intimacy in dual relationship roles increases, so does the potential for harm if problems develop in the relationship. The levels of intimacy range from minimal (as in brief acquaintances or remote professional associations) to moderate (as in friendships or business partnerships) to high (as in sexual relationships and many long-term therapeutic relationships).

Each role in the dual relationship must be evaluated, considering both social and professional intimacy. For example, occasional social acquaintances who also interact as professionals may have little concern about the duality of their relationship. At the other end of the spectrum, a sexual component in a professional dual relationship greatly increases the risk potential. Some professional roles also involve a high level of intimacy; massage therapists and other somatic practitioners often interact with clients on a deeply personal, though not sexual, level.

A dual relationship that combines an intimate professional role with a sexual role carries so much risk for harm that it's never justified by the perceived benefits. Indeed, a sexual relationship with a client is a violation of helping professionals' codes of ethics, and in many states is illegal. One technique used by practitioners to foster an atmosphere of safety and clarity for their clients is publishing a straightforward policy statement about the inappropriateness of sexual contact between the practitioner and the client.

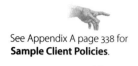

See Appendix A page 338 for **Sample Client Policies**.

What Is the Impact of the Power Differential?

When a professional helping relationship shifts to a dual relationship, both parties need to be as aware as possible of the effects of the power differential in every facet of their interactions. In a relationship between a practitioner and client, the power differential favors the practitioner. The helping relationship is an authority relationship because the client has a need and the practitioner has mastery, skill, or knowledge that may help the client meet that need. The practitioner holds the authority. The client brings openness and some vulnerability to the relationship.

Professional practitioners are expected to use the power differential to serve the client's needs, not their own. Practitioners must be well trained to recognize the shifts transference and countertransference make in the power dynamics and assure that abuse of the power differential doesn't occur.

See Chapter 1 page 5 for details on the **Power Differential**; and page 3 for information on **Fiduciary Responsibility**.

Two important factors within the authority relationship help determine whether duality in the relationship might work. First, can the person with more power be trusted to not abuse that power? Second, and of greater importance, is the person with less power capable of handling two different roles simultaneously with the authority figure?

Even an experienced practitioner can't always judge a client's ability to handle a dual relationship. It is advisable to err on the side of caution when it comes to dual relationships. Refrain from initiating a request to create a complication of the professional relationship. If the client asks the practitioner to engage in a new role with her, ask if that client is capable of handling the complexity of a dual relationship. Or does the pre-existence of the power differential make the client's consent questionable? A new role may present a considerable and difficult challenge for the client. If the power differential looms large in the client's perception, that very perception prevents the client from communicating freely in the relationship. The key question to ask if a client wants a dual relationship is, "How clouded is the client's judgment?"

To What Extent Does Mutual and Equal Consent Exist?

The answer to this question depends on who initiates the dual relationship. When a practitioner initiates a dual relationship, it's hard to determine whether there can truly be mutual consent due to the power differential. When a client initiates a dual relationship, mutual and equal consent can certainly exist, although the power differential can be at work within the client without the client having any understanding or perspective on it. Also, the responsibility if anything goes wrong will never be equal and always be the practitioner's. Friendships that become therapeutic relationships are more likely to do so with mutual and equal consent, since it's less likely that a power differential existed in the initial relationship.

Who Is Accountable for What in the Relationship?

Careful examination of all aspects of the relationship is needed to answer this question. Nevertheless, from an ethical—and often a legal—standpoint, whoever is acting in a professional role is held accountable for negative consequences of a dual relationship, whether those consequences are professional or social. The idea of accountability rests on several assumptions: the practitioner is aware of complexities and ethical considerations; the practitioner is trustworthy in maintaining the focus of the therapeutic relationship on the client; the client is in a position of greater vulnerability in the helping relationship.

Even if the client is the one who suggests adding a new role to the relationship, the professional is still the one to be held accountable. The decision to enter a dual relationship with a client demands integrity, consistency, and authenticity in all roles—hopefully from both persons involved, but most assuredly from the one who holds the professional power.

What Is the Relative Maturity Level?

This question speaks to the issue of why some dual relationships work and why others fail. Psychological maturity enables a person to navigate the uneven terrain of dual relationships. The mature person shifts easily among changing levels of intimacy and changing power dynamics, distinguishes reality from transference and countertransference, and accepts responsibility for the consequences of her behavior. When this person is a professional, she acts ethically and in the best interests of the client at all times. When this person is a client, she uses the therapeutic relationship to maximize her wellbeing without compromising the practitioner. When this person engages in a personal relationship in addition to a professional one, she allows boundaries to adjust appropriately.

Such maturity is usually a function of age and experience. If both parties in a dual relationship exhibit such maturity, the relationship has a better chance of success. Difficulty arises when the ability to make intelligent judgments is compromised by desire. Most people aren't good at making these kinds of judgments about themselves. Very few individuals say, "I am not mature enough to handle this complex dual relationship." Instead, the common internal thought is, "Maybe most other people couldn't handle this multi-layered relationship, but we can. No problem." If you think you're that rare individual, watch out! And if you find yourself talking to yourself in this way, it's a good time to seek a professional consultation from someone who is thoroughly impartial and with whom you have no other relationship. If we're developed enough to think we can handle something that most people can't, then we should be mature enough to tell it to a third party with the particular expertise to help us make that judgment.

How is the Therapeutic Relationship Affected?

Answering the previous questions brings the answer to this question into view. Consider whether the therapeutic nature of the relationship will be enhanced, hindered, or unaffected. Often creating a checklist, like a pros and cons list, is sufficient. What are the therapeutic benefits to the client? Is there any possibility of hindering the therapeutic treatment plan? Is it possible to have a dual relationship that can leave the therapeutic relationship unaffected?

What Are the Consequences of Non-Participation?

This final question is a litmus test when all other aspects of the potential dual relationship have been examined. If refusal to participate in a given aspect of a dual relationship brings negative consequences, it's likely that mutual and equal consent to the relationship doesn't exist. It is even possible that whoever suggests the dual relationship is attempting to manipulate or control the relationship to his advantage. In such cases, there may be tremendous pressure on one party to accept the proposed dual relationship.

Consider the possible consequences to a professional relationship if one person wants to initiate a more personal interaction and the other person refuses. Ideally, both the invitation and the refusal are dealt with maturely, and the original professional relationship remains intact. However, in some circumstances the invitation carries with it a threat that refusal will damage the professional relationship. This threat might impact the decision to refuse.

If a practitioner asks a client to a social function, what happens in the mind of the client? Questions and alarms begin to sound. "What does this invitation mean? Is this a date? Is she interested in me? What happens if I say no? Will she be mad at me? Will it alter this great professional relationship I have with her? Well! I knew she was interested in me; I should've asked her out myself first."

If the client asks the practitioner to a social function or out to coffee, what happens inside the mind of the practitioner? "Is this casual or is this client asking me out? It's kind of flattering that he is interested in me. What will happen to our professional relationship if I say no? Will he be upset with me and never return for treatment? I shouldn't have accepted those gifts. I should've made this clear in my policy statement the way that book said I should. This is awkward, what should I do now?"

Accepting a dual relationship is often very enticing. It takes character strength to decline the travel agent client's offer of free tickets to your favorite get-away in return for keeping him company on his trip. It is very attractive to hire an A+ student who graduated last week to teach at your school when you're hiring new teachers: he may know the material, be a great person and understand the culture of your school, but it's usually too quick a transition from student to teacher without an intervening year or two to develop professional distance.

In such situations, refusing the dual relationship requires skill and sometimes a great deal of courage. When the invitation comes from a client, the practitioner needs to refuse even if doing so risks loss of income, loss of referrals or loss of a professional relationship. Similarly, when the invitation comes from a practitioner, the client needs to refuse even if doing so risks loss of the therapeutic relationship. Clear statements of professional ethics, which every client should read before the beginning of the professional relationship, support both practitioners and clients in finding the courage to do the right thing in difficult circumstances. This is helpful because the boundaries of the relationship have been laid out and stated beforehand.

 To Dual or Not To Dual?

- List which relationships are so important to you that you wouldn't risk them by entering into a dual relationship.
- Think of a time when a relationship you were involved in had the opportunity to become a dual relationship, but did not. Whose decision was it to refuse? What reasons were given for the refusal? What were the results of refusal?
- In what situations might it be useful to have a written contract, however informal?
- Why is it always the healthcare practitioner's responsibility, rather than the client's, to ensure that dual relationship issues are discussed openly?

Sequential Relationships

Sometimes a relationship undergoes a change that is clearly acknowledged and publicly recognized: students graduate and are hired by their schools; classmates meet after graduation and form business partnerships; a former student joins the faculty and becomes a colleague; a former employee and employer marry. When one set of roles completely ends before a different set of roles begins, it's called a sequential relationship. However, although the change in sequential relationships may be clearly one-way (e.g., the school employee never returns to being a student), the former relationship may still exert an influence. The influence may be problematic if there has been a significant shift in the power differential. For instance, when a student or employee, who clearly has less power than the teacher or employer, begins to relate as a colleague of equal status, both parties need to transform their previous ways of relating. Therefore, people experiencing a relationship in transition must consider many of the same issues as those involved in dual relationships.

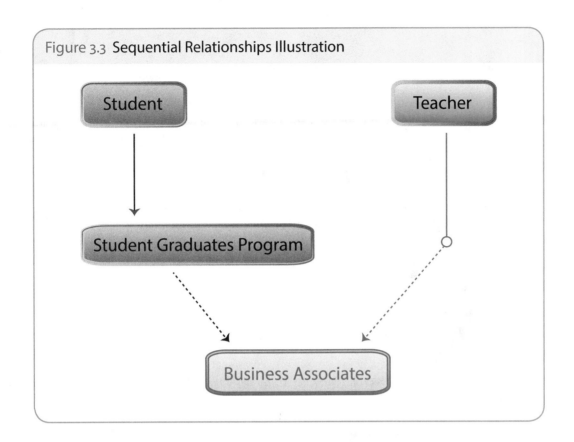

Figure 3.3 **Sequential Relationships Illustration**

Student

Teacher

Student Graduates Program

Business Associates

Sequential Relationships Exploration

Describe a sequential relationship you've experienced. What adjustments, if any, did you or the other person have to make when the relationship changed?

Dating Former Clients

Many practitioners haven't given much thought to the issue of sequential relationships, and may be unaware of the potential risks. A heavily publicized court case made it clear that these risks sometimes include legal liability. One Minnesota massage therapist risked losing her right to practice for having sex with a man who is now her husband.[6] Although this occurred months after their professional relationship ended, the couple didn't wait the two years mandated by state law, and were subjected to a three year ordeal including interrogation and psychological examination. This sparked the ACLU-MN to challenge the constitutionality of this type of law that holds alternative healthcare providers to a more rigorous standard than other healthcare providers. This standard, similar to that of psychotherapists, may be appropriate in cases where practitioners work with clients as they journey into deep emotional, mental, and spiritual healing. The Minnesota Department of Health rescinded its order for discipline.

When the topic of practitioners dating clients comes up in an ethics discussion, the focus is usually on sexual relationships with current clients. There is consensus throughout the field that such dual relationships are never appropriate; combining a professional role with a sexual role carries too great a potential for harm. But not all situations are so black and white. When it comes to dating *former* clients, legal and ethical codes often don't provide clear and consistent guidelines.

What's at Stake?

When a practitioner dates a former client, the client is the person most obviously at risk, as a result of issues relating to power and transference. All therapeutic relationships involve a power differential. The practitioner is the authority figure, and has the power to directly affect the client's wellbeing. In the shift to an intimate personal relationship, there's a risk that the therapeutic power dynamic will continue, so that the individuals can't relate as equals in a balanced partnership.

Additional risks arise around the issue of transference. The transference may be positive (e.g., adoration or idealization of the practitioner) or negative (e.g., feelings of anger or a sense of betrayal similar to a betrayal experienced in a previous relationship). Some anecdotal evidence suggests that physical contact (particularly intentional, caring touch) can stimulate regressive experiences, which may make transference more likely.

See Chapter 1 pages 8-11 for details on **Transference and Countertransference**.

When a professional relationship involving a wellness practitioner turns into a personal one, such responses leave the client highly vulnerable. As Dr. Sonia Nevis, psychotherapist and educator, explains, "The danger is that the person might not be doing what's necessarily best for them, because they want to please you."[7]

A further complication is countertransference. Like clients, practitioners have unresolved feelings and needs from their past that may be stirred up in the course of treatment. As with transference, countertransference creates serious complications for intimate relationships—significantly increasing the risk that one or both individuals will reenact their early traumas, conflicts, or family dynamics.

The risks of sequential relationships apply not just to clients, but also to practitioners. Issues related to transference or countertransference may cause just as much emotional distress for the practitioner as for the client. Moreover, it's the practitioner who's held liable for any legal or ethical violations or complications that may occur. Psychologist Gary Schoener, a respected expert in the field of ethics, boundaries, and sexual abuse issues, states the following:

> Although the literature, ethics codes, and licensure standards have focused on the danger to the former client, professionals need to be aware of their own liability and vulnerability. If something goes wrong in the eventual relationship, the professional may be liable civilly and criminally, and stand to lose a great deal… Once lines are crossed, the professional is at considerable risk if the former client becomes angry or frustrated, and especially if the relationship ends.[8]

Even if the client was the one who initiated the relationship, the practitioner is fully accountable for whatever happens. As we mentioned earlier, the individual may be violating state laws or professional codes of ethics, and could risk losing her license or expulsion from a certifying organization. An interesting twist is that the complainant doesn't have to be the client. For example, in the Minnesota case noted above, it was the ex-wife that filed charges against the massage therapist.

In addition to the personal liability involved, dating a former client could damage the reputation of an entire spa, multi-practitioner center, or other healthcare facility. Gossip travels quickly. Research has shown that negative information travels three to four times faster than news of positive experiences. For any organization that provides somatic therapy, having an impeccable reputation is essential. People looking for wellness services have many options to choose from, and doubts about a business's integrity can easily drive them to seek other alternatives.

A further risk of dating former clients is the potential to strengthen old negative stereotypes about a profession. For instance, although massage therapy has gained increasing acceptance as a reputable healthcare profession, that perception isn't universal; the image of the "massage parlor" mixing massage with sexual services still persists in the public imagination.

Complicating Factors

What makes this whole issue more complex is the great diversity of therapeutic relationships, with some eliciting much more of a power differential than others. At one end of the scale (generally less risky) is a spa practitioner who works on a client only once. Near the other end would be a practitioner who sees a client for six months or more, performing treatment including somato-emotional bodywork, injury rehabilitation, or lifestyle coaching.

The most straightforward factor affecting risk in a personal relationship is the duration and consistency of the professional relationship. All other things being equal, it's less problematic to transition from a sporadic, short-term relationship (e.g., three or four sessions over the course of a few months) than from a regular, long-term one (e.g., one or two sessions each week for a year).

It's also important to consider the quality of the professional relationship, including the depth of the therapeutic work and any dependence or intimacy that has developed in that context. Gary Schoener identifies several warning signs that indicate an increased risk of harm if the relationship turns personal:[9]

- The therapist has become a key figure in the client's life.
- The therapist talks to the client about the client's personal life, relationships, and psychological struggles—not just physical issues.
- There is significant emotional involvement or dependency.
- The therapist breaks her own rules with the client.

A relationship between mature peers would be quite different from one between a middle-aged practitioner and an emotionally vulnerable college student. Nina McIntosh, author of *The Educated Heart*, points out the following:

> In any circumstances, you must take into account the emotional stability of the client. For instance, does the client have solid self-esteem, or is she prone to depression, easily influenced, in crisis, or facing any other situation that would make her emotionally fragile? Some clients may never see themselves as equals with their practitioners.[10]

Prior relationships also play a role. For instance, the power differential could be lessened if the practitioner and client previously knew each other as equals.

Another key consideration is the client's history. Of particular concern is any prior experience of sexual, physical, or emotional abuse. Abuse often has silencing, self-doubting impacts on a person. Clients may have difficulty discerning and communicating their true feelings, which, in turn, doesn't allow for clear, mutual, and equal consent. Clarity can be especially challenging for a client when surrounded by confusing and intense feelings of attraction to and from a person who has been in a position of power.

When there is residual power differential as a practitioner engages in a romantic relationship with a former client, the practitioner is creating a dynamic of abuse parallel to that of incest.[11] For a survivor of abuse, the violation of trust through a former practitioner's engagement in a romantic relationship can evoke an intense, devastating period of crisis. During this time, the client needs much assistance to heal from the present day wounds that are inflicted alongside the ripped open scars of past violations.

When a practitioner's former work with a client involved any deep emotional healing, it's wise to follow guidelines for psychotherapists. The American Psychological Association's code of ethics gives two years as the waiting period before sequential relationships; however, caution is expressed, "even though sexual relationships that occur at least two years after therapy ends may be technically acceptable, they can still be harmful."[12]

On the positive side, some clients with abuse histories develop relationships with their previous practitioners to no ill effect; typically these individuals have worked through their prior traumas over many years of psychotherapy. There's no hard and fast rule to apply here; the appropriateness of personal involvement depends on the context and the individuals involved. When in doubt, get supervision and err on the side of protecting former clients.

> " A decision is made with the brain. A commitment is made with the heart. Therefore, a commitment is much deeper and more binding than a decision.
>
> —Nido Qubein

Guidelines for Navigating Romantic Relationships

The decision to enter a romantic relationship with a former client demands integrity, consistency, and authenticity. It isn't always easy to determine whether a romantic involvement is truly in the best interest of the former client. The shift from a therapeutic to a personal relationship should never be initiated by the practitioner. Taking such action is unprofessional and reflects negatively upon the somatic professions.

If you ever find yourself considering a romantic relationship with a former client, we strongly recommend you follow these five guidelines:

1. Familiarize yourself with the relevant laws in your state and with the codes of ethics of your professional organizations.

2. Consider each of the complicating factors mentioned above to make an informed judgment about the client's vulnerability with you. How large has the power differential been? Did the sessions with the client involve potent emotional states? Has there been any transference? Keep in mind that the client could one day wake up and be more aware of the impact of having had a romantic relationship with a former practitioner. The client may recognize that intentionally or unintentionally, you've taken advantage of his vulnerability. These issues aren't easy to assess by yourself. It is often useful to discuss them with a psychotherapist or supervisor.

3. Consider your own level of involvement and vulnerability. Has there been any countertransference? Do you have trouble maintaining boundaries or find yourself breaking your own rules with clients? It is difficult to evaluate your own feelings and actions from a rational, objective point of view. Tell the facts to a trusted colleague and get that person's opinion. Notice if you're reluctant to tell anybody—that, in and of itself, could be a sign of trouble.

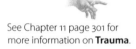

See Chapter 11 page 301 for more information on **Trauma**.

4. Wait before taking any steps toward a relationship. This gives both you and the former client some time to think more clearly. There isn't fixed consensus on how long the waiting period should be. Nina McIntosh suggests waiting six to nine months. She says, "Most people don't know how to judge if a client is too vulnerable. There needs to be time for reality to set in."[13] Few experts would advocate a blanket two-year rule, as previously instituted in Minnesota. ABMP President Les Sweeney has called the Minnesota rule "unrealistic and excessive." However, in some circumstances the two-year time period may make sense, such as with long term clients or when emotional or trauma healing has been a part of the sessions. Caution is advised here as well, since a practitioner may not be aware of, and therefore a poor judge of, just how deeply the work affected the client's mind, body, and soul. Sonia Nevis advises waiting at least two years in any case where there's a power differential. When there isn't a power differential, she suggests waiting six months and then reevaluating the situation. Keep in mind that there is always a power differential with a current client.

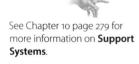

See Chapter 10 page 279 for more information on **Support Systems**.

5. Get some counseling and supervision. As a person interested in a relationship, the practitioner is always biased and needs assistance. The questions that come up are often complex and difficult to answer by oneself. Evaluating the magnitude of residual power differentials with former clients can be most reasonably accomplished with outside counseling and supervision. No matter how long the waiting period, both parties should get individual counseling to help make a healthy, well-informed decision. For those who decide to pursue a sexual relationship, we recommend ongoing couples counseling to help balance any remaining power differential and build healthy boundaries.

Figure 3.4 Guidelines for Navigating Romantic Relationships

- Know relevant state laws and your professional code of ethics.
- Consider complicating factors.
- Ascertain your level of involvement and vulnerability.
- Wait before forming a relationship.
- Get counseling and supervision.

▌ Minimizing Concerns

For a dual relationship (or sequential relationship for that matter) to work well, both parties must share a clear understanding of the complexities, especially the risks, involved. Furthermore, both parties must allocate equal responsibility for the establishment, continuation, and, if necessary, termination of any part of the dual relationship. Mutual and equal consent to all aspects of the dual relationship must be shared by both parties. Although this sounds reasonable, it's incredibly difficult to do. Even social relationships are often not equal or mutual in power.

It is the practitioner's responsibility to fully educate the client of the risks to the client and to the therapeutic relationship. In doing so, practitioners support the client's capacity to give informed, mutual, and equal consent or non-consent when contemplating dual relationships.

> ❝ Any change, even a change for the better, is always accompanied by drawbacks and discomforts.
>
> —Arnold Bennett

Sharing excerpts from this book can be a part of this education. The practitioner who educates the client about both potential positives and potential negatives of the duality provides the client with the tools he needs to make an informed decision. This education is important whether the suggestion for the dual relationship comes from the client or from the practitioner. If, for example, the client suggests attending a social event together, the practitioner helps the client recognize how adding personal dimensions affects an established professional relationship.

The practitioner who offers to hire a client to do some work should encourage the client to think about the invitation and to discuss it with a trusted friend or colleague before responding. The client must consider the risks to the therapeutic relationship if the added relationship is unsuccessful. The risks of that loss are very real and shouldn't be minimized.

1. A practitioner hired a long time client to do some renovations to her kitchen. The practitioner found herself a bit uncomfortable with her client being in her private space and interacting with her family. Essentially everything went along fine until the kitchen caught on fire and was destroyed. The fire also damaged many irreplaceable objects of sentimental value. After the fire, the practitioner found herself feeling resentful toward the client wondering if the fire was caused by negligence or if it was just an accident. She was also upset with herself for entering into this exchange of services with the client. The client felt devastated, depressed, and guilty. The practitioner felt she could no longer see him as a client and terminated the relationship.

2. A client approached her practitioner about walking his dog in exchange for treatment. This bartering arrangement continued for six months without any problems. The client and practitioner were very happy with the situation. It seemed ideal to the practitioner who never seemed to have enough time to walk his beloved dog. One day the dog pulled so strongly that the client lost her grip on the leash. The dog had seen another dog across the street and was running to visit

and play with the other dog when it was hit by an oncoming car. The owner was grief-stricken and couldn't bring himself to continue seeing the client.

Points to Ponder

Are there any boundaries that could be set in the above scenarios to minimize the risks for negative outcomes? When is it okay for practitioners to enter into these types of agreements with clients?

It would be unethical for a practitioner to offer a client blanket assurance that the addition of other roles has no effect on their professional relationship. If it's of primary importance to either party that the professional relationship remains unchanged, then a dual relationship should not be initiated. Sometimes merely suggesting a dual relationship, much less entering into one, causes an immediate change in how two people relate.

When dual relationships develop more fully (e.g., into a friendship), the initial professional relationship may take on a lesser role and even perhaps end by mutual consent. It is impossible to know whether what can be gained is more valuable than what might be lost. The richness of our lives is often enhanced through our complex, growing, and changing relationships. When both parties bring maturity and a sense of responsibility to the decision about developing a dual relationship, there is a good chance for each person to feel empowered and enriched by the experience no matter what may happen to the relationship itself in the future.

 Role-Play Adding a Relationship

Role-play with a partner: one of you is a practitioner, the other a client. In the first interaction, have the client suggest to the practitioner an added role to their relationship, and allow the practitioner to respond. Then, in the same roles, have the practitioner suggest to the client an added role, and have the client respond. Switch roles and repeat the exercise. After the experience, discuss the following questions: What did you feel while playing each role? How easy or difficult was it to respond to the suggestion that the relationship change? How did your partner's reactions affect your perception of whether the dual relationship would work?

Seek Supervision

Professional supervision is invaluable if a practitioner is trying to decide about engaging in a dual relationship or working to evaluate one in which he already participates. The questions are often difficult to answer alone and many of the answers depend heavily on interactions involving complex factors. Consulting someone else outside the relationship enables the practitioner to gain perspective and to better see the whole picture. This is usually not easy to do by yourself.

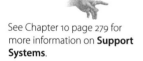

See Chapter 10 page 279 for more information on **Support Systems**.

Often the person in the power position of a dual relationship doesn't perceive the relationship doing any harm, while the person in the vulnerable position experiences negative consequences. No matter which role you find yourself in, supervision helps re-orient you to a position of responsibility and positive decision-making. Consider the following scenarios:

1. A client asked a practitioner to barter some artwork for treatment because she was low on cash and didn't want to stop treatment. The practitioner was aware that this client often had financial problems and wanted to help if he could. He told the client that he wanted a few days to think about it. The practitioner then took this issue to his professional supervision advisor to help him decide what to do. The supervisor had the practitioner explore how his desire to help others at his own expense, his issues with money, and the difficulties he had earlier in his career, all related to his desire to help this client at any level of risk. The client had said that the practitioner could view her work and decide what he wanted to pay for the paintings. The supervisor pointed out that this arrangement could lead to enormous problems if the practitioner didn't like the client's work or if he offered a price that was too low or even too high.

    The practitioner and the supervisor came up with a plan that included informing the client of the risks to the relationship if he wasn't interested in any of his client's artwork and the dangers of the practitioner choosing a price. After this discussion with the client, the practitioner would ask the client to take a few days to think about the risks and decide if she wanted to pursue this idea further. If she did, she would have to set the prices for her artwork and understand that the practitioner might not be interested based on the type of art and the price.

Points to Ponder

Could the practitioner have simply refused the offer, rather than propose an alternate plan? Does the alternate plan account for all the possible pitfalls of this type of agreement?

2. A practitioner treated a friend for a shoulder pain and the friend didn't like the service that she received. She felt physically hurt and in pain for a couple weeks after treatment and immediately stopped seeing the practitioner professionally and personally. Not only did the person lose a client, but also a friend. The practitioner and the friend were very upset about this turn of events. It seemed reasonable enough at the time; the friend had a need and the practitioner/friend seemed to have the expertise. The practitioner took this issue to supervision to understand what happened and what thinking errors she had made. She learned that she didn't fully appreciate or understand the risk she was taking by the following: treating her friend for a pain problem without informing the client/friend of the possibility that her treatment might not work; not acknowledging that the client/friend might not like her work; and forgetting the fact that the treatment might cause soreness for many days. She took it for granted that the friend would understand. It was a hard lesson to learn, and she never entered into a dual relationship lightly again.

Points to Ponder

Who are the people in your life who can give you clear, knowledgeable advice in the area of dual relationships?

Supervision helps you ethically manage your practice and is even useful in analyzing dual relationships after an error in judgment has already been made.

The Special Case of Schools

For touch practitioners in training, the school setting is an important context in which to learn and practice the principles surrounding dual relationships. All the dynamics mentioned throughout this chapter can exist between teachers and students who consider adding social or other roles to their interactions. Indeed, one dual relationship in this setting often affects the dynamics of an entire class or faculty group, and may even affect the reputation of the school as a whole.[14] In addition, the process of learning (particularly touch therapies) can elicit deep healing processes within students, bringing them to places of vulnerability, similar to that of clients.

Precise, published policies are crucial in school environments to lay the groundwork for ethical behavior around issues of dual relationships between students, teachers, and administrators.

Consider the example of a teacher and student who begin dating. Is it possible for a teacher to obtain mutual and equal consent from a student, when a power differential is so obviously at work? Can the teacher remain objective when he has to evaluate and grade the student's work? How do other students in the class respond to their own evaluations if they feel the teacher is biased in one case? How does knowledge of the relationship affect the class's interactions in partner and group activities? If a different teacher has to fail or sanction the student, how does this influence the faculty relationship? If the social relationship ends badly, might the student bring charges against the school?

All of these examples have happened numerous times in many school settings, often with disastrous results for the student, the teacher, or the school. A conservative stance, like that taken by most educational institutions, is worthwhile in this setting because the consequences can be far-reaching. Many schools have strict non-fraternization policies in place to avoid just these situations. These non-fraternization policies can vary: from simply prohibiting sexual relationships between teachers and their current students; to prohibiting all social interactions between teachers and active enrolled students, including social media sites. Because some schools view the risks of dual relationships as just too great, many of them don't allow teachers to treat students in their private practices.

> A teacher tutoring a student after class made advances to the student. The student felt in awe of the teacher's knowledge and charisma. An intimate relationship followed, and the other students became aware of it. Gossip was stimulated at the school, and considerable tension in the class resulted because the student was called on frequently in class and received high grades. The relationship ended after a few months. The student was devastated and felt awkward about staying in school.
>
> After making a complaint to the school administrators, no actions were taken to discipline the teacher or formulate new policies to protect students. Even with ongoing emotional repercussions including anxiety and insomnia, she summoned the courage to initiate a lawsuit against the school and the teacher. The teacher was fired (and sued the school) and the school's reputation suffered. Eventually the school implemented non-fraternization policies for its faculty.
>
> ### Points to Ponder
>
> Should a school have the authority to set non-fraternization policies? What would you suggest be included in these policies? Could these issues have been avoided if the school in this situation had such policies?

When boundaries about dual relationships between students and teachers aren't clearly stated and enforced by a school, painful consequences often follow. In this example, there were devastating effects on the students, the faculty, and the reputation of the school. Everyone in this situation was upset and hurt for a long time: sides were taken; students felt betrayed, angry, and unsafe; faculty felt shamed; and there were severe financial consequences for the school.

A female teacher and a male student became friends. The teacher needed to find someone she trusted to stay with her kids and the student needed to earn money, so she hired him to babysit her children. The student developed a close relationship with the teacher's children. He also had an unrecognized transference on the teacher and idolized her. This continued for a year until the student got upset with an interaction the teacher had with her children. The student felt betrayed and never saw the children or the family again. Everyone concerned experienced a great deal of pain in this situation: the student, the children, and the teacher.

Points to Ponder

Is it possible for teachers and students to safely form friendships? What was the biggest mistake that the teacher made in this situation?

The point is that creating friendships between teachers and students can have negative consequences. The teacher should never have befriended the student in this manner. The teacher was ultimately responsible for exercising very poor judgment in this situation. Bringing the student into the teacher's family was, by far, the biggest mistake in this situation.

A school director, who was also a somatic practitioner, had a client who expressed an interest in attending the school where she was the director. He enrolled, and, for a short period of time, was a client and a student. After a few weeks, the practitioner/director discussed dual roles with the student/client. They mutually agreed to stop the client/practitioner relationship. A year later this same student asked to become a temporary office worker in the school. It was agreed that he could but that he wouldn't directly work for the school director. The student graduated from school and a year later became a teacher in the school. After several years, the school director began seeing her former client/student/employee for occasional treatments. Their relationship lasted more than 10 years.

If this sounds complicated, that's because it was. Often, the two would consciously and overtly state which roles they were in. They wouldn't mix roles in their conversations and interactions. Although there were elements of a dual relationship along the way, it was also a sequential relationship where one role was left and another begun. What made this relationship work was clear, honest communication and deliberate acknowledgment of which roles they were in at the time.

Points to Ponder

What formal situations at school or at work have you been in that had specific policies regarding dual relationships? How did it appear to affect relationships in that setting? Overall, was it a positive, safe experience, or was it uncomfortable in any way?

In this last example, both parties talked openly and communicated effectively about the transitions in their relationship. They moved quickly out of dual relationships and into sequential ones. Their ability to change roles and reverse positions of authority as well as the lasting nature of the relationship demonstrates how one can successfully navigate the complexities of human and professional relationships.

Conclusion

Dual relationships are a natural aspect of human interaction. They hold the potential to enrich our lives. They also hold the potential to cause great pain. As a somatic practitioner, you must be especially aware of the dynamics of these complex relationships. With mature self-awareness and responsible choices, you can safeguard the therapeutic relationship and enjoy appropriate overlapping connections with clients.

4
Dynamics of Effective Communication

"The single biggest problem with communication is the illusion that it has taken place."
—George Bernard Shaw

Communication Barriers
- Noise
- Defense Mechanisms
- Power Differentials

Challenging Topics of Conversation
- Strong Emotions
- Boundaries
- Feedback
- Managing Your Negative Feelings

Communications Beyond the Treatment Room
- Ambiguity
- Privacy
- Professionalism

Key Terms

Aggressive Language
Ambiguity
Assertive Language
Conflict
Consistency
Contradictory Communication
Defense Mechanisms

Denial
Feedback
Mind-Reads
Noise
Passive Language
Privacy
Proactive Discussions

Professionalism
Projection
Rapport
Redundant Messages
Repression
Self-Disclosure

It is difficult to overstate the importance of clear communication for a successful and ethically responsible practice. Communication is the primary way in which we build professional relationships; set, maintain, and negotiate boundaries; empower clients to take an active role in their treatments; and resolve any conflicts that arise. All the best intentions and principles are of limited value if you can't put them into practice through what you say and how you say it.

We begin this chapter by discussing various barriers to effective communication which range from the ambiguity inherent in our language to the specific difficulties posed by defense mechanisms and power differentials. We then go on to explore four particularly challenging topics of conversation: strong emotions, boundaries, feedback, and managing negative feelings. Later, we address communications that occur outside the treatment room through writing, phone conversations, electronic messages, and social media.

Learning to communicate effectively is no easy task. It requires a great deal of study, time, and patience, as well as good teachers and a safe educational setting. However, it's one of the most worthwhile investments you can make in establishing and maintaining healthy long-term relationships with your clients. Be patient with yourself as you begin to incorporate new ways of communicating into your work. You may need to practice for quite a while before they begin to feel natural and automatic. Nevertheless, the payoff is well worth the effort. Mastering the skills in this chapter can bring about significant positive change not only in your therapeutic work, but in every aspect of your life.

▊ Communication Barriers

At one time or another, we've all had the unpleasant experience of trying hard to express ourselves clearly, and still being misunderstood. No matter how carefully we organize our thoughts and choose our words, we sometimes fail to get our message across. And, of course, this may happen in reverse as well: someone else tries hard to communicate a message to us, but we mishear or misinterpret what they're saying.

In addition to causing frustration, these problems may lead to a host of other complications, particularly in a healthcare context. For example, a variety of research studies have found that there are often large gaps between what patients really want and what their doctors think they want. As a result, healthcare providers may believe they're following a patient's wishes, when in fact they're doing the exact opposite.[1] In the following sections, we look at some of the most common causes of communication breakdowns and consider what we can do to prevent them.

Noise

At the heart of all communication is a single purpose: to transfer information from one person, or group of people, to another. No matter what content is being discussed—test results from a doctor, questions from a client, deep feelings expressed to loved ones, or worries shared with a friend—the goal is to get a message across. Unfortunately, we often communicate in ways that make it harder for this to happen; something about the way we talk tends to interfere with the transfer of information. The term for this type of interference is *noise*. (Note: The discussion of noise that follows is drawn from the *System for Analyzing Verbal Interaction* (SAVI®), developed by Anita Simon and Yvonne Agazarian.[2, 3, 4] Simon and Agazarian built on Claude Shannon's and Warren Weaver's concept of noise; the SAVI grid organizes all communication into noisy and non-noisy categories of behavior.[5]) The three forms of noise are *ambiguity*, *contradiction*, and *redundancy*.

AMBIGUITY. Ambiguous comments are vague or unclear, subject to multiple interpretations. For instance, if your clients tell you, "Your office decor is very unusual!" or "You have an interesting style of working," it isn't clear whether they're criticizing you or paying you a compliment. This ambiguity makes it less likely that you'll understand what the clients really mean and respond appropriately.

CONTRADICTION. Contradictory communication sends two conflicting messages at the same time. Often the words say one thing, and the voice tone says just the opposite. For instance, a therapist talking about a practitioner she doesn't like might use sarcasm: "Oh, yeah, he's a great person to interact with." Her words say that this person is great, but her tone says that he really isn't. In some situations, the contradiction comes through body language; we sense a lack of congruity when someone expresses irritation or anger with a smile on his face. (Please note that the SAVI framework addresses only the verbal aspects of communication, but the concept of contradiction can easily be extended to body language as well.) Another example of contradiction is yes-butting, which is essentially saying yes and no simultaneously. A teacher may tell a student, "Yes, your paper was interesting, but you didn't write about the topic I assigned you." Contradiction creates problems in a conversation because it's difficult to take in two conflicting pieces of information at once.

REDUNDANCY. Redundant messages are so repetitious that the people on the receiving end tend to stop listening. This may happen in a classroom setting, when an instructor keeps explaining the same idea over and over again. It can also happen in a therapeutic session when a practitioner has a favorite saying, story, or piece of advice that she repeats to the point where her clients are sick of hearing it.

> " No one would talk much in society if they knew how often they misunderstood others.
> —J. W. von Goethe

Noise in Your Communication

Take a moment to reflect on the noise in your own communication. Which of the three types of noise do you use most often? Can you think of specific examples of ambiguous, contradictory, or redundant things you sometimes say?

Which type of noise tends to bother you the most when it comes from other people? What are some ambiguous, contradictory, or redundant comments you hear from clients, colleagues, or other people in your professional or personal life?

The Ambiguity of Language

The ambiguity in our language isn't limited to obviously vague words like "interesting" and "unusual." Words are generally imprecise vehicles of communication. The 500 most frequently used English words have 12,078 separate and distinct meanings in *The Oxford English Dictionary*. On average that's 24 meanings per word!

The biggest problem with language is that the meaning of words is in people, not in dictionaries. Each of us projects our own meanings onto the words we say and hear, based on our unique personal history—which includes our perceptions, beliefs, emotional patterns, sensitivities, personality, likes and dislikes, educational training, and so forth. What you mean when you say something may be quite different from the meaning that the listener takes away. Suppose that you ask clients to call you only "in an emergency," and they agree. The communication appears at first to be perfectly clear. However, you and your clients may have very different ideas of what constitutes an emergency. This becomes clear if, for instance, a client calls you at all hours of the day with questions that you don't consider to be emergencies.

Reducing Noise

Each of the three forms of noise makes communication more difficult, and also tends to increase stress; when information isn't getting through, people typically start to feel frustrated.

Figure 4.1 Noisy Communication Behaviors

Behavior	The Problem	Example	More Useful Alternative
Yes-But	Saying yes and no at the same time sends a contradictory message and emphasizes disagreement rather than common ground.	"Sure, it costs more to come twice a week, but it's critical for your healing process."	Three builds plus a broad (open) question: "Increasing sessions from once to twice a week can be a real financial challenge. It isn't something you would have budgeted for. And I know this is a tough time for you, with all the medical expenses you have now. Do you have any thoughts on how to give your injury the attention it needs, while still keeping your expenses manageable?"
Mind-Read	By talking as though you know what someone else thinks or feels, you act on assumptions rather than reality.	"I can tell you're not really comfortable discussing this topic."	Statement of your thought plus a yes/no question: "I'm thinking you might be uncomfortable discussing this topic. Is that true?"
Negative Prediction	Assuming that a bad outcome is inevitable can lead to hopelessness and failure to take action.	"If I talk to this client about the strong perfume she wears, she'll get offended."	Broad questions to identify facts and plan for a better outcome: "In my past communications with clients about similar issues, what factors have contributed to the discussion going well or going poorly? What can I do to increase the chances that this conversation will go well?"
Leading Question	Questions that pressure the other person to agree with you tend to elicit either resentment or inauthentic agreement.	"Aren't you uncomfortable in that position?"	Your opinion plus a yes/no question: "That position looks uncomfortable to me. Is it uncomfortable for you?" Or ask a broad question: "How do you feel with your body in that position?"
Complaint	A hopeless, passive outlook blocks you from actively moving toward what you want.	"This new intensive work I'm doing is just killing my back, but it's all people seem to want now so I'm stuck with it."	A statement of what you want followed by a proposal to help you get it (repeated as necessary): 1. "I want to start doing less of this type of treatment." (want) "I could limit the number of appointment slots I allot for these treatments each day." (proposal) 2. "I actually would rather stop doing this type of work." (deeper want) "I could gradually start referring some clients to other therapists who provide this treatment, while working to attract new clients seeking less physically demanding modalities." (proposal)
Attack	Venting anger or irritation at others damages relationships and distracts from the underlying problem that's upsetting you.	"There's no point in working hard to help you heal if you're going to keep taking crazy risks and re-injuring yourself."	Combination of facts, feelings, proposals and/or questions: "Twice before, you've healed from an injury and then been injured again within a month." (fact) "I care about your health and wellbeing, and I worry about what might happen if you return to extreme sports." (feeling) "Would you be open to discussing steps you might take to prevent future injuries?" (question)

The converse is also true. Stress tends to increase noise, because when people are frustrated, they're more likely to communicate in noisy ways. The result is a vicious cycle. Noise in the conversation generates frustration, which in turn generates more noise, and so on.

The first step in reducing noise is to shift your awareness from *what* you're saying (your content) to *how* you're saying it (your behavior—the combination of your words and your voice tone). Often we think a great deal about the ideas we're trying to get across, but fail to notice the particular ways we're expressing them. The same basic message will come across very differently depending on the behavior you use to express it. For example, suppose you're trying to tell a client how her lateness is affecting your work with her. You might ask, "Don't you think you'd benefit more from this work if you arrived on time for a full session?" (a leading question); or snap, "You make it impossible for me to give you a proper treatment!" (an attack); or whine, "It's just *so hard* to do what I need to do in less than an hour" (a complaint). Each of these behaviors is inherently noisy; in other words, they automatically increase the level of ambiguity, contradiction, or redundancy in the communication. As a result, talking in these ways tends to make your conversation more difficult and stressful than it needs to be. More useful behaviors in this situation might include giving a fact ("For the past three weeks, you've arrived 15 minutes late for your appointment") or a feeling ("When I don't have time to give you a full treatment, I feel disappointed and frustrated").

From time to time, we all communicate in ways that make it more difficult for our message to get through. Figure 4.1 gives examples of six very common noisy behaviors (drawn from the SAVI grid), together with suggestions of alternative behaviors that are likely to be much more constructive. (For more detailed strategies for managing each of these troublesome behaviors both in yourself and in others, as well as a discussion of the SAVI framework from which all of this material is derived, see *Conversation Transformation*.[6])

Visit the **SAVI Communications** website, for more information on the SAVI framework, a copy of the SAVI grid, and a more extensive bibliography.

http://www.savicommunications.com/

Defense Mechanisms

Defense mechanisms are psychological strategies of relating to the world around us that we develop unconsciously to protect us from fear, pain, shame, anxiety, and other emotionally painful experiences. At the time when a defense develops (often early in life), it serves a very useful purpose—shielding us from feelings that we're unable to handle. However, if the defense persists long after the original difficult experience has ended, it may limit our ability to respond to future challenges in an appropriate, functional way. Three defense mechanisms that often affect communication in a therapeutic context are *projection*, *repression*, and *denial*. (For a more detailed discussion of defense mechanisms, see *Therapeutic Communications for Health Care*, by Carol Tamparo and Wilburta Lindh.[7])

Projection

One way in which people defend against an uncomfortable thought or feeling is to *project* it onto someone else, seeing it as the other person's issue. When a practitioner projects her own experiences onto a client, she may end up giving the type of session that she herself needs, rather than addressing the actual needs of the client. Often the individual who is the object of projection ends up feeling frustrated, confused, or irritated. Consider these examples:

1. A practitioner recently lost a loved one and has been grieving for several weeks. When one of her clients isn't as animated as usual, she assumes that he is feeling sad. During the session, she offers words of comfort such as "Don't worry; everything will be okay" and "It's okay to feel sad," and gives him a reassuring pat on the shoulder. The client says, "What do you mean? I feel fine." The practitioner responds, "It's normal not to want to admit it when you feel sad, but this is a safe environment for you." The client leaves feeling perplexed, disconcerted, and less trusting of this practitioner's judgment.

2. A practitioner is feeling a great deal of unresolved anger about a recent breakup. In a session with one of his clients, the client makes several requests—asking for more pressure, more attention to certain body areas, and so forth. After each request, the practitioner feels uneasy and hurt. He concludes that the client is dissatisfied and angry with him, and he begins to withdraw. As a result, the client experiences him as not being present and becomes more demanding. The treatment ends with the client feeling dissatisfied and the practitioner feeling disrespected.

Points to Ponder

In each of these two situations, how could the practitioners increase awareness of their own emotional states? What clues might they have noticed, either in their own state of mind or in the client's reactions, that suggested they were projecting?

Notice that the type of thinking associated with projection ("She's feeling sad," "He's angry with me") is one of the noisy behaviors listed in figure 4.1: Mind-Read. If you notice yourself having a strong emotional response to something one of your clients says or does, ask yourself whether you're making any assumptions about what that person thinks or feels. Could those assumptions be projections of your own mental state?

Projections also happen in the opposite direction, from client to practitioner. An individual who tells her practitioner, "It's obvious that you're angry" or "I can tell you're attracted to me" may (among other possibilities) be projecting her own experience.

Repression

In *repression*, feelings or memories that are too painful to bear are blocked from conscious awareness. For example, an adult who experienced a trauma in childhood may have no recollection of the event. This is frequently the case in incidents of sexual abuse. Note that repression results not from a conscious decision to forget an experience, but from a purely automatic, instinctive reaction to trauma.

It isn't uncommon for repressed memories to surface spontaneously during hands-on therapeutic sessions. Practitioners working in this field need to be aware of that phenomenon and know how to respond appropriately, within their scope of practice. Often it's wise to refer the client to a psychotherapist who specializes in working with traumatic memories.

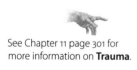

See Chapter 11 page 301 for more information on **Trauma**.

Practitioners should also be aware of the possibility that their own behavior could be influenced by unresolved repressed experiences. As psychologist and bodyworker Dr. Ronan M. Kisch explains in *The Hidden Dimensions of Bodywork*, "Repression may lead bodywork practitioners to seek personal gratification from professional contacts…or attempt to avoid the clients with whom the issue arises and anxiously hope that they never come back."[8] Repression by the practitioner can have physical consequences as well. Repressed awarenesses, Kisch explains, don't simply go away. "They are translated into somatic tension lodging in the body tissues, covertly robbing the practitioner of peace of mind and precision in work." In some cases that tension may be somatically transferred to clients.

Denial

Denial is an active refusal to recognize or acknowledge the full implications of an undesirable reality. Denial bears some similarity to repression, but requires the collaboration of the conscious mind. Although the person realizes the truth of the situation, at least at some level, he insists on a distorted interpretation of the facts.

The classic example is a person who suffers from alcohol or drug addiction and insists that he doesn't have a problem and can stop anytime he wants, despite a mountain of evidence to the contrary (failed relationships, lost jobs, car accidents, and so forth).

As a practitioner, you may encounter clients who are in denial about how their body is being affected by a variety of lifestyle choices, from overwork to unhealthful eating to participation in extreme sports. It is also possible for denial to follow the retrieval of repressed memories of abuse; victims may, for a time, speak of the traumatic events as though they were unimportant, thus denying the impact of the trauma on their lives.

Power Differentials

As we discussed in Chapter 1, all therapeutic relationships involve a power differential. The practitioner's knowledge and status place her in a position of authority in relation to the client. This aspect of the relationship can have a negative impact on the client's ability to communicate effectively. In particular, clients may often be hesitant to raise concerns about boundary issues. They may worry that these concerns will seem foolish, trivial, or cowardly; that the practitioner will see them as being disrespectful or insulting, resulting in poorer service; or that the positive connection they have with the practitioner will be lost. Alternatively, clients may resent the practitioner's power and become angry, challenge the practitioner's competence, and undermine their treatment.

> The right to be heard does not automatically include the right to be taken seriously.
>
> — Hubert Humphrey

In some therapeutic relationships, the practitioner actually feels less powerful than the client, and this creates difficulties as well.

A physical therapist had a client who was a well-known surgeon. The therapist was in awe of this client's training and expertise, and her work with him was tentative. She found herself reluctant to point out the lifestyle stresses that were contributing to his low back pain or to strongly recommend exercises for him to do at home. She felt relieved when the surgeon stopped booking appointments with her.

Points to Ponder

What were the needs of the client in this situation? How did the physical therapist's experience of the power differential make it harder for her to meet those needs?

Problems can also arise when practitioners are uncomfortable with the very existence of a power differential and have difficulty speaking with the authority that is appropriate for their role. These individuals may find themselves being lax in communicating about boundaries in an attempt to put themselves and their clients on an "even footing." If you find yourself frequently deferring payments for sessions, extending session times even when your schedule is tight, booking outside your regularly established hours, and making home visits you would prefer not to make, consider whether you're fully comfortable with the power associated with your professional role.

- Are you comfortable with the power dynamic of your role as practitioner? Are you perhaps too comfortable?
- How might your feelings about the power differential affect your communication with clients?
- How might you use skillful communication to help diminish any negative effects of the power differential?

Challenging Topics of Conversation

As in any other area of life, our communication with clients includes some conversations that are effortless and enjoyable, and others that are much more stressful and difficult. Topics of conversation that are frequently challenging for practitioners include strong emotions, boundaries, feedback, and managing negative feelings.

Strong Emotions

Hands-on techniques can elicit strong emotions in some clients. Sometimes just touching a particular area triggers an emotional response. In the course of a session, a client may cry or become fearful, anxious, or angry. Many practitioners discuss this possibility prior to beginning work with a client, particularly if the type of treatment is prone to eliciting emotions or if the client's history suggests emotional volatility.

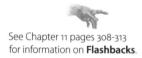

See Chapter 11 pages 308-313 for information on **Flashbacks**.

Take great care to remain within your scope of practice. The boundary between the roles of somatic practitioner and psychotherapist can easily get blurred, particularly when clients experience emotions that are associated with events in their past. Keep in mind the significant difference between 1) assisting a client in letting go of a thought, memory, or feeling that has surfaced spontaneously, and 2) actively promoting an emotional reaction or release. While the former may be useful and appropriate, the latter typically is not. (Note: Traumatic flashbacks are a special case and require a specific course of action.)

In situations where clients want to talk to you about their experiences, it's usually fine to let them express themselves. However, be sure to avoid making your own interpretations, encouraging them to divulge more details, or probing into the causes of their emotions. See figure 4.2 for several examples of questions that are almost always inappropriate to ask in a somatic therapy session.

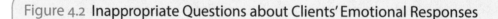

Figure 4.2 Inappropriate Questions about Clients' Emotional Responses

- Do you know why you felt sad when I touched your leg?
- Were you thinking of someone in particular when you began to feel anxious?
- Do I remind you of someone in your family or your past?
- Do you remember the first time this ever happened to you?

For any practitioner who hasn't had training in working with clients' emotional reactions, or who isn't highly skilled at communicating about these issues, the best response is a simple one: defuse the situation and change the focus of the session. Begin by making subtle technique changes (e.g., work on a different area, change the stroke or pressure). Consider saying something like, "This seems to be an area in your body where a strong experience is being held. Let me move to a different area." This may also be a good opportunity to mention that emotional experiences are often held in the body and that psychological counseling can be beneficial in processing emotional issues that come up in touch therapy.

If at any time the magnitude of a client's emotional expression becomes overwhelming—either to you or to the client—it's your responsibility to bring at least temporary closure to that interaction. Depending on the situation, it may be appropriate to stop the session or take a time-out, either remaining in the room or (if the client prefers) stepping outside. In such circumstances, achieving some physical and emotional distance helps to ensure a safe environment for the client and enables you as the practitioner to maintain professional and ethical behavior.

The following sections offer more specific guidelines for responding to several common emotions that often cause confusion or stress for practitioners: sadness, fear, anxiety, annoyance, and anger.

Sadness

When a client begins to cry during a session, gently check in with her. Ask whether she would like to take a short break, end the session, or have you continue working. Most sessions can proceed if a client is gently crying. If you do continue working, keep the client focused on the present moment. You might suggest that she breathe into the area where you're working, and perhaps open her eyes. If the client is uncomfortable with the experience, let her know that it can be a normal part of the treatment process.

> What is necessary to change a person is to change his awareness of himself.
>
> —Abraham Maslow

If the client wants a short break, ask whether she would like to have you stay in the room or would prefer to have some time alone. If she wants to be alone, leave the room, letting her know you'll check back in five minutes or so. If she wants you to stay in the room, refrain from conversation and make physical contact only if the client requests it.

Fear and Anxiety

Fear and anxiety are related, but not the same. Fear is one of the most basic emotions; it's what we feel when we perceive an immediate threat. A client may experience fear if hands-on work in a particular body area brings up memories of a frightening situation. Anxiety is a more generalized state of apprehension. It can arise from a thought, a feeling, a sensation, or the uncertainty of the unknown.[9] For example, clients may feel anxious if:

- they realize they forgot to pay their parking meter and worry about getting a ticket
- they experience an emotion, such as grief or anger, that they aren't comfortable with
- they feel an unusual tingling or twitching sensation
- they have no prior experience with your type of work and don't know what to expect

Possible signs of anxiety or fear include clenched fists, tightening in the jaw, involuntary shaking, feeling numb, holding one's breath, skin discoloration (going white in the face), sweating, nausea, erratic movements, and avoidance of eye contact.

If you suspect that a client has become anxious or afraid, slow down or stop the session and check to see whether your suspicion is accurate. You might say something like, "I'm having a sense that you might be getting a little anxious. Is that true?" If the client answers yes, temporarily stop the session, and maintain gentle contact while refraining from doing any more hands-on work until the client's anxiety has diminished. It may be helpful to simply take a short break or to have the client sit up (either giving him a chance to get dressed or making sure he's fully covered with the sheet). Being fully clothed and sitting face-to-face often lessens the power differential and diminishes the client's feeling of vulnerability and anxiety.

Another option is to pose a series of questions that help the client track physical sensations. (Note: If the person's anxiety is triggered by a particular sensation, have him begin by noticing the sensations in other areas of his body.) Ask the client if he's willing to try something that might help him feel better, and try this method only if he says yes. You can do it with the client lying down or have him sit up first. Here's an example of what such a dialogue might sound like:

Practical Application: Tracking a Client's Physical Sensations

PRACTITIONER:
Are you more comfortable sitting up than when you were lying down?

CLIENT:
Yes, I'm definitely more comfortable, but I still feel anxious.

PRACTITIONER:
Where do you feel the anxiety in your body?

CLIENT:
I feel it in my chest and my abdomen.

PRACTITIONER:
Is the sensation getting more intense or less intense?

CLIENT:
It's getting a little stronger.

PRACTITIONER:
Is the sensation moving anywhere?

CLIENT:
Yes, I feel it down my arms as well.

PRACTITIONER:
Do you feel the sensation in your legs?

CLIENT:
No.

PRACTITIONER:
Do you feel it in your neck?

CLIENT:
No.

PRACTITIONER:
Is the sensation getting larger or smaller now?

CLIENT:
I only feel it in my chest now.

PRACTITIONER:
Can you describe exactly what it feels like?

CLIENT:
It's like a cold wind running up and down in my chest.

PRACTITIONER:
How are you feeling now, compared to the way you felt when you first sat up?

CLIENT:
I feel much better; the sensation seems to be fading.

Points to Ponder

How do you know that you're helping clients to track physical sensations without the influence of your own thoughts and feelings? What other types of questions can be helpful to direct the client in describing physical sensations?

Make sure that when you help clients track physical sensations, you don't end up playing armchair psychologist. If the situation develops into something beyond your scope of practice, you should be prepared to refer clients to appropriate healthcare providers.

Annoyance and Anger

For the majority of practitioners, the most challenging emotions to respond to are anger, annoyance, and similar negative feelings. A client may express these emotions directly (saying, "I'm angry!") or indirectly (blaming you for something or using a hostile, edgy, or sarcastic voice tone). When this happens, the first thing to do is to listen very carefully. Do your best to set aside your own reactions and interpretations, and just hear what the person is saying.

What happens next depends on your own state of mind. If you find yourself feeling upset, defensive, or immobilized, try to keep the conversation short. Tell the client you want to take some time to think about what was said and continue the conversation later. As soon as you can after the session ends, talk through the issue with a supervisor or trusted peer.

See page 102 for information on **Receiving Feedback**.

If you can stay grounded and not take the client's comments personally, the next step is to verify you heard the message accurately. Say back what you heard the client say, using either the same words he used or your own words. In addition to clarifying your own understanding, this lets the client know that you're really listening to him. That alone can help him to calm down.

When responding to a client who has been raising his voice, it's best to keep your own voice strong and clear; think about reflecting back his energy, without the edge or hostility. If he yells, "I'm really angry!" and you reply in a calm, quiet tone, "I'm hearing that you're angry," he is likely to get even more upset. Someone who is extremely upset may not feel heard until you've reflected back his message, with feeling, for several minutes or more.[10]

See Chapter 1 pages 8-10 for more information on **Transference**.

Once you're clearer about what the client is saying, it may be possible to resolve the underlying cause of his anger or annoyance, provided that:
- The client is now calm enough to have a rational discussion.
- You feel calm enough to have a rational discussion.
- The client's emotional response is directly related to you, rather than to a flashback or memory that has surfaced from the person's past.
- You have sufficient time to discuss the issue fully.

If either of you is still feeling upset, if you're pressured for time (for instance, if you've reached the end of the session and another client is waiting), or if you'd like more time to think things over, make plans to continue the discussion later. If the client's emotion seems way out of proportion to the issue at hand, it's wise to seek supervision; the person may be experiencing a strong transference reaction. Supervision is also advisable if the client's emotion is related to one of your own past experiences and you're unsure how to respond.

See Chapter 10 page 281 for more details on **Supervision**.

In some situations the resolution may be fairly straightforward. If the client has raised valid concerns—for instance, you made a mistake or inadvertently crossed a boundary—you can apologize and take any necessary steps to correct the problem. If the client was mistaken about the facts or misunderstood something, you can give clarification (provided, again, that the client is sufficiently calm to consider these facts rationally). Later in this chapter we give more detailed recommendations for responding to clients' feedback and managing your own negative feelings.

Client Emotions

- Create a list of questions designed to help keep clients present when they're feeling extreme sadness or grief.
- Identify the types of emotional expression that might make you feel uncomfortable in a therapeutic context. Role-play these situations.
- Brainstorm options for 1) responding to clients who seem overwhelmed by their emotions, and 2) responding to clients when you feel overwhelmed by how much emotion they're expressing.

Boundaries

As we emphasized in Chapter 2, our ability to maintain a successful and ethically responsible practice is dependent upon having clear boundaries. Clear boundaries, in turn, are dependent upon effective communication. We must be skilled at clearly communicating our boundary needs to others and at listening and responding to others who communicate their concerns to us.

Since boundary issues often bring up strong feelings for people, talking about these matters can be extremely challenging. Of course, some conversations about boundaries are simple and straightforward. Few practitioners have serious difficulty setting a boundary about not wearing perfumes that may cause an allergic reaction, or complying with a client's straightforward request to avoid working on a particular body area. However, discussions about emotionally charged issues such as money, repeated lateness, or intrusive questions can easily generate stress and conflict. The sections that follow provide guidelines for approaching these sorts of topics with clarity and sensitivity.

Communicating Respect for Client Boundaries

In flagrant boundary violations, the practitioner's communication skills play at most a minor role. A therapist who engages in insurance fraud or has sexual relationships with clients demonstrates not a lack of skill, but a blatant disregard for professional ethics. It is in the less clear-cut, gray areas of ethical practice that effective communication about boundaries can make a great positive difference. You can support your clients in maintaining healthy boundaries by treating each client as a person, not an object; admitting your mistakes; fostering appropriate self-disclosure; and encouraging the client to speak up.

Treat the Client as a Person, Not an Object

This concept may seem too obvious to mention, but to varying degrees many practitioners and organizations treat clients in depersonalizing ways. The procedures in healthcare offices are often designed to make things easier for the organization or the practitioners, rather than to help put clients at ease. As a result, clients may be subjected to bureaucratic intake processes, needlessly long waits for service, and perfunctory responses from receptionists and other administrative staff, as well as detached, impersonal care from the practitioners themselves.

> A client arrived for an appointment at a holistic clinic known for its technical excellence, and was shown to a private room to wait. When the practitioner entered the room, she walked right past the client without acknowledging him, and read notes about his health history from his file. Finally, after several minutes, the practitioner began the assessment. The client answered her questions, but never raised any of his own concerns. He didn't make a second appointment.

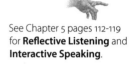

See Chapter 5 pages 112-119 for **Reflective Listening** and **Interactive Speaking**.

Points to Ponder

While the practitioner was silently reading the client's file, what might the client have been thinking and feeling? What conclusions might he have drawn about his role in the therapeutic relationship?

It isn't easy for any caregiver to be engaging, truly interested, and responsive day after day, year after year. Nobody does it perfectly. However, it's only with sincere and clear communication that we can empower clients to actively participate in their own treatment. Unless a client can talk openly to his practitioner, he is unlikely to be comfortable raising concerns about boundary issues.

The bottom line is that good rapport—a harmonious relationship marked by trust, openness, and mutual understanding—is good for the client's boundaries. Of course, good rapport is also good for business. After you've made a good first impression, rapport is often the single most important factor in determining whether a person sees you once or becomes a long-term client. (See figure 4.3 for simple steps you can take to help build rapport.) In Chapter 5, we give detailed explanations of two specific techniques that foster open, two-way communication: reflective listening and interactive speaking.

Figure 4.3 Tips for Building Rapport with Clients

- Be punctual
- Greet the client
- Smile
- Shake hands
- Maintain good eye contact
- Give the client your full attention
- Allow ample time for clients to talk, and listen carefully to what they say

- Demonstrate genuine concern
- Speak with enthusiasm and conviction
- Use the client's name frequently, being sure to pronounce it correctly
- Use language that the client can easily understand, avoiding unnecessary jargon and complex technical terms

---

 What Constitutes Good Rapport?

- Think about your own experiences as a healthcare patient or client. What are some of the specific ways in which you've been treated in a depersonalizing manner?
- When you've experienced good rapport with a practitioner, what has contributed to making that relationship work well?

Admit Your Mistakes

As we mentioned in the section on power differentials, clients are often hesitant to raise boundary concerns because they're afraid that the practitioner will respond negatively. One of the most effective ways to counteract this worry is to admit your mistakes. All practitioners have moments when, through no fault of their own, their best attempts to honor the client's boundaries fail. Drapes slip, hands fumble, and accidents happen. Or, despite our best intentions, we inadvertently overcharge, overbook, or run late for an appointment. The best response in these situations is to immediately and clearly communicate with the client about what happened.

1. While working on a male client's thigh, a female polarity therapist leaned across the table and accidentally brushed the client's testicles. The therapist straightened up and placed both her hands on the client's arm near his shoulder; "I'm sorry," she said. Her reassuring touch and simple apology allowed the session to continue without incident.

2. A male chiropractor started to work on a prone female client who was wearing a gown opened in the back. He placed one of his hands on her lower legs and the other hand on her upper back. All of a sudden, with a cry of shock, the client said, "Doctor, what's going on?" The chiropractor looked down and saw that his tie had fallen between the client's thighs. In an even and professional voice, he said, "I'm sorry; my tie slipped and is touching you. Let me keep my hands where they are while you turn your head to see for yourself." The client saw that the chiropractor was telling the truth. Because of his clear and honest communication, she relaxed and the treatment continued.

Points to Ponder

If you were the practitioner in either of these scenarios, how might you have reacted? What thoughts or feelings might be triggered by the realization that you'd accidentally crossed a physical boundary? What could you do to help keep yourself grounded and focused on reassuring the client?

Foster Appropriate Self-Disclosure

Self-disclosure refers to the personal information that gets exchanged between a practitioner and a client. It's appropriate, and important, for clients to disclose personal information that is directly relevant to the condition for which they're seeking help. This information guides the practitioner in providing an accurate assessment and proper treatment. However, clients sometimes engage in excessive self-disclosure, sharing details about themselves that the practitioner doesn't need to know and isn't qualified to interpret. Excessive self-disclosure is particularly likely to happen if clients are socially isolated and have no one else to talk to, have very loose boundaries around communicating personal information, or are uncomfortable with silence and tend to fill it with the first thoughts that come to their mind.

Excessive self-disclosure can also be an indication of transference. Clients often view their practitioners as all-knowing, and expect advice and input that is beyond their scope of practice. It is common for somatic therapists to be asked questions that cross into the realm of psychotherapy. When this happens to you, it's your responsibility as the practitioner to set a boundary. Be gentle, to avoid embarrassing or shaming the client for asking an inappropriate question, but also be firm and clear. For instance, you might say, "That sounds like a really challenging situation. What you're asking me is outside my field of expertise, so it would be unethical for me to give you any type of advice. I would be happy to refer you to a good counselor or psychotherapist who can help you think through this issue."

The other side of self-disclosure—the personal information revealed by the practitioner to the client—can have an equally strong impact on the therapeutic relationship. Sometimes making a personal disclosure can be a powerful therapeutic intervention, or simply an act of kindness. For example, if a client begins to cry as he tells the practitioner that his teenage daughter is using drugs and failing in school, causing enormous pain and stress, the practitioner might respond by saying, "My son had a similar problem, and it was one of the most painful and difficult things I have ever had to go through." With this brief disclosure, she communicates to the client that she really understands what he is going through. Many clients report that instances of appropriate self-disclosure by the practitioner have been among the most important moments in their therapeutic relationship. When done well and expressed at the right moment, they help to establish trust and safety.

When you're trying to decide how much of your personal experience to disclose to a client, remember the principle of client-centeredness. Ask yourself why you wish to reveal the information. Is it because you believe it will be helpful to the client? Or is it because of a personal reason that has nothing to do with the client? Suppose that the practitioner who disclosed her difficulty with her son had gone on to tell a 15-minute story about how the son dropped out of school, stole money from her, and ran away from home. In this case, her self-disclosure would primarily have been for her own benefit. Instead of feeling supported, the client would probably end up feeling overloaded and invaded by the practitioner's problems.

Effective Use of Self-Disclosure

- What types of self-disclosure might be useful from the practitioner to the client?
- What types of practitioner self-disclosure might be destructive?
- What types of client self-disclosure make you uncomfortable?
- How might you handle excessive client self-disclosure?

Encourage the Client to Speak Up

From the very beginning of your work with clients, let them know that you want to make the experience as safe and comfortable as possible. Describe your policies on confidentiality, lateness, cancellations, payment, and other issues, and invite questions or comments. Close by saying that while you'll never knowingly do anything to make them feel ill at ease, everyone has different levels of comfort with various aspects of hands-on treatment. You might say something like, "Let me know if you ever feel uncomfortable about anything that happens in a session."

Communicating About Your Own Boundaries

Clients aren't the only people with boundary concerns. Clear, healthy limits protect you as a practitioner as well. Some clients may become so absorbed with their own needs that they become oblivious to yours, overrunning your boundaries in numerous ways: missing appointments; showing up without an appointment; calling you at home late at night; attempting to develop a friendship; being delinquent on payments; making overtures for physical intimacy; and using verbally or physically aggressive behavior. Maintaining your own boundaries is essential to preserving not only your quality of life, but your professional competence as well. Practitioners suffer burnout when they fail to shield themselves from excessive client demands. Keep in mind that because you hold the position of greater power in the therapeutic relationship, the ultimate responsibility for managing boundaries always lies with you, not with the client.

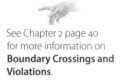

See Chapter 2 page 40 for more information on **Boundary Crossings and Violations**.

Be Proactive

Boundary-wise practitioners are proactive in addressing boundary issues. They make many of their limits clear in the initial phases of working with a client. There are two advantages to doing this. First, it prevents many boundary crossings and violations from occurring, since the boundaries and consequences are made clear up front. Also, proactive discussions are usually far less stressful for the client. If you wait until a client crosses your boundary before speaking about the issue, the client is likely to feel guilty, hurt, angry, or even betrayed because she broke a "rule" that was never explicitly stated. After-the-fact discussions often trigger negative feelings that not only make the boundary discussion more difficult, but also make your work harder by straining the therapeutic relationship.

Before a problem arises, it's helpful to figure out both where your boundaries lie and why. In his book, *Back to One: A Practical Guide for Psychotherapists*, Sheldon Kopp discusses where he draws the line on several boundary issues and explains his rationale for each choice. For example, Kopp doesn't take emergency calls from clients: "The only time the switchboard operator is to buzz through for me is if there is an urgent call from my wife or from one of my kids. That's my boundary." Here's the rationale. Kopp works with "well-functioning people… for whom the focus of therapy is more a matter of growth than of problem solving." In this context at least, Kopp says,

> *There are no other emergencies in my profession. I only run the therapy; my clients run their lives. Should clients attempt to make their emergencies mine, I accept no responsibility for intervening in their crises. At such times of distress in their lives, just as I do, they must turn to family, to friends, or to community crisis intervention services (such as the police, the fire department, the local hospital emergency room).*[11]

You might not draw the line where Kopp does or agree with his rationale. Different people in the same profession often have significantly different boundaries. We cite this example because of the mental clarity Kopp demonstrates, not only about his boundaries, but also about the personal and professional reasons why those boundaries make sense to him. When you carefully think through the reasoning behind the boundaries you set, it becomes much easier to explain and maintain those limits.

A massage therapist had a history of injury to her hands from working too deeply. After her recovery she practiced her communication skills to set a clear boundary when clients asked for deeper work. "The kind of work I do doesn't become deeper through pressure," she would say. "I've found that slow and gentle work allows most of my clients to relax in a deeper way. We can try this method and if you don't like it, I'll be happy to give you a referral."

Points to Ponder

In what ways does the massage therapist's clear boundary help to protect her as a practitioner? How might that boundary be helpful to her clients?

One aspect of being proactive is taking time for self-reflection and analysis on an ongoing basis. All practitioners have experiences from time to time when their conversations about boundaries don't go as well as they'd like. Learn from these experiences to hone your skills and change your future behavior.

Be Assertive

Earlier in this chapter, we emphasized that how you express yourself is just as important as what you say. The particular combination of words and voice tone you use has a strong influence on what your clients hear and how they respond. When you're discussing a boundary issue, it's best to communicate in a way that is assertive, rather than passive or aggressive.

ASSERTIVE LANGUAGE communicates clearly, with minimal emotional content. The voice tone is neutral—not a monotone, but a natural intonation free from hostility, whining, hesitation, and anything else that might potentially distract or upset the person who's listening. Common examples of assertive language include direct instructions to the client ("If your schedule changes and you can't make this appointment, let me know right away") and "I" statements about what the practitioner will or will not do ("If you cancel with less than 24 hours notice, I will charge you for a full session").

PASSIVE LANGUAGE, on the other hand, communicates a lack of self-confidence or self-esteem. The tone of voice may be whiny, hesitant, or self-deprecating. Passive statements are generally ambiguous, failing to clearly specify what the practitioner wants, or expects, to have happen and what the consequences are if the client doesn't comply. When a client says that his work schedule is unpredictable and he might need to cancel, a practitioner speaking passively might say, "Oh... well, then, try to let me know, if you can, okay?"

AGGRESSIVE LANGUAGE communicates undertones of anger through the words, the voice tone, or both. Often, the message that comes across is subtly blameful or threatening. A practitioner might say, "Don't get lazy and wait to call until the last minute like you did last time. You're not my only client, you know." Clients hearing this type of communication tend to react less to the substance of the practitioner's message, and more to the anger beneath it, and they may feel defensive, hurt, angry, or ashamed.

Practical Application: Passive, Aggressive, and Assertive Communication

A PRACTITIONER DECLINING A TIP:
- Oh, gosh, why did you have to do that? (passive)
- What do you think I am, a waitress?! (aggressive)
- I've chosen not to accept tips, but I appreciate your thoughtfulness. (assertive)

A PRACTITIONER REQUESTING PAYMENT FROM A CLIENT WHO FORGETS TO PAY:
- It would be really good if you could remember to bring your checkbook. (passive)
- You'd better bring your checkbook next time. I can't just keep treating you for free. (aggressive)
- Please put a check in the mail to me tomorrow. My policy is to expect payment at the time of the session, so please be prepared for our next appointment. (assertive)

Points to Ponder

Which type of communication best describes your natural responses to these types of situations? What are some additional assertive statements you could use under similar circumstances?

Assertive language provides the foundation for the Assertion Sequence, a detailed protocol designed to help protect a practitioner's boundaries in response to any challenge that might arise in working with clients. In Chapter 5, we'll discuss that protocol in detail.

 Defining Assertive, Passive, and Aggressive Language

In your own words, describe the differences between assertive, passive, and aggressive language. Come up with examples of each type of communication, applied to the following client behaviors:
- Talking loudly on a cell phone in your waiting room.
- Eating in your waiting room, leaving crumbs.
- Gossiping about another practitioner who works in your office.
- Asking personal questions about your children.
- Parking in an area reserved for residents of your building.
- Other behaviors you can think of that cross a boundary in some way.

Be Consistent

In addition to being proactive and assertive, effective communication about boundaries must also be consistent. That means you give the same clear message about your cancellation policy to all clients, regardless of how much you personally like them or how much money they make. And you stick to that policy throughout the duration of your work with all clients, regardless of how strongly they argue with you or how generous and understanding you might be feeling on a particular day.

Of course, consistency must always be balanced with reason. Take care not to be too rigid, at the expense of common sense and consideration for your clients. For example, if a client got into a car accident on the way to an appointment with you, it would be unreasonable to charge for a cancellation.

Feedback

Feedback has developed a bad reputation. If a client, teacher, or co-worker (or anyone else) tells you that they'd "like to give you some feedback," chances are you cringe inside while you prepare yourself to hear something negative. This response is often justified—the term is widely misused and misunderstood, so that what many people call feedback is actually criticism, blame, or a personal attack. In contrast, genuine feedback can play a very useful and constructive role in our personal and professional lives.[12]

Feedback is critical to the proper functioning of a wide range of mechanical, biological, and social systems. The classic example is a thermostat, which requires feedback on a room's temperature to determine when the heat should be turned on and turned off. An important type of biological feedback is hunger, which provides information about our need for food at any given moment. Feedback can be a matter of life and death. For instance, animals that never receive internal cues that food is needed (or that enough has been eaten) wouldn't survive very long!

In the context of a therapeutic relationship, feedback gives us insight into how what we're doing affects our clients—what they observe, think, or feel when we act in certain ways. This can include anything from our hands-on techniques and professional advice to the way we dress, answer the phone, or schedule appointments. We're often in a position to give feedback to clients as well. We might discuss how their ways of eating, exercising, and using their bodies in their jobs are affecting them, or how various behaviors related to their treatment (e.g., arriving late, asking personal questions, missing payments) affect us.

The ability to solicit honest feedback provides therapists with several distinct advantages. Often, clients who are dissatisfied with some aspect of their treatment don't directly express their concerns; they just stop booking sessions. By opening the door to feedback, we can learn on an ongoing basis what is and is not working for each person. This continuing dialogue helps us retain the clients we have and work more successfully with others in the future. Another benefit is increased receptivity on the part of our clients—the better we are at receiving their feedback, the more open they are to hearing our observations and suggestions.

Most of us never received training in ways to exchange feedback and have observed few models for doing this effectively. Fortunately, however, these skills can be learned at any stage in life.

Giving Feedback

Giving feedback can be a stressful process, as we balance our desire to get our concerns addressed with our wish to maintain positive and healthy relationships. The following three-step strategy helps you maximize the chances that the other person will hear and understand your feedback, and do something useful with it. The examples we give are mainly from practitioner-client interactions, but the same basic strategy works equally well in other contexts.

Step 1: Set a Goal

The first step in giving feedback is something that happens well before you open your mouth: clarifying your intention. What is the goal of the feedback you're planning to give? When working with a client, there are a variety of goals that can lead to useful feedback. These include:

- Correcting misinformation (*"Actually, ice isn't an effective treatment for stomach pain."*)
- Helping the client to perform an activity more safely or effectively (*"If you bend your knees a little more as you do this exercise, you'll protect your lower back."*)
- Informing the client about the effects of certain behaviors on them (*"When you were eating more healthfully, your injury was healing more rapidly."*)
- Informing the client about the effects of certain behaviors on you (*"When you didn't arrive for your appointment and didn't call, I was worried about you."*)

In contrast, some goals—such as trying to make the person change, feel guilty, or understand that she is wrong—are unlikely to lead to a useful outcome. Before you give feedback about something that you think isn't working well, stop to consider what your purpose is; this may dramatically change what you want to say, and how you want to say it.

Step 2: Select Your Facts

After you've identified your goal, notice what type of information you're planning to offer in your feedback. Are the things you want to say your personal opinions, or are they facts? There's a big difference between the two. An opinion is subjective—it's your judgment, evaluation, speculation, or interpretation of the situation. A fact, on the other hand, gives concrete, objective data. Feeling statements are a type of fact, giving direct information about your experience. In general, facts are much more likely to provide helpful information that listeners can use to make decisions or guide their actions. Consider a situation in which your client hasn't been doing the exercises you recommended. Here are a few different types of facts you could give:

- Facts about the situation (*"The last three times you came in, you told me that you didn't do your exercises."*)
- Facts based on research (*"Studies have shown that patella tendon injuries heal 40 to 50 percent more quickly when this exercise is done regularly."*)
- Facts from your own observations (*"Among my clients, the people who have done their exercises regularly have healed more quickly."*)
- Facts about your feelings and concerns (*"I really care about your health. I'm worried about the possibility that your knee won't heal properly before you begin running again."*)

Notice that the following are not facts, but opinions:

- *"You really ought to do your exercises."* (Your judgment about what the client should do)
- *"I can tell that you think these exercises aren't important."* (Your interpretation of what the client is feeling or thinking—a mind-read)
- *"You're being so irresponsible!"* (Your evaluation of the client's character, in the form of an attack)

The preceding examples all involve feedback about something that isn't going the way you'd like. However, the distinction between opinions and facts also applies to feedback about things that you think are going well. Giving an opinion such as "You're such a great client to work with" may make clients feel good, but it doesn't provide any substantive information. You could be referring to their punctuality, how many questions they ask, the nice things they say about you, or any number of other things. Without more details, they can't know what you're basing your opinion on, and therefore they can't know whether they agree or disagree with that assessment. It may turn out that once they learn what you mean by a "great client" (perhaps, someone who never questions the therapist's advice), they don't want to be one after all!

When you give facts, clients have the chance to use them however they wish. They can make their own decisions about what the information means to them, and they can find ways to use it that are consistent with their own beliefs, priorities, and goals. Options for responding to opinions are much more limited. Clients will either agree or disagree with you, or perhaps just suspend judgment until they learn more. For instance, if you say, "Massage therapy is a better option for you," clients might agree or disagree based on how much they trust your judgment, but they won't understand why you believe this is true. In contrast, when you provide concrete

> While you can learn much by listening carefully to what people say, a great deal more is revealed by what they do not say. Listen as carefully to silence as to sound.
>
> — Dee Hock

facts—such as the average healing time, rate of success, and likelihood of complications with each type of intervention—you give clients tools to make their own choices about treatment.

Back Up Opinions with Facts

Identify 3 to 5 strong opinions you have that are related to your work. (For instance, "The most effective treatment for chronic tension headaches is…" or "Nutrition is an essential consideration when helping clients to heal from injuries" or "Aromatherapy is a useful complement to hands-on work.") For each opinion, come up with at least 3 supporting facts. These facts may be based on research or your own observations, or they may relate to your personal feelings and concerns.

Step 3: Deliver the Feedback

Once you've determined what your goals are and what facts you'd like to give, the final step is speaking directly with the person. Below is a basic protocol for giving feedback that helps to foster receptivity, understanding, positive feelings, and problem solving:

1. **ASK PERMISSION TO GIVE FEEDBACK.** (*"I would like to talk to you about… Is this a good time to do that?"*) If the person doesn't want to hear the feedback right away, for any reason, set another time to discuss it.
2. **STATE YOUR GOAL.** (*"I wanted to have this conversation with you because…"*)
3. **SOLICIT QUESTIONS.** (*"Please ask me questions if anything I say isn't clear."*)
4. **EXPLAIN THE SITUATION.** Remember to use facts, rather than opinions, whenever possible. Give small amounts of information at a time so the person can process it.
5. **CHECK FOR UNDERSTANDING.** (*"What are you hearing me say?"* *"What message are you taking away from this?"*) Express agreement with the person's summary or correct any misunderstandings.
6. **ASK FOR A RESPONSE.** (*"How do you see what happened?"* *"What are your thoughts about what I said?"* *"What was going on for you?"*)
7. **IF APPROPRIATE, DISCUSS POSSIBLE SOLUTIONS.** You might talk about ways in which one or both of you could change your behavior, as well as any appropriate follow-up steps you could take.

See the following Practical Application for a sample feedback dialogue that applies this protocol to a situation with a colleague.

Practical Application: Sample Dialogue

Giving Feedback to a Practitioner Sharing Your Office

PRACTITIONER:
I'd like to talk to you about our office space. Is now a good time to do that? [Asking permission]

COLLEAGUE:
Sure.

PRACTITIONER:
Great. We've never really talked about the maintenance and organization of the office, and I'd like for us to come to some agreements about that. [Stating the goal]

I will start off by telling you what my thoughts are and what I've observed. Let me know if you have any questions. [Soliciting questions.]

A couple of things happened this past week that I wasn't expecting. On Monday, there was a fishy smell in the room, and a client complained. I didn't figure out where it was coming from until after her appointment when I found a food container on the window sill that had been there since Friday. Also, this morning I noticed that the cloth under the oil dispenser was gone, and there was a ring of oil on the table. I want to find a way to stop these sorts of things from happening in the future. [Explaining the situation]

Let me stop here and make sure we're on the same page so far. What message are you taking away from what I'm saying? [Checking for understanding]

COLLEAGUE:

I'm getting the message that I need to do a better job of cleaning out the office before we switch off.

PRACTITIONER:

If you could clean up really thoroughly, leaving everything the way you found it, that would be great. Does that sound reasonable, and like something you could commit to doing? [Asking for a response]

COLLEAGUE:

I'll definitely be more careful. But it's possible that I won't remember exactly how everything is supposed to be arranged. I'm not always good about keeping track of those sorts of things.

PRACTITIONER:

Why don't we check in every week or two about how things are going? If there's something that's bothering me, I'll let you know, and you can let me know if there's anything that isn't working well for you. What do you think? [Discussing possible solutions]

COLLEAGUE:

Sure, that sounds good.

Points to Ponder

How might this conversation have been different if there had been no request for permission and the colleague was distracted by an upsetting event in his personal life? Which statements in this dialogue give facts? Given those facts, what opinions might you have about the colleague and the colleague's behavior? How might this conversation have been different if the factual feedback were replaced with opinions?

 Difficult Feedback in Your Experience

Think back to a time when you've given someone feedback and the conversation that followed didn't go well. How did the approach you took compare to the protocol we're suggesting here? Fill out the checklist below, either in your head or on paper.

In my difficult feedback conversation, I did the following:
- ❑ I asked permission to give the feedback.
- ❑ I clearly stated my goal.
- ❑ I solicited questions.
- ❑ I used mainly facts, rather than opinions.
- ❑ I gave small amounts of information at a time.
- ❑ I checked for understanding.
- ❑ I asked for a response.
- ❑ I discussed possible solutions.

For any steps you didn't take, consider how those actions might have changed your conversation. If you had a chance to have that discussion over again, what would you do differently?

Receiving Feedback

Receiving feedback can be a stressful experience for all of us. There's always a chance that we'll be told something that hurts or surprises us or that we don't want to hear. While you don't have full control over the way feedback is given to you, you can still take steps to help move the conversation in a positive direction. If the feedback is unsolicited, notice whether you feel comfortable receiving it in the current situation. Ask to postpone the discussion if you feel rushed, distracted, or upset.

As you receive feedback, make an effort to gather the information that is most useful to you. If the person isn't providing all the facts you'd like to hear, ask for them. For instance, suppose you ask a client for feedback on your work with her, and she responds with an opinion: "You give a great treatment." While this may feel good to hear, it's unclear exactly what she means. Try asking for more specific details about what she felt or observed. You'll learn much more from facts such as, "I like your treatment because you give exactly the amount of pressure that I feel I need, when you work deeply you don't hurt me, and I'm never sore after I leave."

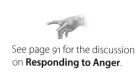

See page 91 for the discussion on **Responding to Anger**.

When the feedback is critical, work to fully understand what the client is saying before sharing your own thoughts on the issue. Ask the person to give you small amounts of information at a time, and paraphrase what she says to verify that what you're hearing is what she intended. If she is really upset, be sure to reflect her emotion as well.

Once you've heard and acknowledged the client's point of view, there are a variety of different responses that might be appropriate, depending on the situation:

- **Thank the client.** Remember that the power differential makes it particularly challenging for a client to give critical feedback to a healthcare professional. Taking a risk to say what she doesn't like takes a good deal of courage, and often warrants an expression of gratitude (provided you can give it sincerely).
- **Clarify facts.** If the client is mistaken about any of the relevant facts, provide clarification. Be sure to keep your voice tone neutral, without any defensiveness or hostile edge.
- **Apologize.** If you've made a mistake, big or small, it's always a good idea to say you're sorry. Even if you acted with the best of intentions, and even if you never could have predicted that the client would react negatively, you can still apologize for the unintended consequence of your behavior. Apologizing for having a negative impact on the person doesn't mean admitting to having bad intentions.
- **Discuss possible solutions.** If the client doesn't volunteer a suggestion for what you might do differently in the future, ask for her ideas, or share your own ideas and ask for her input. Work together to find a solution that works well for both of you.

Practical Application: Receiving Feedback from a Dissatisfied Client

Client:

Oh no, is that it?

Practitioner:

Yes, that's the end of the session. It sounds like you're disappointed. Is that right? [Clarifying what the client said]

Client:

Well, yes. I had asked you to focus on my back, and you didn't spend much time on my back at all. You just kept working on my feet.

Practitioner:

You're right, I did focus more on your feet, and I didn't explain why or ask whether that was okay with you. I'm very sorry about that. [Apology] I was using a reflexology technique that's designed to relieve back pain through certain points on your feet. [Clarifying facts] Does your back feel any better?

CLIENT:

Actually, I guess it does. I don't know if it was that foot thing, though.

PRACTITIONER:

I'm hearing that you're not sure whether my work on your feet was helpful. Is that right? [Clarifying what the client said]

CLIENT:

Yeah, I can't really see how that would affect my back.

PRACTITIONER:

I felt the same way when I first learned about reflexology; it's very counterintuitive to think that working only on your feet could affect a part of your body that's so far away. There are a number of different ways I could work on your back, and I want to be sure you're comfortable with the methods I use. Would it be helpful for me to give you something to read about reflexology, as well as the other techniques I offer? Then you can make a fully informed decision about the type of treatment you receive. [Proposing a possible solution]

CLIENT:

Yes, I'd like to look at that information.

PRACTITIONER:

Great. I'll gather some articles for you. And I want to thank you for speaking up when the treatment wasn't what you expected. [Thanking the client] If anything about a session is ever disappointing to you or doesn't feel right, please let me know and I'll do my best to address it.

Points to Ponder

How might you respond if the client in this scenario were very angry? If this client had not given any feedback, how might her unspoken dissatisfaction have affected the therapeutic relationship?

Managing Your Negative Feelings

In the preceding sections, we've covered a variety of situations that might elicit negative feelings for you:

- responding to a client who is angry with you.
- asserting your boundaries, particularly when clients challenge them.
- giving challenging feedback and receiving challenging feedback.

In this section, we discuss what you can do when you're feeling angry or irritated—whether it's with a client, a colleague, or anyone else you encounter in your work.

We've all had the experience of having a challenging conversation while our emotions are running high. Typically, when that happens, we fail to get the results we want. We're so upset that either we say things we regret or we shut down and fail to express what really matters to us. As a result, the underlying problem that's bothering us remains unresolved, and often the relationship gets damaged as well.

Whenever you recognize that you're too upset to talk rationally, it's always wise to take a break from the interaction. If you're in the middle of a conversation, you might tell the other person directly that you're feeling upset, or simply say you need some time to think about the issue before saying more. Plan another time to continue talking, whether it's half an hour later or a week later. (Allow at least 20 minutes to let your nervous system calm down.) During that break, we recommend that you 1) clarify your feelings and 2) clarify your goal. It's often best to ask a trusted friend or colleague who isn't involved in your conflict to coach you through this process. If that's not possible or convenient, you can do it by yourself.

Clarify Your Feelings

To clarify the feelings that are triggered by a particular issue, think briefly about that issue and notice what you experience. Try to identify one or more feeling words that capture that experience. Be careful to identify true feeling words, such as *angry, ashamed, disappointed, fearful, overwhelmed, sad,* or *uncomfortable*. Avoid words like *abandoned, betrayed,* and *criticized* that sound like feelings, but actually are blameful judgments about the other person. (Essentially you're saying, "He abandoned me" or "She criticized me," rather than naming what's happening for you.) If you're working with a coach, she can help you with this. Whether working with a coach or on your own, state each feeling out loud, with as much authentic emotion in your voice tone as possible—for example, "I'm angry!" or "I feel really scared."

There are several benefits to clarifying a strong negative feeling. First, noticing your own internal state helps to shift your focus away from the person with whom you're angry or irritated. When someone has done something upsetting, it's easy to get caught up in repetitive or escalating angry thoughts, fixating on what's wrong with him and his behavior. That type of thinking is likely to leave you feeling even angrier, and less able to communicate effectively.

In addition, clarification can be valuable in deepening your self-awareness. For instance, after a client makes sexual comments to you, you might immediately know that you're angry, but require further reflection to realize that you're also feeling embarrassed and a little fearful.

A third benefit of clarifying your feelings is that it helps you calm down. Research shows that simply naming a negative feeling can help to reduce its impact.[13]

Clarify Your Goal

Once you're clear about your feelings, ask yourself what you'd like to get out of talking with the other person. What is your goal, and is it likely to lead to a useful conversation? Remember from our discussion of feedback that it makes a big difference whether your goal is productive (e.g., letting someone know how their behavior has affected you) or unproductive (e.g., trying to make the person feel guilty). Again, getting feedback from a coach or a clinical supervisor can be extremely helpful.

Next Steps

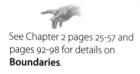

See Chapter 2 pages 25-57 and pages 92-98 for details on **Boundaries**.

Once you identify a productive goal, think about the type of conversation that would help you reach that goal. Odds are good that whatever you have to say will fit into one of three categories: giving feedback, responding to feedback, or talking about boundaries. Review those sections of the book for detailed guidelines on structuring your discussion.

If, despite your coach's help, you can't think of a productive goal, it may be best to skip the conversation entirely. For example, if you realize that you've been projecting your own feelings onto a client, that issue is best discussed not with the client, but with a supervisor or psychotherapist. In some cases, you might find that after you've talked things through and expressed your feelings with your coach, the issue feels resolved and you can simply let it go.

Working with an Upsetting Conflict

Think of an upsetting conflict in your personal or professional life that brings up strong emotions for you. Clarify your feelings and set a clear, productive goal for talking to the other person.

Communications Beyond the Treatment Room

Up to this point, we've been focusing on communication that happens in person, face to face. But of course, practitioners also communicate in a variety of other ways, including written letters, phone calls, emails, texts, and social media messages and posts. These types of interactions raise a set of concerns that differ somewhat from the issues surrounding face-to-face interactions. The primary issues to consider are ambiguity, privacy, and professionalism.

Ambiguity

As you may recall from earlier in this chapter, one of the major sources of trouble in conversations is *ambiguity*; when a communication isn't clear, the message received by the listener can be very different from the message the speaker intended to send. Electronic forms of communication (e.g., emails, texts) are inherently ambiguous because they don't capture voice tone. Suppose you send a message to a client saying, "Your appointment is at 3pm. Remember to leave plenty of time to get here, and park in the side lot." If you were to speak those words, your tone might be friendly and conversational. But the client who simply reads that message may hear it as snide, hostile, or threatening.

Even talking by telephone adds a certain amount of ambiguity, because you can't see any facial expressions or body language. Silence is particularly problematic on the phone. If you make a comment or ask a question and get no response, you have no physical cues to suggest what might be happening for the other person. He may have been very upset by what you said, may just be thinking quietly, or may have gotten distracted and simply stopped listening. If you had bad reception—which can often happen with cell phones—there's a good chance that he didn't hear, or misheard, what you said, or that he actually replied and you didn't hear him.

Whenever you need to make a choice about which communication method to use, keep in mind the potential complications of ambiguity. For straightforward, factual exchanges, electronic messages often work perfectly well. However, for more complex or emotionally charged interactions, it's typically best to speak in person or at least on the phone. Figure 4.4 gives more detailed guidelines on the situations in which electronic messages typically are, and are not, useful.

Privacy

When you and your clients share information in the context of a treatment session, maintaining privacy is relatively straightforward. So long as nobody outside the room can overhear your conversation, the two of you have full control over what happens to the information. With less direct methods of communication, things can get a lot more complicated. Medical records that you print out in hard copy or save in electronic files must be carefully protected to ensure that they never get viewed by any unauthorized individuals. Voicemail messages may also raise privacy concerns—for instance, if you have an assistant who checks messages that clients leave for you, or if you leave messages on voicemail accounts that clients share with other members of their families.

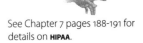

See Chapter 7 pages 188-191 for details on **HIPAA**.

Figure 4.4 Electronic Messages

Electronic messages include emails, text messages, tweets, and other social media postings.

ELECTRONIC MESSAGES CAN BE EFFECTIVE AND EFFICIENT WHEN:
- the purpose of the message is clearly stated
- making a request for specific actions (provided that those actions are spelled out clearly, and aren't likely to elicit an emotional response)
- passing along facts or links
- making appointments (so long as minimal back-and-forth negotiation is required)
- a written copy would be useful for later reference

ELECTRONIC MESSAGES CAN BE INEFFECTIVE AND INEFFICIENT WHEN:
- you're concerned about the privacy of your comments
- you're trying to resolve a conflict
- you're frustrated, irritated, or upset
- you want to express your feelings about something
- you say things you wouldn't say in person, including talking negatively about other people
- you need to ask questions or negotiate issues (too much "back and forth")
- you're giving bad news or other information that may upset the recipient (make a call or talk in person instead)
- voice tone would provide you with additional key information (make a call or talk in person instead)

BE AWARE:
- It is easy to lose control of information when communicating via email. Attend carefully to who's copied on each email before hitting "reply all."
- Humor, joking, and sarcasm often don't travel well over email, and sometimes don't travel well to other countries and cultures.
- Any of these (particularly emails and texts) can be used as legal documentation.

Identify Appropriate Communication Modes

Make a list of various pieces of information you might communicate to clients outside the context of a standard treatment session—anything from special offers to boundary concerns. For each one, identify which mode of communication you think would be best, and why.

Professionalism

See Chapter 7 pages 168-170 for a more detailed explanation of **Professionalism**.

Another issue to consider is the way your communications affect your professional image and credibility. Any information that people receive from you, or about you, will shape the way they view you and your work. While there's no direct relationship between editorial skill and therapeutic skill, sending out messages with misspellings, incorrect grammar, or other errors reflects poorly on you as a professional. Similarly, while your social life in college isn't directly relevant to your competence as a practitioner, you can damage your reputation by connecting with clients or colleagues through social media sites that show old pictures of you at wild parties.

Figure 4.5 provides guidelines for communicating professionally by telephone, written communication, electronic messages, and social media.

Figure 4.5 Do's and Don'ts for Professional Communication

	Do	**Don't**
Telephone	• Have a set greeting you use every time you answer your phone • Return calls in a timely manner (and if you can't for some reason, give a clear explanation for the delay on your voicemail message) • Record a voicemail message that is clear, professional, and friendly	• Allow individuals who don't know your greeting (including your children) to answer your phone • Answer your phone when you're feeling upset, or when you're in a loud or distracting environment • Mumble or have distracting background noise on your voicemail message • Forget to change date-specific messages (e.g., "Today is Monday, July 4th, and I'm out of the office.")
Written Communications	• Manually check for typos and misspellings, in addition to using computerized spell checking and grammar checking • Have another person proofread any important documents, particularly if grammar or spelling is a challenge for you. • Use professional letterhead or include your contact information at the top or bottom of the page	• Type the main body text in a font that is hard to read or very informal (err on the side of standard and conventional, rather than cute and quirky) • Hand-write notes if your handwriting is hard to read
Electronic Messages	• Review the guidelines in Figure 4.4 to ascertain if an electronic medium is appropriate for the message you're sending • Type your message into a word processing program first, to check the spelling and grammar, and then copy and paste • Create a subject line that is relevant to your message (e.g., Appointment change, Referral information) • Include a greeting (such as "Hi John," or "Dear Dr. Lewis:") • Include your name or an email signature with additional contact information • Check your inbox regularly and respond in a timely manner	• Hit "Send" without re-reading your message first • Fill in the "To" line until you've finished your message (in case you accidentally hit "Send") • Leave the subject line blank, or use a generic subject like "Hi" • Use an email address that sounds unprofessional or suggestive in any way (janedoe@gmail.com is always preferable to hotjane@hothands.com)
Social Media	• Read the discussion of social media ethics in Chapter 9 • Use privacy settings to limit the visibility of any information or photos you want to keep private • Separate your personal online presence from your professional online presence (e.g., have both a personal and a professional Twitter account, or make professional connections through LinkedIn and personal ones through Facebook)	• Post confidential information or details about clients (ever) • Post complaints about a client, colleague, employer, or employee (ever) • Forward links to any articles or videos that you haven't thoroughly reviewed first

- List the aspects of your communication that you think show the highest level of professionalism.
- List the aspects that are the least professional.

Conclusion

Human communication is complex, and all of us at times have conversations that don't go well. Within the context of therapeutic relationships, added complications such as power differentials and boundary concerns make the communication process even more challenging. In many situations, you can use the concepts and strategies discussed in this chapter to prevent confusion, stress, and misunderstanding. And in those situations where problems still occur despite your best intentions, you can use this information to figure out what went wrong and make better choices in the future.

5
Communication Techniques and Strategies

"What you do speaks so loudly that I cannot hear what you say."
—Ralph Waldo Emerson

Reflecting
- Beyond Reflection: Clarifying Unspoken Concerns

Inviting Input
- Interactive Speaking
- Informed Consent Discussions

Responding to Body Language

Educating
- Learning Styles

The Assertion Sequence
- Assertion Sequence Stage I: Agreement Discussion
- Special Cases: After-the-Fact Agreement Discussions
- Assertion Sequence Stage II: Follow-Up
- Assertion Sequence Stage III: Confrontation
- Assertion Sequence Stage IV: Termination

Key Terms

Assertion Sequence
Body Language
Confrontation

Informed Consent
Interactive Speaking
Learning Styles

Multiple Intelligences
Nonverbal Communication
Reflection

I n Chapter 4, we discussed a wide variety of factors that can make communication more difficult, from psychological barriers to challenging topics to the specific issues raised by electronic messaging and social media. This chapter focuses on specific ways of communicating that work well—techniques and strategies that can promote mutual understanding, strengthen the therapeutic relationship, and help you overcome any challenges you may encounter. We cover five types of interactions that are essential for practitioners to manage effectively: reflecting, inviting input, responding to body language, educating, and asserting and maintaining boundaries.

▌ Reflecting

One of the key components of effective communication is listening. Individuals who communicate well are frequently described as being "good listeners." On its own, however, simply listening isn't enough to have a positive impact on a conversation. Typically, people perceived as "good listeners" don't just sit back and passively absorb what someone else says; they show that they've heard and understood what was said by *reflecting*. Reflection is an integral part of several communication methods discussed in this chapter, and is also an important skill in itself.

In reflecting another person's message, you capture the essence of that message in your own words. You don't need to reflect every individual idea; the goal is to succinctly distill the core meaning. The description of reflection that follows is drawn, with some adaptations, from Robert Bolton's discussion of reflective listening in *People Skills*.[1] Useful starter phrases for reflection include:

- You feel…
- You're saying…
- You're thinking…
- Your point of view is…
- Your concern is…

The purpose of rephrasing what the other person said, rather than repeating it verbatim, is to drive yourself to go beyond hearing the words to getting a clear understanding of what the person meant. This also gives you an opportunity to verify that your understanding is accurate. Imagine that a client says, "I'm worried that if my shoulder doesn't heal soon, everything is going to start falling apart." You reflect, "You're worried that if your shoulder injury persists, you'll start to have problems in the rest of your body." The client may say, "Yes, that's right," or else, "No, I'm worried that I can't do my job, and the rest of my life will start falling apart." Had you simply repeated, "You're worried that everything is going to start falling apart," the client might never have provided that clarification. Note that if the person doesn't volunteer an agreement or disagreement with your reflection, it's useful to ask for one: "Is that accurate?" "Did I get that right?" "Have I heard you correctly?"

Throughout the conversation, give your physical attention to the other person by facing her, leaning slightly into the conversation, and maintaining eye contact. While she's talking and you're silently listening, nod your head from time to time and briefly acknowledge what she's saying (e.g., "Mmm hmm," "I see," "Go on"). When you're reflecting a feeling or other emotionally charged content, attune to the person's mood and resonate with her through your tone of voice and facial expression. (This is advisable to do when responding to any strong emotion, from joy to fear to rage.)

Reflecting a client's communication helps her to say what's on her mind and encourages her to finish a train of thought, rather than jump from topic to topic. It also creates a safe, empathetic climate where she feels freer to discuss difficult topics such as boundary concerns.

Have a conversation with a friend or colleague where you take turns practicing reflection. First, have the other person talk to you about something important to him (e.g., goals and aspirations, career concerns, beliefs about health and wellness), and reflect what he says. Then switch roles, so you discuss something important to you and he practices reflecting. At the end, talk together about your experience. What was it like to reflect another person's point of view? What was it like to have your point of view reflected? What did you learn about the process of reflection?

Beyond Reflection: Clarifying Unspoken Concerns

In some situations, you may suspect that a client isn't being direct, or isn't saying everything that's on his mind. Possible clues include hesitation or wavering; vague, ambiguous comments; a sudden change in his voice tone or body language; or voice tone or body language that contradicts what he is saying (e.g., the words "Yes, that pressure is fine," accompanied by a grimace and sudden tightening of the muscles you're working on). Be alert for these sorts of signals, particularly if you're discussing a potentially sensitive or upsetting topic.

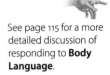

See page 115 for a more detailed discussion of responding to **Body Language**.

A male acupuncturist who took a "whole person" approach to health care was conducting an annual physical with a female client. After discussing her diet and exercise habits, he asked, "Do you have a satisfactory sexual life?" She flushed and replied, hesitantly, "I don't know if that's relevant." The acupuncturist proceeded to explain why the question was indeed relevant, and then asked it again. The client mumbled, "Yes, yes, it's fine."

Points to ponder

How might this communication affect the therapeutic relationship between the acupuncturist and the client? In what way is talking with a client about sexual issues different from discussing these issues with a peer? Which ethical principles are at stake?

When discussing an issue as personal as sexual activity, any indication of discomfort (in this case, hesitation, flushing, and an ambiguous, indirect answer) is a clear cue to check in with the person. If the acupuncturist had heeded those signs, he might have made the reasonable guess that the client was uncomfortable answering his question. Instead of persisting and pushing for an answer, he could have reflected her reply and given her a chance to opt out of this line of discussion.

CLIENT:

I don't know if that's relevant.

ACUPUNCTURIST:

This doesn't seem like something I would need to know?

CLIENT:

No, it doesn't.

ACUPUNCTURIST:

I ask about sexual activity because it helps me to guide some aspects of my treatment. But it's perfectly okay to skip this topic. Would you prefer to do that, and move on to other issues?

CLIENT:

Yes, thank you.

Points to Ponder

What role does reflection play in this brief exchange? Is it important? If so, then how? If a client resisted answering a question that you believed was essential to their treatment, how would you respond?

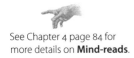

See Chapter 4 page 84 for more details on **Mind-reads**.

Notice that the offer to move on to other issues was phrased as a question, not a definitive statement. It would be presumptuous of the practitioner to say, "I can tell that question made you uncomfortable" or "You'd rather not talk about this subject." (You may recall from the previous chapter that these are mind-reads.) Be careful not to rely on your own assumptions about what's going on for someone else. If you find yourself speculating about a client's unspoken thoughts or feelings about your work with them, get a reality check. Suppose you ask a client how she felt after her last treatment, and she says "Same as usual," in a flat tone of voice; you suspect she is disappointed that she didn't leave feeling better. After reflecting her comment, you might say, "I'm thinking you might be feeling disappointed that the session didn't make more of a difference for you. Is that true?" In this way, without claiming to know what a client is feeling, you gently encourage her to share a concern that she might be reluctant to volunteer.

▌ Inviting Input

A general rule of communication is that dialogues are more effective than monologues. When one person does all the talking, there's no way to know whether the other person heard and understood what was said—not to mention whether the person agrees, disagrees, or has something important to add. In a therapeutic context, two-way communication is essential for helping clients to feel comfortable bringing up boundary issues or other concerns.

Unfortunately, all too often there is a preponderance of one-way communication from the practitioner to the client. It is easy to see how this can happen. Clients seek hands-on work to address problems they can't solve on their own; they're likely to expect practitioners to run the show. Practitioners, quite naturally, want to be helpful. From their perspective that often means developing solutions that they then impart to their clients. As a result, despite good intentions on both sides, the practitioner ends up dominating the conversation, and the client is left feeling passive and disempowered.

If a client takes the initiative to start a conversation, you can keep two-way communication going simply by reflecting. However, in many cases clients don't do that, as a result of their experience of the power differential or for other reasons. In those situations, it's your job to maintain a collaborative dialogue by inviting their input.

Interactive Speaking

You can make it a habit to invite input by incorporating a technique known as *Interactive Speaking* into your conversations. Interactive Speaking is a simple, straightforward approach that is appropriate to use whenever you're communicating important, meaningful, challenging, or complex information. It consists of a three-step cycle:

Speak ⇒ Invite ⇒ Reflect
(Repeat the cycle as needed)

SPEAK: Say what you have to say. Keep it short, preferably 30 to 60 seconds. You can add to your statement in later cycles.

INVITE: After you've made your point, invite the other person to respond. Simply pause and wait, or ask a checking question such as:

"What's your reaction?"
"Does that sound okay?"
"Do you have any problems with this?"
"What do you think so far?"
"How does this sound to you?"

REFLECT: From time to time, as the other person responds, succinctly restate the essence of his message. Once he's finished saying what he has to say and you've finished reflecting, the ball is back in your court.

Exploring Interactive Speaking

In what specific situations would Interactive Speaking be particularly useful? In what situations might it not be useful? When have you experienced one-way communication in your personal or professional life, either as a speaker or as a listener? What impact did that communication have on your relationship?

Informed Consent Discussions

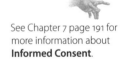

See Chapter 7 page 191 for more information about **Informed Consent**.

One very useful application of Interactive Speaking is the *Informed Consent Discussion*. In this type of conversation, the practitioner invites the client's input on an aspect of their treatment that may potentially raise concerns for the client. The practitioner provides three pieces of information:

1. *What* she proposes to do in the next session or next part of the current session.
2. *Why* she believes this technique or procedure will be beneficial.
3. *How* it might affect the client (e.g., how uncomfortable it's likely to be).

This information is divided into small segments, with each segment initiating a Speak/Invite/Reflect cycle.

A client is receiving a series of Rolfing® treatments. One of his concerns is jaw pain.

PRACTITIONER SPEAKS:
I think it would be helpful to do some work inside your mouth. That is the most effective way to manipulate the fascial membrane of the jaw muscles.

PRACTITIONER INVITES:
Would this be okay with you?

CLIENT RESPONDS:
I'm not sure.

PRACTITIONER REFLECTS:
You're not certain whether you want to receive this type of treatment. Is that right?

CLIENT RESPONDS:
Yes. My main concern is hygiene. Also, is this going to be painful?

PRACTITIONER SPEAKS:
I always wear sterile gloves while working in the mouth. Some people do find this technique to be uncomfortable, but you shouldn't feel pain. If at any point the discomfort feels like too much, you can just raise your hand and I'll stop immediately.

PRACTITIONER INVITES:
[Pause]

CLIENT RESPONDS:
That sounds okay. If you think this will help me, let's try it.

Points to Ponder

Did the practitioner use the what, why, and how method? What might the client have said that would lead the speak/invite/reflect cycle to continue?

Within the broader healthcare field, the issue of informed consent typically comes up in the context of surgery, anesthesia, and other interventions associated with direct physical risks. However, it also plays a critical role in innumerable less consequential procedures. For example, when a practitioner believes that a client would benefit from treatment in a particularly vulnerable area (such as the upper inner thigh or a strained muscle just below the female breast), an informed consent discussion is invaluable.

By keeping clients informed about exactly what you're planning to do and how they're likely to be affected, you give them a background for agreeing to go forward, expressing concerns, or saying no. Moreover, you make it easier for them to speak up about any future boundary issues that may arise. Clients are more likely to discuss their concerns when they're engaged early and often in low-risk conversations about their treatment. As a further benefit, clients' active participation in the treatment process makes it more likely that they'll do their part to make it a success.

 Informed Consent Discussion Script

Write up a script of an Informed Consent Discussion that incorporates the what, why, and how. Include at least three cycles of Speak ➡ Invite ➡ Reflect.

Responding to Body Language

Establishing a two-way conversation is particularly challenging when the impetus for that discussion isn't your idea or in response to a client's comments, but your observation of the client's body language. You may notice that the person suddenly frowns, squirms, or tenses up, and want to be responsive to what's happening for the client. You can't simply provide a reflection because there is no explicit verbal content to reflect. What you can do is tell the person what you've observed and ask him to share what's going on. For example, if the client squirms and tightens up, you can say, "I noticed you jumped a little there and tensed up the area I was working on. Can you tell me what happened for you in that moment?" This method of clarifying the nonverbal message from the client gives you a way to address what you're seeing without relying on mind-reads. You may find yourself doing this frequently with some individuals. Clients are often hesitant to express themselves in words, particularly around sensitive or upsetting boundary issues. Nonverbal cues may be the only signs you get of a significant problem or worry.

> A male client who was training for a long-distance bicycle race talked to a practitioner about having bi-weekly massages to assist in the process. The practitioner explained that she would need to pay special attention to his hips, buttocks, and legs, and would use special stretching techniques for these areas.
>
> With one particular stretching technique, the practitioner sat on the table and used her body weight to stretch the client's legs apart. The client tensed and drew in a quick breath, but said nothing. The practitioner asked if everything was okay, and he nodded silently. As the client was ready to leave, the practitioner asked about booking the next session. The client looked away, mumbled something about his busy schedule, and left.
>
> A few days later, the practitioner placed a follow-up call. The client admitted that during the session he'd been concerned about the way she was hovering over him and separating his legs, but he didn't feel able to say anything. Although he believed that the work she did was appropriate, he didn't like being so openly exposed. He told the practitioner that he didn't want to have another session if that type of technique would be used. He then said that he really respected her expertise and didn't mean to question her judgment; he hoped that his comments hadn't offended her.
>
> ### Points to Ponder
>
> Why might the client have felt unable to speak up in the middle of the session? What could the practitioner have done to reduce that difficulty—either in that moment or earlier in the session? If you were the practitioner in this situation, how would you respond to the client's concerns about questioning your judgment or causing offense?

Note that the practitioner in this scenario didn't ignore the client's body language; she did ask him whether everything was okay. The problem is that a single, very general question wasn't sufficient to empower him to voice his concerns. To make it easier for him to express his concerns, the practitioner might have taken a break from the stretching and—with the client in a less vulnerable position—engaged in Interactive Speaking.

PRACTITIONER SPEAKS:

Let's take a break for a moment. I noticed that as I began that last stretch, your body became tense. If that movement makes you uncomfortable in any way, I'm happy to skip it and move on.

PRACTITIONER INVITES:

Would that be best?

CLIENT RESPONDS:

Yes, thank you.

PRACTITIONER REFLECTS:

Okay, so we'll leave that stretch out and move on to something else.

Once the client was off the table and fully dressed, another round or two of Interactive Speaking could provide additional clarification:

PRACTITIONER SPEAKS:

I want to check in about that stretch that we skipped. Some clients choose to opt out of particular techniques, either because the sensations are too intense or because the positions feel too awkward or uncomfortable. Always feel free to speak up if anything doesn't feel okay to you.

PRACTITIONER INVITES:

Is there anything else you'd like me to avoid going forward?

CLIENT RESPONDS:

Everything else you did was fine. It just felt like too much, having my legs splayed like that with you right over me.

PRACTITIONER REFLECTS:

Okay, so the problem was that particular combination of how your legs were positioned and how I was sitting. Everything else felt okay. Is that right?

CLIENT RESPONDS:

That's right.

PRACTITIONER SPEAKS:

Thank you for letting me know. I'll be sure to avoid doing anything like that in the future. And please do speak up as we go along if anything else ever bothers you.

PRACTITIONER INVITES:

[Pause]

CLIENT RESPONDS:

Okay. I will.

[No reflection necessary in this instance.]

Points to Ponder

Why was it important for the practitioner to allow the client to decide whether they should move on, rather than simply moving on without discussion? Why was it important for the practitioner to revisit the subject after the client was off the treatment table and fully dressed?

When responding to body language cues, you may find it useful to state any of the following in the first ("Speak") portion of the conversation:

- **DIRECT OBSERVATIONS, OFTEN TIED TO A CONTEXT:** "When I lifted your leg" (context), "your breathing sped up and your facial expression changed" (observation).
- **THIRD-PERSON STATEMENTS:** "Some clients disrobe fully, and others prefer not to remove their underwear. Either is fine." (This less-direct alternative to an observation is sometimes preferable when addressing sensitive boundary issues.)

- **EXPLANATIONS OF CHOICES OR ALTERNATIVES:** "It's okay to leave that portion of the history form blank if you prefer." "I can work on this area directly, through your clothes, or not at all. It's your choice."
- **EXPRESSIONS OF OPENNESS TO THE CLIENT'S INPUT:** "Please don't hesitate to raise any concerns that come up during a session." "I'm always open to hearing suggestions on what I could do to help make you more comfortable."

Whenever you make an observation, do your best to give facts (e.g., "I noticed that you hesitated and looked away") rather than interpretations ("I noticed that you seemed uneasy"). Remember that any form of nonverbal communication can signify a variety of different things (see Figure 5.1); any conclusion you draw about the cause of a particular sound, facial expression, gesture, or other physical reaction can only be a hypothesis.

Figure 5.1 Potential Causes of Nonverbal Reactions

Nonverbal Communication	Examples of Possible Causes
Breaking eye contact	Anger, nervousness, difficulty thinking while making eye contact, respect for the practitioner (in many cultures it's inappropriate to look directly into another person's eyes)
Collapsing chest	Fear, depression, meditative breathing
Crossing arms or legs	Defensiveness, feeling cold, cramping, a need to urinate, habitual posture
Gasping	Shock, surprise, pain or discomfort, difficulty breathing, attempts to hold back tears
Grimacing	Disapproval, discomfort, attempts to prevent a sneeze, itchy nose
Laughing at odd moments	Discomfort, embarrassment, unusual ticklishness, suppressed feelings of sadness, irritation, thinking about something funny
Looking down or away	Embarrassment, shame, feeling shy, not knowing how to respond, being lost in thought
Sighing	Boredom, impatience, relaxation
Squirming	A full bladder, sexual arousal, uncomfortable positioning, discomfort with the treatment, tight clothing
Tensing up	Pain or discomfort, feeling cold, an unpleasant memory or emotion, defensiveness, attempts to restrain a belch
Tilting one's head	Confusion, disbelief, hearing problem, neck stretch

Understanding Body Language

Read through the examples in Figure 5.1. For each type of body language, identify as many other possible causes as you can. Then think up several additional types of body language that aren't listed here; consider facial expressions, sounds, gestures, and whole-body reactions. Then match those with as many different causes as possible.

Educating

All wellness practitioners are educators. Whether you do relaxation massage, acupuncture, movement therapy, or injury rehabilitation, you're implicitly educating clients—increasing their physical awareness and teaching their bodies how to relax and heal. Many practitioners also engage in more explicit education which might include: explaining relevant aspects of anatomy and physiology; demonstrating stretches and other self-care techniques; sharing information on related wellness topics; providing reading materials; or assigning homework.

Keeping your clients well informed is beneficial in several ways:

- By reducing the amount of relevant information that you understand and your clients don't, you decrease the power differential.
- Education may reveal choices that clients wouldn't otherwise know they had (e.g., a more uncomfortable treatment promising faster results vs. a gentler approach for a longer period of time).
- When clients have a greater understanding of the different factors contributing to their health issues, they can take a more active role in their own healing—which in turn can speed their recovery and help them stay well.
- As a nice side benefit, deeper knowledge of your work can enhance clients' ability to explain and recommend your services to their friends and colleagues.

Like any other important conversations you initiate with clients, educational discussions benefit from Interactive Speaking. Inviting and reflecting clients' responses helps to ensure that they've taken in and integrated what you've taught. However, speaking alone often isn't the most effective way to provide education. People have varied learning styles and different preferred ways to take in information.

Learning Styles

Most people prefer to take in information by one of three methods: auditory, kinesthetic, or visual. If you use only the auditory channel (speaking), some individuals understand perfectly and others immediately forget what you said. If you use a demonstration or written materials to show the information, you assist the visually oriented segment of the population. To reach someone who is kinesthetically oriented, you can tell a story that makes a visceral or emotional connection for them, or else have them physically perform an exercise or role-play a situation to learn it from the inside out.

Related to the concept of learning styles is the theory of multiple intelligences, which holds that people possess a variety of different intellectual capacities that operate relatively independently from one another. Howard Gardner, the author of *Multiple Intelligences: The Theory in Practice*[2] identified eight major intelligences: Verbal/Linguistic; Logical/Mathematical; Visual/Spatial; Bodily/Kinesthetic; Music/ Rhythmic; Intrapersonal; Interpersonal; and Naturalist. (Since the publishing of his book, he has added the Existential intelligence and has speculated about

> It is better to know some of the questions than all of the answers.
>
> — James Thurber

adding a Pedagogical intelligence.) Each intelligence is associated with a specific set of abilities and strengths, and can be accessed through specific types of teaching methods.

Without extensive training in communication and learning theory, it's often difficult to know what another person's learning style is, or which of the various intelligences are strongest. Therefore, it's safest to communicate using as many methods as possible. For instance, if you're teaching an exercise to a client, you might explain it verbally, demonstrate it yourself, give the client a handout, and then have the client ask you questions, explain his understanding of the movement, and perform the exercise in front of you. In his next session, you can verify that he retained the information by asking him to explain or demonstrate what he's been doing. It is common to use several methods of communication and still have the person show or tell you something completely different at your next meeting. In this case, you may have missed his primary method of communication, or the individual may simply need more repetition to learn and retain information.

See http://TheEthicsOfTouch. com/pdf/client-education. pdf for more information on **Tailoring Client Education** to these Intelligences.

Multiple Intelligences Exploration

- Visit http://surfaquarium.com/MI/inventory.htm to take Walter McKenzie's "Multiple Intelligences Survey" to learn more about the strengths of your own intelligences.
- Identify several pieces of information you'd like to teach to one or more of your clients (anything from instructions for a relaxation technique to the details of recent research supporting your work). For each of those, list the possible teaching methods that utilize the different intelligences.

The Assertion Sequence

In the previous chapter, we discussed the importance of clarifying your boundaries in your own mind and expressing them clearly to others. In an ideal world, this would be all you'd ever need to do to maintain your boundaries. Unfortunately, in reality, things tend to get a lot more complicated. Sometimes you think you have an agreement, but the client has misunderstood what you said. At other times your meaning is crystal clear to the client, but the intensity of the client's own needs overrides the client's desire to respect your boundary. With some clients, this may happen repeatedly.

The Assertion Sequence is designed to minimize misunderstandings in boundary discussions and help you respond skillfully to any challenge you may encounter from a client. It consists of four stages of increasingly forceful conversations.

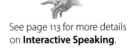
See page 113 for more details on **Interactive Speaking**.

The more effective you are in the early stages, the less likely you'll need to use the later ones. With many clients, the Agreement Discussion is the only conversation you need to have. However, when a client isn't honoring your boundaries, it's generally appropriate to move stage by stage through the sequence. With very serious boundary violations, it may be appropriate to skip a stage or two. Throughout the sequence, make a conscious effort to be clear and concise. Use assertive language and Interactive Speaking.

> **Figure 5.2 Assertion Sequence Stages**
>
> - Stage I: Agreement Discussion
> - Stage II: Follow-Up
> - Stage III: Confrontation Meeting
> - Stage IV: Termination

Assertion Sequence Stage I: Agreement Discussion

The Agreement Discussion has five steps:

1. What
2. Why
3. Consequences
4. Obstacles
5. Recap

Depending on the particular boundary you're discussing, you may wish to do all of these steps, or skip one or more.

Step 1: What

Let the client know what you expect in the form of a single, compact sentence. State the issue positively: focus on the specific behavior you want rather than what you don't want (for example, "I expect payment at the end of each appointment," not "I expect you not to be late with your payments"). Sometimes, for the sake of clarity, it helps to distinguish those behaviors you want from those you don't. In these cases, describe the desired behavior first ("Please turn your cell phone off completely, rather than setting it to vibrate").

Phrase your statement as a specific fact or request ("I begin each session promptly at the start of the hour," "Please arrive in time to begin right at 2 pm"), rather than a general opinion ("It's important for you to be on time"). Keep your body language open and centered, rather than confrontational or submissive, and use a firm, clear tone of voice that conveys that you mean what you say and expect it to happen. Once you have spoken, pause or invite the other person to speak. You might ask, "Is that something you feel comfortable with?" Then listen carefully, reflecting any concerns the client may have.

Step 2: Why

Research in social psychology shows that people are much more likely to comply with a request if it's accompanied by a rationale.[3] You can increase the chances that a client will do what you ask by explaining why that behavior matters to you. For instance, you might say, "I have four children and have only five hours to work each day. Also, it's important to me to show respect for my clients' time by not keeping anyone waiting." Keep your explanation brief. Share just one or two reasons, even if you can think of many others. If you ramble on and give too much detail, the client may get annoyed.

In some situations, there's no need to state your rationale. If you sense that the client grasps the reason behind your request without your mentioning it, skip this part of the conversation. You can always bring it up later in the discussion.

Step 3: Consequences

When you're discussing a boundary that's important or meaningful to you, establish consequences that follow logically from a transgression. In phrasing the message, you may wish to use the formula, "If you [description of the behavior you wish to prevent], I will [statement of the consequences].” For instance, you might say, “If you cancel an appointment with less than five hours of notice, I will charge you for the treatment.”

Keep your statement short and matter-of-fact. An edgy voice tone or emotionally loaded words can turn a straightforward statement of consequences (“When clients come in wearing a fragrance, I ask them to wash it off”) into a threat (“When clients come in reeking of cologne, I refuse to tolerate it”). After you've explained the consequence, provide an opportunity for the client to respond. Ask, “Does that sound reasonable to you?” or “Do you have any questions or concerns about this?”

Step 4: Obstacles

If you think the client might have difficulty sticking to the boundary you've set, ask him to identify possible obstacles (“Can you think of anything that might prevent you from giving me enough notice if you need to cancel an appointment?”). When the client identifies a potential problem, resist the temptation to solve it yourself. Wait patiently until the client figures out a way to resolve the situation. Clients are more committed to implementing a solution when they figure it out themselves. If they're struggling, you might ask, “How might you overcome that problem?”

Step 5: Recap

To make sure there's no confusion or misunderstanding, ask the client to summarize what you've just discussed. You could say something like, “Let's be sure you and I are on the same page. What's your understanding of the agreement we've made?”

Once you've finished discussing one boundary issue, you can move on to any others you need to address. Remember that you don't need to go through every step for every issue. Depending on the situation, you may choose to mention only the “what” (step 1) for each issue and then ask the client to recap at the end of the conversation.

> “
> The most important thing in communication is to hear what isn't being said.
> — Peter Drucker

Special Cases: After-the-Fact Agreement Discussions

Not all boundary issues can, or should, be discussed in advance. Although there are many kinds of boundary crossings that occur in a practitioner's lifetime, only a few are likely to occur in any given relationship. It would be offensive to reel off 50 no-no's in the first meeting with a client, or to initiate a conversation about extreme or highly sensitive boundary violations (“I expect that clients don't make sexual advances toward me”).

If a client crosses a boundary that you never discussed with them, get an after-the-fact agreement. An *After-the-Fact Agreement Discussion* is similar to an ordinary Agreement Discussion, with two important exceptions:

1. You include a disclaimer such as, “I know we never discussed this before, so you had no way to know this was of concern to me…” For example, you might say, “I make it a policy never to socialize with any of my clients because I find that it interferes with my objectivity in providing an effective treatment. I realize I never mentioned that before, so there's no way you could have known my policy.”

2. It is rarely appropriate to address consequences in an after-the-fact discussion. Stick to the What, Why, Obstacles (if relevant), and Recap.

By saying up front that you've never discussed the boundary before—so the client couldn't have known about it—you decrease the likelihood that your comments come across as blameful. When people think they're being blamed, they often react with feelings of guilt, embarrassment, or anger—any of which can impede the therapeutic relationship and make the conversation more difficult. Even when you include a disclaimer, after-the-fact agreement discussions can trigger considerable defensiveness. Take time to listen to the client's point of view, and keep reflecting what the client says until she feels heard and understood.

Assertion Sequence Stage II: Follow-Up

The Follow-Up has three steps:

1. Desirable Behavior Reinforcement
2. Ongoing Reminders
3. Broken Agreement Discussion

If you have established clear boundary agreements in Stage One of the Assertion Sequence, the other three stages may not be necessary. In some circumstances, however, it's wise to follow up. If you're concerned that a particular client may break one or more of your agreements, you may choose to reinforce the desirable behavior or provide ongoing reminders. If an agreement has already been broken, discuss any consequences, and then adjust or re-establish the agreement.

Step 1: Desirable Behavior Reinforcement

Reinforce desirable behavior. When the person does as agreed, thank her for it. This affirms the person and serves as a reminder that the issue is important to you. For instance, you might say, "I really appreciated your calling me with plenty of notice when you had to cancel your appointment" or "Thank you for not wearing cologne at your appointments."

Step 2: Ongoing Reminders

There are a variety of ways in which you can tactfully reinforce your policies: you might include a carefully worded reminder of your cancellation policy on your appointment cards; list payment options on your bills; or hang small, tasteful signs that describe your basic expectations. Although it's a more delicate matter to give verbal reminders of agreements that haven't been broken, it's sometimes helpful to do so. For example, suppose a client says, "I have a hard time relaxing after rushing to get here after work." You might say, "It's always best to plan to arrive a little early, so you have time to transition from your day. You can bring a book and catch up on some reading, or just close your eyes and relax for a few minutes."

Practitioners walk a fine line in protecting their boundaries. If they don't focus enough attention on the limits they've set, they increase the risk of boundary crossings. And yet if they focus too strongly on those limits, they run the risk of seeming more concerned with their own needs than with the needs of their clients. If you're thinking about providing a reminder but worry that it might be overkill, run it by a supervisor, mentor, or trusted friend who will give you candid feedback.

Step 3: Broken Agreement Discussion

When a client crosses a boundary that you've discussed with him previously, remind him of the agreement you made and ask for his response. For example, if a client forgets your policy about fragrance and wears heavy cologne, you could say, "I notice you're wearing cologne today. I ask everyone not to wear fragrances because some of my clients are chemically sensitive. Do you remember our discussion about that? Is this something you still can commit to?" Based on what you learn from the client, you might re-establish your initial agreement or adjust it. In this case, you might arrange to see the client early in the morning before he puts on cologne, or else book him in the last appointment slot of the day so the scent will dissipate before any other clients arrive.

If your original agreement included consequences, be sure to apply them. It is essential for the client to understand that any time they violate the agreement, the consequence automatically follows. But keep your communication objective and matter-of-fact. If you become emotional about the infraction and say something like, "I told you what would happen if you missed an appointment," the person is likely to feel he is being punished rather than experiencing a logical consequence. Punishment can trigger a variety of dynamics you want to avoid, including damaged rapport, disempowering submissiveness, increased resistance, or a spiraling power struggle. Head off those problems by keeping your words and tone neutral: "To cover this missed appointment, I am charging your credit card for two sessions."

Assertion Sequence Stage III: Confrontation

The Confrontation has six steps:

1. Explanation
2. Solution Generation
3. Consequences
4. Reflection
5. Refocus
6. Recap

Most of the time, agreement and follow-up discussions are sufficient for managing boundary issues. When problems persist beyond those initial stages, it's time to confront the issue directly. Confrontation is typically used when a client persistently violates a boundary, but it may also be appropriate on a first occasion if the violation is serious. Note that the six-step process described here is a variation on the standard confrontation process, as described in Robert Bolton's *People Skills*.[4] For the current edition of this book, we have broken the process into numbered components, added the second and third components (solution generation and consequences), and expanded upon the fourth and fifth (reflection and refocusing).

Step 1: Explanation

The first step in a confrontation meeting is explaining the problem that is created by the boundary violation. Do this with a single sentence that incorporates three elements—behavior, feelings, and effect:

Behavior	+	Feelings	+	Effect
When you (describe the agreed upon behavior) **and don't,**		**I feel** (state your feelings)		**because** (state the tangible effect on you).

For example:

When you agree to be on time and arrive 30 minutes late, **Behavior** *I feel upset and frustrated* **Feelings** *because there isn't enough time to give you what you deserve in a session and do my best work.* **Effects**

The wording of this explanation is so crucial that we recommend writing it out, editing it carefully, and memorizing it. When you deliver this carefully prepared message, be sure that your voice tone and body language are assertive, not aggressive.

Step 2: Solution Generation

After you've explained the problem, the next step is working toward a solution. Often, it's helpful to ask for the client's suggestions. You might ask, "What can you suggest to prevent this from happening again?" or "What needs to change to enable you to stick to our agreement?" If the client can't come up with any ideas, you can offer your own and ask the client whether it would work for him. However, keep in mind that people are much more likely to comply with solutions that they have generated themselves.

Step 3: Consequences

Just as in your original agreement discussion, it's often important to communicate consequences. If the problem persists, what will you do? Suppose a client has been arriving 30 minutes late on a regular basis, despite the consequence that you've been consistently applying (charging your full fee for a shortened treatment). You may decide that you're not willing to keep working in that way. Give this message clearly: "If you aren't able to start coming on time, I'll recommend that either we take a break from our work until your schedule gets more predictable, or you switch to working with another practitioner." Again, be sure to remain assertive, not aggressive. Your message should come across as a straightforward statement, not a threat. (Note: If the client is already upset or defensive, skip to Step 4—reflection—and wait to talk about consequences until later in the conversation.)

Step 4: Reflection

Sometimes the first two or three steps of confrontation will be sufficient. Together with the client, you'll come up with a solution that works for both of you. If the client can't think of a solution he can commit to, if he objects to the consequences you establish, or if he gives only grudging agreement, shift your focus to understanding and reflecting his point of view.

The client who repeatedly arrives late may say, "When my meetings run long, it's really difficult to get here exactly on time. If there are important people at the meeting, there's a huge amount of pressure to stay." You might respond, "What I'm hearing is that it's difficult for you to leave meetings if they run long, and it's particularly hard when there are important people there. You feel a lot of pressure to stay late. Is that accurate?" Continue reflecting until the client has finished expressing whatever it is he wants to say. Remember to finish by asking a question or pausing and allowing the person to respond, so you can confirm that your reflection is on target.

Courage is very important. Like a muscle, it's strengthened by use.

—Ruth Gordon

One further step that may be appropriate at this point is to join with what the client has said. If you can sincerely agree with or build on any of the points he made, do that. For instance, you might say, "I agree that that's a tough situation to be in" or "One of my previous jobs was in a high-pressure business environment, and I remember having the same sort of difficulty setting boundaries on my time." If you can't join authentically, just stick with reflection.

Step 5: Refocus

In rare instances, the client's objections may reveal a compelling reason to change your agreement. However, after you've made a point of asking about potential obstacles in the Agreement Discussion and Follow-Up, it's unlikely that the Confrontation discussion will surface any substantial new issues. Typically, it's best to follow your reflection with refocusing—circling back to Step 1 (explanation) or Step 2 (solution generation).

If the client has repeatedly told you how difficult his situation is or how good his intentions are, it may be helpful to not just repeat your explanation, but clarify it as well. Make it clear that the boundary you're setting is designed to solve a problem for you (the difficulty you're having as a consequence of their behavior), not to punish him for doing something bad. Regarding the problem of lateness, you might say, "I'm not making any judgment that you're intentionally being difficult or not trying hard enough to get here on time. The problem is how your lateness affects me—there isn't enough time to give you an effective treatment and do my best work, so I feel upset and frustrated. No matter how good your intentions are and how hard you're trying, I still have that problem." This type of clarification can help minimize a client's defensive reaction in two ways: 1) reducing any feeling he may have of being blamed or punished, and 2) demonstrating that a good defense won't solve your problem or change your mind.

The client's explanations of his difficulties can also provide a good opportunity to refocus on solution generation. You might segue naturally from reflection ("I'm hearing that you have a hard time leaving a meeting when important people are present") to joining ("I can see how that would be tough to do, particularly if your company culture doesn't support it") to refocusing ("Given how hard it is for you to transition from meetings, what would it take for you to get to your sessions on time? Is there an adjustment we could make on this end, like changing the time or date of your appointments? Or can you make some kind of change at work?").

Step 6: Recap

Confrontation discussions can be quite lengthy, particularly if the client becomes upset or defensive. Be sure to have the person give a recap at the end to ensure that the two of you have a shared understanding as you move forward. Set a time in a week or two to discuss how the agreement is working.

Practical Application: Sample Confrontation Dialogue for Talking to a Client Who Asks Personal Questions

PRACTITIONER:

When you agree not to ask personal questions about my romantic life, and then don't stick to that agreement, I feel upset and frustrated because it distracts me from the work I'm doing with you. (Explanation) What needs to change to enable you to do what you we agreed to? (Solution generation)

CLIENT:

I don't see what the big deal is. I just tend to talk very openly about things, and I forget you're so sensitive about your personal life.

PRACTITIONER:

I'm hearing that for you these types of questions are no big deal. You're comfortable talking openly about your own personal life, so you just don't remember that I feel very differently about it. Is that correct? (Reflection)

CLIENT:

Yeah. It isn't like I'm intentionally trying to offend you. I'm just making conversation.

PRACTITIONER:

So for you, you're just trying to have a conversation; you're not trying to offend me. (Reflection)

CLIENT:

Right, I'm really not.

PRACTITIONER:

I can see how this could be frustrating on your end, to try to have a conversation in a way that feels natural to you, and keep hearing that it isn't okay with me. There are many other things I do talk about openly, so it makes sense that you might forget about certain topics being off-limits. (Joining) What would help you to remember? (Refocusing on the solution)

CLIENT:

Well, after we've spent all this time talking about it, I'm sure I'll remember now.

PRACTITIONER:

Okay, good. Let's give it a few weeks and see how things go. If it turns out to be too difficult for you to avoid asking personal questions, I'll suggest that you switch to another practitioner. (Consequences)

CLIENT:

Isn't that a little harsh? I swear, I'm really not trying to be disrespectful or make you upset.

PRACTITIONER:

You're saying that you're not trying to disrespect or upset me, and so it seems extreme for me to think about deciding not to work with you. Is that right? (Reflection)

CLIENT:

Yeah.

PRACTITIONER:

I believe you. I don't think you're trying to be disrespectful. (Joining) The problem for me isn't that I think you have bad intentions. It's that no matter what your intentions are, personal questions about my romantic life distract me from the work I'm trying to do and leave me feeling upset and

---

frustrated. I have a policy that if any client can't stop doing that, I don't work with them. (Refocusing) Does that make sense to you?

CLIENT:

I suppose so.

PRACTITIONER:

So just to be sure we're on the same page, would you mind restating your understanding of the agreement we've just made? (Request for a recap)

CLIENT:

I'm agreeing not to ask you any questions about your personal life. If I don't stick to that, you're not going to work with me anymore.

PRACTITIONER:

That's right. I'm very hopeful that from this point on, we won't have any trouble working together. I really appreciate your having this conversation and agreeing to make a change.

Points to Ponder

Did the practitioner in this example use all the confrontation steps successfully? Can you think of any other ways the practitioner could have addressed solution generation or consequences?

Assertion Sequence Stage IV: Termination

If a client repeatedly violates a boundary, even after a well-conducted confrontation meeting, it's time to consider terminating the therapeutic relationship. Using the previous example of a Confrontation Meeting regarding asking personal questions, if the client continues to ask personal questions, the practitioner should move on to the next step of Termination.

A generic approach to terminating a client/practitioner relationship is impossible to define. We suggest that you work with a supervisor or trusted colleague to figure out whether and how to terminate your work with a client.

Practical Application: Termination Dialogue

PRACTITIONER:

Since respecting my request not to ask me personal questions continues to be difficult for you to honor, I have prepared a list of therapists and their contact information that I think do the type of work you need and like, as well as being less reactive to personal questions than I am. Would you like this list?

CLIENT:

I regret that this isn't working for you. I certainly don't mean any disrespect to you. I guess it's just my nature to be a little more familiar and informal than you're comfortable with. I respect you professionally, and if these are people you recommend, I will give one of them a try. Which one do you recommend for me more than the others?

PRACTITIONER:

I suggest starting with the first one on the list.

CLIENT:

Well, thanks. I am sorry again, but I wish you well.

PRACTITIONER:

Same to you. Good luck in the future.

Points to Ponder

Can you think of any other ways the practitioner could have addressed this solution? How would you feel if you were the practitioner? How would you feel if you were the client?

Conclusion

Investing time to enhance your communication skills benefits you personally and professionally. Using the techniques and strategies provided in this chapter helps you manage a wide range of different conversations, from informed consent discussions to educational exchanges to confrontations about boundary violations. As you begin to put your skills into practice, consider that there is no substitute for in-person training and coaching. We highly recommend working with an experienced teacher or mentor who can give you direct feedback and assist you in making your communication as effective as it can be.

6

Sex, Touch, and Intimacy

*"We cannot touch something without being touched by it in the very same instant.
We cannot be touched without touching."*
—Jon Kabat-Zinn

Key Terms

Arousal

Desexualize

Gender Identity

Intervention Model

Intimacy

Psychosexual

Psychosocial

Sensuality

Sex

Sexual Behavior

Sexual Harassment

Sexual Misconduct

Sexual Orientation

Sexual Response Cycle

Sexuality

Sexualization

Touch

SEX. TOUCH. INTIMACY. What feelings and thoughts are conjured by these words? Excitement, shame, denial, ambivalence, pleasure? For humans these words describe experiences at the core of our being. As a wellness practitioner you might be asking yourself, "Why in the world do I need to think about these issues? What do they have to do with my work?" The answer is that clear boundaries around sex, touch, and intimacy create the foundation for safety and trust which is the basis for healing in all therapeutic relationships, especially in somatic therapies.

In this chapter we focus on the sex, touch, and intimacy issues in client/practitioner relationships. These three topics are profoundly present whenever you have physical contact with a client, yet they're rarely explored in educational training programs. These are the areas where clients state that they experience the most boundary violations from their practitioners. The two most common complaints clients make about healthcare professionals are: the practitioner didn't listen to the client; and the client felt violated by the practitioner, most often from unwanted or insensitive touch or personal remarks made to the client.[1] Unfortunately, most clients opt to find a new practitioner rather than discuss their concerns.

As part of this chapter's exploration, we examine cultural and personal beliefs about sex, touch, and intimacy, and how these may relate to both the client's and practitioner's experience during an actual session. We also focus on practical, ethical steps for practitioners to take regarding sex, touch, and intimacy issues to create a safe environment for both client and practitioner.

A Psychosocial Overview

We are born as sexual beings with a need for touch and intimacy. We require a healthy environment that supports our natural development in these areas to thrive as organisms. However, each of our uniquely personal experiences is culturally bound by unconscious, embedded beliefs. How our beliefs develop is more often a product of cultural values than a natural unfolding of one's own biology and identity and the interplay with our environment. This cultural overlay is influenced by religion, family, social mores, and the larger social fabric of the time. Our "unique" selves would most likely look different if we were raised in another place and time.

A society influences the type and volume of information available to its members. Examples from United States history illustrate the problem of getting information about human sexuality. In the 1800s, several "health reformers" (including Sylvester Graham of Graham Cracker fame and John Harvey Kellogg of Kellogg's breakfast cereal) believed sexual feelings, thoughts, and activity debilitated the body. Although these sentiments were based on opinions largely influenced by religious beliefs, they were presented as fact. In that same century, federal laws that made it illegal to send sexual literature through the mail were applied to the mailing of birth control information. In the mid-20th century, during the political era of McCarthyism, "one Congressman insisted that studying human sexual behavior was paving the way for a Communist takeover of the United States."[2] Though we live in a society that considers itself the most accomplished and sophisticated in the world, more recent examples show that we are still struggling with these issues. The editor of the Journal of the American Medical Association was fired by the AMA for publishing an article that reported on a 1991 Kinsey Institute study asking students to define sex. This kind of cultural legacy makes it difficult to obtain sensitive, accurate, complete information about sexuality that might actually help us to become more responsible, respectful, happier human beings.

Psychosexual Effects on the Individual

Why might there be confusion between sex, touch, and intimacy? Did you receive a good sex education? Before you answer that question for yourself, consider this definition. A good sex education is one where:

- the information you received was developmentally appropriate for your age at the time;
- the learning was ongoing throughout your childhood, and you clearly received all the necessary facts;
- the teaching was sensitive to your feelings and needs;
- you were given a model for decision-making rather than a finite set of rules about how to behave;
- you and your body were treated with respect.

How good was your sex education? Did you receive a good touch education or a good intimacy education based on the above criteria? It is just as crucial for us as humans to be "fluent" in discussing touch and intimacy needs, but rarely do any of us get direct education and experience regarding the issues of touch and intimacy.

Most people find it extremely difficult to talk about sexuality. Even if practitioners are comfortable with sexuality, touching, and intimacy themselves, they might still find it difficult to talk to clients about these issues. This is true for several reasons. First, cultural experience tells them that it's usually improper to talk about these topics. Second, if those conversations occurred they were most likely only with sexual partner(s) or in an impersonal, clinical setting. Third, if as youngsters they didn't have role models for open communication, it's often difficult to comfortably discuss sex, touch, and intimacy. And finally, to complicate the matter further, if they weren't respected and if their bodies were violated in any way, their ability to deal with these topics in an open manner is usually severely compromised unless they resolve the effects of those experiences.

> When we truly care for ourselves, it becomes possible to care far more profoundly about other people. The more alert and sensitive we are to our own needs, the more loving and generous we can be toward others.
>
> —Eda LeShan

The Distinction between Sex, Touch, and Intimacy

By definition, sex, touch, and intimacy are three distinct behaviors and experiences. The fact that they overlap at times is what creates confusion. Most people would concur that good sex includes all three. A person who only feels intimate with someone when sex is involved might start to believe that intimacy and sex are the same thing. Men are more susceptible than women because most cultures assert that men aren't supposed to express feelings (a form of intimacy) except during sex.

How is all this related to health care or somatic therapy? Unfortunately, personal and cultural perceptions of sexuality, touch, and intimacy histories also influence how individuals experience health care. As an example, for many years in the United States massage was a euphemism for illegal sex through prostitution. In the 1980s many people made sexual innuendoes or were genuinely taken aback when someone said they were making a legitimate career choice to be a massage therapist. More than 30 years later, although there is much more mainstream acceptance and understanding about the benefits of massage and other bodywork therapies, there is still a profound cultural legacy and taboo in certain segments of the population.

The general public, clients, and somatic practitioners share in the confusion about how touch therapies and sexuality are and aren't related. The intentional misuse of language (e.g., massage as a euphemism for prostitution) has had a profound impact on the public's understanding of touch modalities. The misuse of words isn't just a cognitive problem; it's a personal and cultural issue about how people relate to certain parts of the body and human experience.

▌ Touch

Touch is a basic human need, as well as a sensory process through which we communicate. However, as with any communication, the intended message may be misunderstood by the receiver. Many countries such as the United States are "low-touch" cultures. The kind of touch given to children tends to be more for care-taking, retrieving, and punishing, and less so for nurturing and affection. For example, modern media such as advertising, magazines, newspapers, movies, music videos, and comics most often displays most touch as romantic, sexual, or violent.

Exploring Touch and Culture

Humans need touch. We crave it, we hunger for it, we get sick and can even die for the lack of it. But we still don't know where touch belongs in our lives. In fact, we are often actively discouraged from touching each other. This conditioning begins early: kindergartners are taught to keep their hands strictly to themselves and are chastised for unnecessary and inappropriate touching. Many children learn early on that touching is bad. We lose our childlike innocence and, after a while, non-sexual touch, the most basic form of communication between humans, seems strange and uncomfortable. Only in a few settings is giving and receiving this vital nourishment acceptable: ritual greetings and leave-takings; contact sports; physical aggression; grooming; and professional touching by hands-on practitioners.

This isn't as true, however, outside of the United States. Psychologist Sidney Jourard made a study of couples' behavior in public situations in a variety of different cultures. In a comparison of touching in cafés, he observed that in San Juan couples touched each other 180 times per hour. In Paris they touched 110 times per hour. In Gainesville, Florida it was two times per hour and in London it wasn't at all.[3]

By the time we reach adulthood many of us have actually forgotten how to touch. We have lived through years of "hands off" indoctrination. Naturally we are confused. We have been told all our lives that the only "right" ways to satisfy this intense physical need is through sex, violence, or contact sports. Touch between parents and their children even becomes strained and confused. In the book, *touch*, Tiffany Field, PH.D., quotes Ashley Montagu, "Such alarm is understandable in a society that has so confounded love, sex, affection, and touch. The genuinely loving parents have nothing to fear from their demonstrative acts of affection for the children or anyone else."[4]

What do we do, then, if we just want to be comforted? As often as not, we don't even identify the need as such. We misinterpret the need for touch as sexual desire, or hunger, or depression. We may seek out sexual relationships less out of love than out of a need for contact. Or, in the absence of someone to hug our outer skin, we hug our inner skin by overeating. There are many ways we try to satisfy our need for comfort when all we really need is to be touched. We don't just have "skin hunger;" we often have skin starvation.[5]

Knowing Where Touch Begins

The sensation of touch actually begins in the womb. The skin, derived from the same cells as the nervous system, is a perfect instrument for collecting information about our surrounding environment long before birth. A fetus withdraws from the touch of a probe at less than eight weeks of gestation, showing that the link between touch and survival is one of the first and most important protective mechanisms to develop.

All human babies are born too soon. Our heads are so big that we can't afford to gestate any longer than we do, so we are born before we are physiologically ready. Most other mammals can move around, at least in a limited way, very soon after they're born. Think of newborn foals or deer, which are up and walking a few moments after birth. Humans, on the other hand, are incredibly slow. In fact, the average time between birth and crawling is identical to the average time between conception and birth, nine months. What does all this have to do with touch? Simply this, newborn human infants aren't fully developed. They can't see clearly or differentiate sounds. They communicate with the world almost entirely through their skin. Virtually all mammals, particularly the young, show behaviors of snuggling. Montagu asserts that touch is a basic behavioral need and that the absence of it causes abnormal behavior[6] and abnormal physical development as well.[7]

Consider a newborn baby. One moment it's supremely comfortable in a snug, climate controlled, perfectly shaped uterus. The next moment it's painfully squeezed into a bright, noisy, cold, wall-less world. All babies benefit from regular touch—from perfectly healthy ones to those who suffer from colic, cocaine exposure, or abuse. Touch reduces stress (as measured by chemicals in the blood). Babies cry less, sleep more, and are generally easier to soothe when touched. The messages we receive through our skin, particularly about our safety and wellbeing, have resonating effects on our behavior for the rest of our lives. Research findings document evidence that the cause of failure to thrive or to mature psychologically can be linked to the lack of demonstrative love.[8]

Even older babies who aren't yet crawling use their skin as a way to get information about the world. Watch a baby explore a new toy: the first place it goes is into the baby's mouth. This baby isn't really interested in how the rattle tastes. It happens that a huge number of sensory neurons are located in the skin of the lips and tongue and this is where a baby gets information. A baby puts a new toy into his mouth to find out what it feels like! Many other cultural statistics show that children who are welcomed with lots of physical touch and tactile stimulation usually grow into well-adjusted, capable, and loving adults. Children who are touch-deprived in infancy show tendencies toward aggressiveness and violent behavior. This has been well-documented in cultures throughout the world.[9]

Naturally, there are countless other variables that influence human behavior besides how we are touched as babies. It makes sense that during this most vulnerable time of our lives we form patterns and expectations about how the world works, specifically about how safe and valued we are in the world, through our skins. Numerous studies show that for lower and higher mammals, receiving touch that is pleasurable, safe, and appropriate reduces sickness, depression, and aggressive behaviors. In fact, as we learn more about this phenomenon every day, we may find that touch holds more answers than we ever imagined.[10]

Babies aren't the only people who suffer from touch deprivation; nor are they the only ones who benefit from adequate touch in their lives. Touch in infancy aids all areas of development: physical; mental; and psychological. Touch in adulthood is equally beneficial. It stimulates immune system function, reduces stress, and keeps us literally "connected" to our community. That sense of connectedness turns out to be a major factor in long-term health. Research shows that adults who have a life-partner live longer, healthier lives than people who live in isolation. For both genders and all races in the United States, people who live alone have death rates anywhere up to five times higher than their partnered peers. This is true for lifelong singles, divorced, and widowed people. Rates for all forms of heart disease and a wide variety of cancers, stroke, pneumonia, diabetes, cirrhosis, and suicide are higher across the board for people who live alone.[11] Touch is essential in infancy; it's vital in adulthood.

The Dynamics of Touch

What really happens when one person touches another? How does a hand on your back or your shoulder translate into better health for you? Human touch can completely change the way the body functions. Welcome touch can make the body work better from heart rate to blood pressure to digestive system efficiency. In a 1998 study, the Journal of Applied Gerontology reports that elders received benefits from giving massage to infants. The elders didn't receive massage, yet they benefitted from the touch.[12] In another study, reported in *Massage Therapy: The Evidence for Practice*, "agitated" or aggressive elders, decreased the number of agitated behaviors with the implementation of a 10-minute massage. These behaviors continued to decrease with the number of treatments.[13]

When we receive human touch, or any stimulus to the skin, information races to the brain. The brain receives that information and creates a response in the body (depending on the interpretation). This response is a relaxing, pleasurable one (parasympathetic nervous system response) if the stimulus is soothing and welcome, or an anxiety-provoking, upsetting one (sympathetic nervous system response), if the stimulus is perceived as threatening. A parasympathetic nervous system response from being touched lowers blood pressure, increases digestion, slows breathing, and generally makes us feel more relaxed and at ease.

Generally, studies indicate that touch is essentially a positive experience for the person receiving it, as long as the touch doesn't impose more intimacy than the person desires or doesn't communicate a negative message.[14] Therein lies the challenge: How do you know if your touch is too intimate or sends a negative message for any specific person? You must train yourself to attune to clients' verbal and nonverbal feedback and be willing to discuss sensitive issues with them.

How touch is interpreted is a complex matter. When people receive touch they go through an analytical process (often largely unconscious) to determine the meaning of that specific touch. According to research done by Heslin and Alper,[15] individuals consider the following aspects in this process:

- what part of the other person's body touched me;
- what part of my body is touched;
- how long the touch lasts;
- how much pressure is used;
- whether there is movement after contact is made;
- if anyone else is present to witness the touch, and if so, who;
- the relationship between myself and the person who touched me;
- the situation in which the touch occurs.

In addition to Heslin's and Alper's findings, other components should be considered as well:

- the verbal exchange that accompanies the touch;
- any nonverbal behaviors present;
- prior touch experiences in my life or with the person who has touched me.

We like to be touched by some people and not by others. While one person's touch makes us feel nurtured, warm and safe, another's may make us feel threatened, cold, and queasy. This holds true whether the touch is from friends, partners, co-workers, acquaintances, or healthcare practitioners.

It is a complicated process that humans go through to determine if touch is a positive or negative, wanted or unwanted experience! Add to this equation the familial, ethnic, and even regional differences in norms regarding touch and then combine prevailing cultural and gender differences, and it's easy to see how "touchy" this experience is for us.

Exploring Touch

Explore your own understanding and experiences of touch with the following exercises:

- Find a person with whom you're comfortable and vice versa. Touch that person intentionally at various depths on her forearm. First, just barely touch the skin. Next, distinguish between the skin and the muscle. Continue to the comfort level of each and discuss the experience.
- Describe how you might differently touch a newborn baby, a lover, an elderly person, and a stranger.
- Experience touching as many different textures as possible. What kinds of thoughts and feelings occur with each texture?
- When you receive touch, what aspects do you consider to determine the meaning of that specific touch?
- Identify an experience in which the meaning of your touch was misinterpreted.

Gender and Touch

There are also gender differences around touch. Girls are touched more frequently and less roughly than boys. As boys reach puberty, non-sexual touch decreases just as sexual experiences increase. So for many men, touch and sex become synonymous. Consider the following scenario:

> After receiving weekly bodywork therapy for a few months a client expressed a change he experienced since he was receiving massage therapy on a weekly basis. One day, he said that he wasn't "jumping into bed" with women he was dating since he had been receiving massage regularly. He said, "I realize in retrospect that one of the main reasons for choosing to be sexual with someone was to experience touch." Since he was now receiving touch regularly through massage, he better understands his needs.

Points to Ponder

How can a practitioner help clients realize this need for healthy, appropriate touch? How do you know when the client's needs are being met?

In the scenario the client's experience demonstrates the profound confusion most of us experience in differentiating these very primal, human, and necessary needs, as well as how best to get them met. The confusion isn't limited to men. Women confuse touch and sex as well.

Much fear and misunderstanding about sexual orientation abounds. The prevailing attitude has been that heterosexual sexuality is normal and homosexual or bisexual sexuality is not. Consequently, we become acculturated not only to deny same gender feelings, but to avoid anything that would remotely look like same gender intimacy and sexual activity. Touch has now become suspect. Who is touching whom? And why? Men are socialized to be more wary in this regard than females. Same gender touch for men is virtually taboo because it's automatically assumed to indicate homosexual desire which is culturally unacceptable. For women there is much less stigma around touching one another.

Women are usually less concerned with the gender of a person who touches them but they want to know that person. Given this, in a touch therapy setting some female clients might not choose a male practitioner if they don't know him. Some men may especially avoid male practitioners because they can't imagine being touched so intimately by another male. On the other hand, some men prefer male practitioners because they mistakenly assume that a man is automatically stronger than a female. Some clients choose same-sex practitioners to avoid possible cross-gender sexual tension.

Unfortunately, there are few images of men as nurturers in this society. Related to this phenomenon is an interesting and confusing paradox at play in terms of healthcare practitioners. Men traditionally have been given the power to do things, know things, and fix things. Traditionally health care has predominantly been male-dominated except in direct interaction fields such as nursing, physical therapy, and massage. Consciously, the culture automatically views men as having the information and techniques necessary for healing. Yet the cultural unconscious says that men aren't necessarily a source of comfort or trust. This is exacerbated by a picture of males as perpetrators of violence. Male practitioners might be seen as both powerful and fearsome. This doesn't make for an easy therapeutic relationship.

Female practitioners may need to do more to prove their competency, but they're more easily accepted as someone safe and nurturing. Male practitioners must work harder regarding their professional image but are successful as long as they're attentive to possible touch and gender concerns.

Honoring the Power of Touch

Healthy people seek hands-on therapy because it feels good. Beyond satisfying the need for touch, it strengthens responses to mental and physical stressors. For instance, a good massage, in addition to lowering blood pressure, increasing immune system activity, and helping the body to get rid of wastes, makes the client more alert, emotionally calmer, and more capable of dealing with everyday challenges.

But somatic work can do even more than that. Helen Colton, author of *Touch Therapy*, suggests that people recovering from accident or trauma have greater than normal need for touch and comfort. "Touch may even be the basic need of patients, more vital than medication, so that, when their touch need is satisfied, patients can direct their energies toward dealing with problems and traumas that they have."[16]

A client driving a small truck was rear-ended by a city bus. In her words, "the accident turned her long-bed truck into a short-bed truck." When she began somatic treatment she was a mass of bruises and her pain threshold was very low. But as the treatments slowly proceeded, she realized that what she valued most was the opportunity to feel how much of her body didn't hurt from her accident. This helped her to maintain a good attitude—which was a key factor in her recovery process.

Points to Ponder

How can a practitioner help a client recognize the signs of healing and the benefits of touch after a traumatic event like a car accident?

The power of touch isn't always positive. Physical and sexual violence are prevalent in our society: abusive touch occurs between family members, acquaintances, friends, and strangers. As a culture we are numbed to the effects of such violations. As individuals we may interpret all touch to be a hurtful, powerful tool used against us and therefore avoided. These "accepted" touch taboos and behaviors are reinforced by painful experience. Personal touch histories are very complex and not obvious to others. It is safe to assume that for most people touch has been a mixed experience.

Practitioners need to pay attention to the verbal and nonverbal communication clients give regarding touch. Let clients know why, when, and how you'll touch them. When possible, give clients a choice about this. In training, you may have been taught a specific way to do a procedure or treatment and assume you must do it that way. Demonstrate respect to clients by being creative and finding other ways to work that better meets their needs if necessary. The variety and innovation also helps you stay interested in your work.

A client can experience sexual confusion when receiving touch—even where there aren't overt sexual cues. Touch, in and of itself, is a sexual cue for some people.

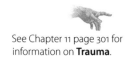

See Chapter 7 page 191 for more information on **Informed Consent**.

An acupuncturist found that three male patients started to communicate with her in ways that felt too personal: one wanted to meet for coffee; another hinted about his openness for a date; the third kept asking her personal questions. She decided to ask for feedback from several trusted female friends who had also received treatments from her. The behavior that each noted was how much this practitioner casually touched each of them above and beyond the treatment protocol. For the practitioner, the amount of touch was normal given her high-touch family background and her intent was to use touch as a reassuring gesture for her clients. But her frequent touch was suggestive to her male patients.

Points to Ponder

Should this practitioner change her behavior? If so, how can she change her behavior to avoid the possibility of suggestive touch?

Addressing Touch with Clients

One way to address the touch component in the client-practitioner relationship is to talk about it directly as part of the first appointment. Let your clients know what kind of touch to expect during each treatment and ask permission to proceed with the kind of touch described. Clients need to have the option of saying no. Keep in mind that clients in the less powerful position can find it difficult to say no.

High-touch practitioners, such as the acupuncturist, might incorporate a clarifying tool with her clients to avoid confusion and mixed messages: add a "touch education" component to her intake interview either verbally or in a written statement; describe her use of touch while letting clients know that it's optional; and limit her touch with clients while they aren't directly receiving treatments.

For client comfort and safety, practitioners must be willing to modify behaviors. You must also be sure that you aren't touching a client in ways based on your own history.

See Chapter 11 page 301 for information on **Trauma**.

1. A massage therapist found that clients weren't feeling his presence or depth in touch. Since he had been physically abused as a child, he was afraid of hurting others which prevented him from making real connection and contact.
2. A shiatsu practitioner, who had been physically abused as a child, was criticized as being too hurtful in her work. She honestly thought that touch was supposed to feel like this since she had no other somatic experience to the contrary.

Points to Ponder

How can practitioners be sure their work has appropriate depth and connection? Is it possible to keep past traumatic experiences from affecting quality of touch with clients?

By addressing the personal trauma, each of the practitioners in the above scenarios successfully learned healthy, connected touch. As a result, appropriate touch became possible for them and client safety was ensured.

█ Intimacy

Our cultural confusion about the meaning of intimacy is revealed through dictionary definitions and how we use these words. "Intimate" is described as: "very personal, private, indicative of one's deepest nature, marked by close association." When you turn to the definition of "intimacy," new meanings are revealed: "having sexual relations" and "illicit sexual relations."[17] Surprisingly, "intimate" and "intimacy" have come to mean very different things and the original meaning of "intimate" transforms to a sexual connotation when the term "intimacy" is used. Culturally we seldom talk about sex in a direct, honest way, so we must create euphemisms for sexual activity and intercourse. Take a moment to think of all the slang words you have heard, or use, to talk about sex, as well as the slang used for sexual body parts. How many people give their elbow or knee a nickname?

Betsy Tolstedt and Joseph Stokes from the University of Illinois used three measures of intimacy for a study they conducted regarding marital satisfaction.[18] Intimacy was assessed in terms of physical, emotional, and verbal factors:

- Physical intimacy entails affectionate and sexual touch.
- Emotional intimacy refers to feelings of closeness, tolerance, and support.
- Verbal intimacy involves disclosure of emotions, feelings, and opinions.

Many people experience sexual encounters without emotional or verbal intimacy. People often complain about the lack of intimacy in their lives, but it's important to consider what the complaints are actually about. Upon examination, a person might feel satisfied with the amount and kind of affectionate touch received from a partner, but wants more sexual interaction. Or the person may feel supported and respected by a partner, but finds the partner uncomfortable talking about her feelings and concerns. It becomes clearer that some intimacy needs are being met in this particular relationship while others are not. When we feel dissatisfied about the level of intimacy in our lives it's helpful to look at each of these three areas and apply them to various relationships including partner, friends, family, and colleagues. The results illuminate not only others' comfort levels with the different types of intimacy but also our own.

Establishing Appropriate Intimacy

The distinctions between physical, emotional, and verbal intimacy also shed new light on therapeutic intimacy for somatic practitioners. In a therapeutic relationship that involves the client's body as the focus of treatment, concerns about intimacy take on greater importance. The appropriate intimacy for any therapeutic relationship is a one-way intimacy. Practitioners physically touch their clients, allow them to disclose thoughts and feelings, and offer both verbal and physical support. The therapeutic relationship's function isn't for the clients to do the same for the practitioner. This seemingly clear-cut protocol is often challenging in practice.

One difficulty with establishing appropriate intimacy in therapeutic touch relationships arises simply from the presence of touch. Touching the client means that the practitioner has automatically violated a cultural taboo. Even if the client is voluntarily present and consents to touch, cultural meanings of touch still exert a strong influence on one's immediate experience. This cultural violation may make both client and practitioner uncomfortable and nervous, especially if clear boundaries haven't been discussed and established.

This context sets the stage for the following possible sequence of events. Once the cultural taboo concerning physical intimacy is overridden, the client needs to quickly create safety. She may therefore attempt to find out as much as possible (and as quickly as possible) about the person doing the touching by asking questions, sometimes more personal than professional. In other words, the movement is from increased physical intimacy to increased verbal intimacy. If the practitioner isn't savvy to the safety or comfort needs of the client, it's easy to fall into answering all the questions even if they aren't appropriate or relevant to the treatment at hand. The focus can then shift from the client's relevant concerns to the practitioner's personal life.

Conversely, a practitioner who feels anxious (often unconsciously) about violating the touch taboo might be the one to initiate chit-chat with the client and either ask questions of the client or reveal personal information unnecessary or inappropriate for the relationship. Once this dynamic is set in motion, it's easy for the client or practitioner to think that, given the physical and verbal intimacy, greater emotional intimacy is now expected or required. This is the point where confusion often abounds about the expectations and boundaries of the relationship: are we now friends; do we socialize; do I act on romantic feelings?

Another factor in this confusion relates to practitioner self-care. As stated earlier, therapeutic relationships entail a one-way intimacy. The appropriate focus is client-centered, meaning the concerns and needs of the client are the focus of the work together. Practitioners who spend their days listening to, helping, and facilitating change in others need a strong support system wherein they receive the same nurturing. Those with a support system who are actively intimate with others usually don't want nor need to solicit intimacy from their clients. Practitioners who don't experience intimacy elsewhere in their lives are vulnerable to using their clients to fulfill personal needs.

Practitioners who don't create avenues for intimacy in their personal lives often jeopardize their professional relationships. Perhaps these practitioners are shy, tired, busy, vulnerable, or in a crisis. Maybe they lack self-confidence or feel uncomfortable with intimacy. A practitioner on the giving end of one-way intimacy occupies a powerful, safe place since it doesn't entail any real risk-taking on the practitioner's part. Being actively involved in relationships with two-way intimacy in one's personal life is a challenge and can feel like a loss of control of self. A common boundary crossing occurs when a practitioner devotes a significant part of the session to discussing his personal problems with the client and essentially uses the client as a sounding board. A seriously problematic situation occurs when a somatic practitioner uses the session to seduce a client to intimacy.

> At a social event, a practitioner becomes attracted to someone and offers a complimentary session. In that session the client talks while the practitioner appears nurturing and emotionally available. The practitioner touches the client physically without any risk of returned touch. The practitioner is in control of the situation since the client is in a more vulnerable position.
>
> **Points to Ponder**
>
> Is this situation inappropriate? How could the practitioner have handled this differently? Is it possible for this session to truly be therapeutic if the practitioner is focused on his own needs and desires?

Aside from the fact that this is hardly the way to start a healthy, equal relationship, it's manipulative, unethical, and undermines one's professional integrity.

▌Sex

Of the three concepts, "sex" is the most culturally taboo to discuss and the most fraught with anxiety. As a culture, we are most comfortable thinking about sex in regard to gender, biology, reproduction, and heterosexual activity. "Sex" in common usage has come to mean heterosexual intercourse. Many people deny sexual feelings, erotic sensations, and a complete range of sexual behaviors that aren't intercourse or heterosexual.

Sexual behavior occurs on a continuum from less intense interactions like holding hands to overtly sexual behaviors like sexual intercourse. What makes a behavior considered sexual

"
To mature is in part to realize that while complete intimacy and omniscience and power cannot be had, self-transcendence, growth, and closeness to others are nevertheless within one's reach.

—Sissela Bok

depends on the intent and the emotional tone, as well as the type of touch and the area being touched. A hug or a kiss may or may not be sexual. It could be merely a way of greeting, or it could be foreplay. Even exchanging a look can be considered sexual if an accompanying sexual feeling or sensation is present. The starting point on the continuum differs from person to person and varies from day to day and year to year.

Historically, a limited definition of sex that only included sexual intercourse created a problem in identifying sexual abuse and incest. Prior to the late 1970s, many women who had been sexually violated didn't identify their experience as sexual abuse because intercourse had not occurred. Though they knew their boundaries had been violated, and though they experienced bodily shame and felt sexually guilty, they didn't make the direct link to sexual abuse. Men are also sexual abuse survivors. Women are used as the example because the first time incest and sexual abuse were taken seriously in the United States was in 1978 with the publication of Susan Forward's book, *Betrayal of Innocence: Incest and Its Devastation*, which focused on girls as victims.[19]

In recent decades, society has witnessed a sexual exploitation rampage. Sex appeal is promoted, advocated, and revered. We are deluged with sex, sexuality, and sex appeal. Michael V. Reitano, M.D., Editor in Chief of *Sexual Health Magazine*, says, "Virtually every advertisement, movie, television show, magazine or book has, either at its core or as part of its appeal, issues of sex: how to achieve it, maintain it, enjoy it, remain safe from it, embrace it, abolish it, prohibit it, exploit it."[20] Even animated characters in children's movies possess sex appeal. Skewed views on sexuality perpetuate the association of sex with the touch professions in the minds of the consumer, despite a growing respect and appreciation for the holistic health benefits of somatic work.

The sex industry has used massage therapy as a front for prostitution, and the word "massage" still summons questionable associations for some consumers. The association between massage and the sex industry is perpetuated by advertisements, movies, and television. Additionally, many telephone directories, as well as the Internet, have inappropriate listing policies. When the average person searches the Internet or printed materials for a legitimate massage therapist and is inundated with suggestive photos and words with sexual overtones inviting him to call, it reflects badly on the entire industry of professional therapists. The attitude of sex for sale and exploitive sex versus healthy sexuality reflects the attitudes of the society.

Examining Cultural Values

Sex is also laden with cultural values. These values may serve a positive purpose: providing group cohesion, group functionality, and group security. Problems arise when cultural myths, which often arise from values, are treated as facts. The following beliefs aren't "true" in and of themselves, but their repetition has given them the aura of fact:

- Boys should get experience.
- Girls need to abstain from sex until in a committed relationship (preferably marriage).
- Girls are passive and boys are aggressive (this appears to be changing).
- Sex and love are the same.
- Same-sex attractions are abnormal and to be avoided.
- Older people are asexual.

Many people believe our sexually permissive culture has created problems such as child abuse and pornography. In fact, pervasive sexual repression in many cultures has produced a sexual-obsession backlash. This obsession occurs in the societal context of sex repression, where even sex education is opposed in schools. For example, Jocelyn Elders, the U. S. Surgeon General, was fired in 1994 for advocating that masturbation should be taught as an alternative to intercourse in an "abstinence-only" curriculum. When people are uncomfortable and feel shame about their own sexuality, they can become focused on the sexuality of others to an obsessive degree. Why? Perhaps they're trying to deflect their own discomfort with sex, or are trying to determine if they're "normal." Unclear social boundaries, mixed messages, fear, and lack of access to truthful information make frank discussions about sex rare.

 Compare and Contrast Sex, Touch, and Intimacy

- Describe the healthy sexual images in your culture.
- What is the relationship for you between sex, touch, intimacy, and love?
- What are the important sex, touch, and intimacy issues for you in relation to your profession?

The Sexual Response Cycle

Prior to the 1950s, we didn't have information about the physiological aspects of the sexual response, mainly because the technology necessary to obtain this information wasn't available. In 1954, gynecologist and researcher Dr. William Masters, with his assistant Virginia Johnson, began studies of the human sexual response. With 694 volunteers, they observed and recorded physiological responses during sexual behavior. Results of this research were first reported in 1959 and later published in the groundbreaking *Human Sexual Response* in 1966.[21]

Masters and Johnson identified a "Sexual Response Cycle" in men and women that consists of four phases:

1. An excitement/arousal phase (lasting several minutes to hours);
2. A plateau phase (30 seconds to 3 minutes);
3. An orgasmic phase (3-15 seconds); and
4. A resolution (with orgasm—10 to 25 minutes; without orgasm—several hours).

Distinct, gender-specific physiological changes occur in each phase. The most relevant information from this research for all healthcare practitioners who touch clients is the "excitement phase" because touch and other environmental cues can automatically trigger the sexual response cycle. As humans, sexual response starts with any stimulus an individual perceives as erotic, and involves the senses or cognitive processes. Being in a familiar place or setting, seeing someone attractive, hearing music, having a memory or fantasy, or receiving touch may stimulate a sexual response.

Isolating the physiological or anatomic functioning aspect is key to understanding the physical associations between the somatic treatment and the sexual response. There are three significant physiological connections, all of which stem from the body's nervous system: the sensory aspect; the parasympathetic nervous system; and the limbic system. The primary sensory aspect is touch. The tactile stimulation of hands-on work provides a central and peripheral nervous system tune-up of sorts, and the client's whole sensory mechanism is stimulated.

Touching certain areas of the body further complicates the matter. For instance, the areas of the abdomen, parts of the lower extremities, and buttocks share the same two nerve plexuses as the genitals—the lumbar and sacral plexuses. Stimulation of these nerve plexuses can affect the genital nerves.[22]

The parasympathetic nervous system provides the second vital link between touch and the sexual response. This aspect of the autonomic nervous system is responsible for the body's regulation of the "rest and digest," or the restorative responses. It also counterbalances the effects of the sympathetic division, which regulates the "fight or flight" dynamic. Furthermore, parasympathetic influences regulate both the relaxation response induced by hands-on treatments as well as the physiological changes that occur during sexual arousal. When methods such as slow, rhythmic, repetitive stroking, passive movement, slow, broad compressions, reflexology, and acupressure are used, the relaxation response, under parasympathetic control, is induced. The parasympathetic nervous system also controls the primary and secondary bodily responses that occur during sexual arousal. These are vasocongestion, or the increase of blood supply to the genitals, and myotonia, which is the increase in muscle tension that is the result of sexual stimulation.[23]

The third link is the limbic system. The limbic system is a group of structures that form a curved border around the brain's core. This complex aspect of the brain controls emotional and sexual experiences.[24] Stimulation of the body by therapeutic touch influences the limbic response. This not only serves to be another physiological connection between sex and touch, it may also explain why emotional responses occur during or after a treatment.

Sexuality

What is sexuality? Some think that sex and sexuality are synonymous. Because sex is most obviously biological and physiological, oftentimes sexuality is viewed solely as a physical process. However, most sources agree that sexuality is greater than the sum of its parts—that sexuality encompasses biological (anatomy and physiology), psychological (thoughts, feelings, and values), and cultural (family, society, and religious) influences.

The Sexual Health Network describes sexuality as the following:

Sexuality spans the biological, psychological, social, emotional, and spiritual dimensions of our lives. It begins with us and our relationship with ourselves and extends to our relationships with others. Our relationship with ourselves includes how we feel about ourselves as a person, as sexual beings, as men and women, and how we feel about our body, and how we feel about sexual activities and behaviors.[25]

The ways in which we express our sexual nature are as different as the number of human beings on this planet. How we integrate our sexual nature into our personality is greatly influenced by genetics, upbringing, health status, and cultural, social, and religious influences. While we don't have control over possessing a sexual nature, we can learn to choose when and how we express it.

Sexuality is innate. Human sexual-erotic functioning begins immediately after birth and continues until death. Contrary to popular belief, those who choose to not act sexually still possess sexuality. Although sexual feelings can be ignored or we can decide not to act on them, sexuality isn't something we can excise from our being. There are people who have chosen a religiously celibate lifestyle who celebrate their sexuality as a vehicle for personally connecting with their god(s). Sexuality is complex because it includes the multiple meanings we give it; it's a uniquely subjective experience for each of us.

Three specific aspects of sexuality are essential to consider: sexual orientation; gender identity; and sexual behavior:

- **SEXUAL ORIENTATION** refers to which gender(s) we are attracted romantically and sexually.
- **GENDER IDENTITY** is our personal concept of self as male, female, or neither. Most people develop an identity that matches their biological sex. However, some experience their gender identity as different from their biological or assigned sex.
- **SEXUAL BEHAVIOR** is what we actually do sexually.

Sexual orientation is misunderstood and feared because of cultural beliefs that say there are two orientations, heterosexual and homosexual. These same beliefs place a value on each, most commonly that heterosexuality is "good" and homosexuality is "bad." In the 1940s, research by Alfred Kinsey shed light on sexual orientation and the reality of human sexual experience.[26]

Kinsey's researchers asked people about their sexual orientation in two ways: what were the psychological responses (attractions, fantasies) they had to others; and what were the overt sexual behaviors in which they participated. The research results (later known as the Kinsey Scale) showed that sexual orientation actually falls on a continuum rather than on the extreme

Create a gender sensitive and inclusive environment for all children and teens.

http://www.genderspectrum.org/

"
I was brought up to believe that how I saw myself was more important than how others saw me.

—Anwar el-Sadat

ends of an exclusively heterosexual or homosexual scale. Not only was bisexuality a viable orientation, but when both psychological responses and overt behaviors were considered, most people fell within a range on the continuum. Making this concept even more interesting is the fact that it's "impossible to determine the number of persons who are 'homosexual or heterosexual.' It is only possible to determine how many persons belong at any particular time to each of the classifications on the scale."[27]

With gender identity, as in sexual orientation, we seem stuck again in a binary paradigm: that of male and female. The traditional thinking is that an individual's gender self-concept develops in such a way to match one's secondary sex characteristics and how that person is raised. However, recent research has shown that gender identity development is influenced by such factors as genetic triggers, prenatal and puberty hormones, and brain anatomy.[28] This supports the reality that human experience is much more fluid and individuals are identifying themselves in evermore non-binary ways. The continuum includes those who identify as transvestites (those who like to wear clothing of the opposite gender), transsexuals (individuals whose gender identity doesn't match their assigned birth gender), androgynes (those who aren't distinctly masculine or feminine in appearance or behavior), and genderqueers (those who reject cultural labels and identify with more fluid concepts of gender identity and sexual orientation), to name a few.

When we look honestly at human sexual experience, it becomes clear that sexual orientation and gender identity can shift; they aren't necessarily a permanent or fixed reality. In fact, other studies show that in cultures where variations in sexual orientation and gender expression are acceptable, more people act within a wider range.

Touch practitioners and all healthcare providers need to attune to these realities of sexuality in several ways. First and foremost is the issue of making assumptions about the sexual orientation and gender identity of clients and colleagues. Such assumptions don't create safety for clients and peers, and, if assumptions cause clients to leave a core part of themselves out of the therapeutic experience, practitioners miss the opportunity to facilitate the client's healing. Secondly, if practitioners are uncomfortable with orientations and gender identities other than their own, it's their professional responsibility to look at their biases so that they don't inadvertently cause harm to clients. Given the cultural legacy, initial discomfort about these issues is inevitable. People who are comfortable with this issue have examined their inherited fears and beliefs and learned new ways to respond appropriately and with care.

Recognizing the Family as Sex Educator

How do people learn all these sexual myths and scripts? Books, friends, religions, subgroups, and experience are all part of sex education. In this century, the media bombards us with sexual messages. Recent research of sexual content on television in the United States revealed that more than half to two-thirds of prime-time shows contain sexual content, yet less than 10 percent refer to risks or responsibilities of sex. In one week, 88 scenes of intercourse were depicted with almost half (47 percent) of these interactions between characters with no prior romantic relationship.[29] However, despite these other factors, the most influential teacher of sexual concepts and attitudes is the family.

Although many people report that sex was never discussed in their family, the family still conveyed many beliefs and messages about sex and sexuality through example and by what was left unsaid. Authors Miriam and Otto Ehrenberg describe four family sex types that illuminate the sex education styles predominant in American culture.[30] In reading the descriptions, keep in mind that there are few "pure" nuclear families, stereotypically seen as headed by a mother and a father. The definition of family can expand to include all those people who influence a child's upbringing. All family systems influence our sexual development, regardless of the family configuration—including single parents, step-parents, or extended family as caretakers.

> To put the world in order, we must first put the nation in order; to put the nation in order, we must put the family in order; to put the family in order, we must cultivate our personal life; and to cultivate our personal life, we must first set our hearts right.
>
> —Confucius

What many people find when working with these models is that although different types might be represented in their family, usually one parent had more influence than the other and therefore shaped the predominant experience. Another common experience is that the family type shifted at different points in the family's life cycle or at different stages of a child's development.

SEX REPRESSIVE: Sex is seen by parents as inherently immoral, dirty, and evil, so the family actively squelches sexuality in their children. Ironically, research has shown that children from these families are more likely to become sexually active than their peers but are less likely to use birth control and take other precautions since they feel ashamed and guilty.

SEX OBSESSIVE: Focuses on sex as a main issue to discuss, flaunt, and emphasize. Rather than letting their child's sexuality unfold naturally, there's a tendency to propel children into precocious sexual behavior. This family doesn't respect children's boundaries, rationalizes uninhibited behavior, and projects adult needs into the parent/child relationship.

SEX AVOIDANT: Is intellectually accepting of sex as a positive life experience, but emotionally uncomfortable with sex and sexuality. Generally, negative input isn't present but neither is any real discussion. Typically, children may be given reading materials or permission to attend sex education class in school but parents don't follow up with their own input. As a result, their children receive a double message about sex: it's okay but probably dangerous since no one wants to talk about it, and they're left to their own devices regarding decision-making.

SEX EXPRESSIVE: Understands sex as a life-enhancing force that is neither ignored nor emphasized. Parents are willing to talk openly about sex and set reasonable limits around their children's behavior. These children gain respect for their bodies and their sexuality, and because of this they tend to be sexually responsible.

The Impact of Family Patterns in a Therapeutic Setting

The categories above described by the Ehrenbergs are useful in making connections between practitioners' behaviors and their own family system patterns. Practitioners must understand how sex education affects the ways in which they relate to others, especially clients. Conversely, a client's background and history directly affects how she understands, communicates about, and feels about the therapeutic experience.

Family patterns are important to recognize as a factor influencing the practitioner and client. Knowing the possible impact of family patterns can be useful in understanding the sexual dynamics in the therapeutic relationship. Consider the following possibilities:

- Practitioners from sexually obsessed family environments might be overly focused on sexuality and engage clients sexually.
- Those from sexually repressed backgrounds might judge sexual feelings they experience while giving or receiving treatments to be unacceptable and shameful; or, they might project, needlessly shaming a client who has legitimate sexuality concerns that need to be discussed.
- Practitioners from sex-avoidant backgrounds might notice, but choose to ignore, sexual aggression from clients and put themselves at risk.
- Sex-expressive backgrounds might help practitioners feel comfortable talking about a client's bodily responses to touch and set appropriate boundaries.

Through an awareness of family patterns, practitioners can respond consciously, professionally, and ethically concerning sexuality in the treatment setting.

Sex and Touch Therapy

All humans are, by nature, sexual beings, therefore it isn't possible to entirely keep sex and sexuality out of the treatment room. Biology equips people with a sexual nature to preserve and propagate the species. Every client and every practitioner brings their sexual nature and background with them into the therapeutic setting. The ultimate ethical challenge is to acknowledge the role of inherent sexuality in a milieu where sex is absolutely inappropriate. In other words, practitioners must allow sexuality and at the same time, desexualize the experiences of both giving and receiving hands-on therapy.

Cultural beliefs and personal experiences manifest in somatic therapy. By its nature, it breaks the cultural and personal taboos of touch. An ethical touch therapy treatment could be misinterpreted by a client because of her prior touch history. Physical intimacy may be confused as a prelude to sexual activity. If touch has been experienced only in sexual situations for a client, then touch therapy may mean sex to that person.

The location and atmosphere of a touch therapy session holds many potential cues. Depending on the treatment, the specific factors that could allude to sex include: degrees of nudity; the manner of draping; the positioning of the client; the type of touch; lubricants such as oils and creams; certain lighting; and the setting (professional office versus someone's home). As one student aptly noted, the kind of smile on the practitioner's face can make a client aroused or scared or both.

Typically, the sexual nature of the client or practitioner is regarded only if something sexually inappropriate happens that requires ethical intervention. A reactive stance is insufficient. Diligence in ethical efforts requires that practitioners be proactive in understanding human sexuality (both their own and that of their clients) and acting appropriately. Practitioners must always appreciate the impact that treatments can have on the sexual response, take full responsibility for how they're affected when performing their work, and remain keenly aware of the potential effects of touch on clients.

Male somatic therapists are sometimes avoided by both men and women clients because of homosexual fears or perceived danger. Additionally, male therapists may be susceptible to subtle and overt seduction from female clients and may find themselves inappropriately responding to these clients. One reason for this stems from the cultural myth that women aren't sexually aggressive so their overtures should be discounted and ignored. Another reason has to do with the socialization that men and women have received about how they relate. In a culture that assumes everyone is heterosexual, many of us were raised to see the other gender only in terms of romantic and sexual potential instead of as human beings. This dynamic pervades many daily non-sexual interactions. Women have also been told that their sexuality should be hidden and indirect and that flirting is permissible to express both interest and power. Men often unconsciously feel they must respond to a woman's flirting because otherwise their masculinity and sexuality might be questioned. Given all this, it's very possible for a male

What we see depends mainly on what we look for.

—John Lubbock

practitioner to discount a female client's sexual behavior as part of the cultural norm, neglect to set appropriate boundaries with her, and then find himself in a compromising situation.

Female practitioners complain about sexual innuendos, provocative jokes, and aggression from their male clients. This may be due to sexual scripts men are taught. The social pressure to "act like a man" is interpreted by some men to mean they must project a secure, aggressive, and sexual image. One way for men to assert a semblance of power is to appear sexually powerful, whether or not they actually feel this way. Joking and bringing up sexual topics is, for some men, a form of flirting and an enactment of a cultural script. Male clients who have no harmful intent often use sexual jesting as an attempt to tolerate the intimacy of the therapeutic relationship and to garner some control in a vulnerable setting. Because humor is often used socially to diffuse tension, in a situation where the tension is sexual, the humor often becomes sexualized.

Consider these situations: in most massage sessions, the client is either nude (underneath the sheets/towel) or partially naked; in a shiatsu or acupressure session, the client is fully clothed but is often lying on the floor, rather than on a table, and the practitioner leans over and even straddles the client's body during the session; in acupuncture the client may be wearing varying degrees of clothing with the practitioner sticking needles into vulnerable places; in a physical therapy session, the client is usually partially unclothed and in a vulnerable position; in some energy treatments there is more than one practitioner involved at a time; in an osteopathic session, the client may be fully clothed or asked to wear an open-backed hospital gown; and many chiropractors set up their clinics with several tables in one room and the client receives a treatment in full view of others waiting for their appointments.

Many clients are surprised at, and unprepared for, the high level of intimacy (physical, emotional, and verbal) that occurs in the therapeutic setting. Practitioners must be aware of the impact of the setting on the client. They must also consider reactive behaviors in that context.

Sexual Feelings During Treatment Sessions

Consider the following three observations:
- Clients often experience sexual feelings when receiving treatments.
- Practitioners often have sexual feelings when giving treatments.
- Many clients and practitioners are confused, ashamed, and embarrassed, and sometimes behave inappropriately in response to these feelings.

Sexual talk, sexual relations, sexual acts and activities, sexual pleasures, sexual intercourse, or being involved in a sexual manner, is always unethical and must never occur in the professional relationship.

Many types of touch therapy provide a sensual experience. Unfortunately, while sensual originally meant "connection with the senses as opposed to the intellect," the concept has become associated with "indulgence in the baser pleasures of the senses, licentiousness, brutishness, and grossness."[31] Sensuality incorporates the awareness of bodily sensation, taking pleasure in sensation and utilizing sensation to be more fully present in our bodies. However, because of the family, cultural, and religious beliefs discussed earlier, most people learn to tune out their body's sensations. Touch therapy often reawakens this awareness in clients and practitioners.

Sensuality and sexuality aren't the same although they can occur on the same continuum. Sensual and sexual feelings are part of being a vital human being and are normal. Denial of sensual and sexual feelings is pervasive and dangerous. Staying personally (and culturally) unconscious, individuals are more likely to act in ways that are harmful to themselves and others. Ethical behavior, however, includes the ability to be self-aware, to recognize sexual feelings within yourself, to take steps in the moment to shift the feelings to a non-sexual nature, and never to act on these feelings with a client.

Given the nature of the sexual response, some clients experience sexual arousal regardless of the practitioner's behavior. Sexual arousal is, in some ways, distinct from attraction. Arousal is at times disembodied—not related to the particular individual a person is with at the moment but more as a result of other cues. Other times, the arousal is based on a specific attraction to the individual. Sorting out this distinction is helpful in understanding what is happening in the moment with a client. The practitioner's ethical responsibility is to respond non-sexually to the client and to eliminate any misunderstanding on the client's part as to the intent of the practitioner.

A practitioner is also likely to experience sexual arousal because of the personal nature of the work. Sometimes practitioners are personally more in tune with their physical responses.

> One practitioner in supervision shared that he had experienced several attractions in one week: one with a client, one with his doctor, and another with a salesperson. He was concerned about his lustiness. As he talked, it was clear that none of his behavior was unethical and the feeling was probably in response to his ending a relationship in which he had felt sexually shutdown.
>
> **Points to Ponder**
>
> What is the point when sexual feelings can be considered unethical? What are the parameters? How does potential sexual behavior influence unethical behavior? How can this practitioner be sure that his feelings don't instigate those behaviors?

A sexual response can be completely bypassed under most circumstances. Or, if a sexual response does occur, as long as the erotic energy isn't entertained and it's short-lived, the treatment can continue with ethical safety. Regardless of the situation or circumstances, if sexual arousal does occur, on the part of either the practitioner or the client, it's always the practitioner's responsibility to establish and maintain appropriate boundaries.

Sexual Attraction to Clients

It is normal for sexual feelings to occasionally arise during a session or for practitioners to feel attracted to a client. Unfortunately, many professionals react to the feelings with fear, shame, judgment, guilt, and projection. Having a sexual feeling is part of the normal range of feelings that is possible to occur during a session like sadness, irritation, frustration, or joy. The problem comes when we judge our self or think we need to act on the feelings we have. Rare, fleeting sexual feelings in themselves aren't unethical behaviors. Allowing these to remain, become stronger, or evolve into fantasies is unethical. When you become aware of *any* feeling that takes your attention away from the fact that a human being is in your care, the most ethical response is to acknowledge the feeling(s) to yourself, refocus on the client's needs, and after the session process the feelings by yourself or with a trusted colleague or supervisor.

Between stimulus and response, one has the freedom to choose.

—Stephen Covey

Fantasizing about a client during a session or between sessions objectifies the person and results in being out of relationship with him in that moment. If this happens, not only is the practitioner using the client for personal gratification, but is also at risk for unethical behavior. Once the practitioner stops relating to the client as a person, it's easy to see the client as someone who can and should take care of the practitioner's needs.

Figure 6.1 Processing Your Thoughts and Feelings

- What is the quality of the feeling I'm having?
- Do I treat this client differently in session than other clients?
- Is this attraction so strong that I want to pursue a relationship?

One reason most practitioners avoid acknowledging sexual arousal and attraction is that it leads them into unfamiliar territory that the culture presents as dangerous and not to be explored. But it's more dangerous for both the client and practitioner to avoid these feelings. If sexual feelings or attractions occur, it's critical to distinguish what underlies the attraction and how to respond. These are some questions to ask yourself:

1. **WHAT IS THE QUALITY OF THE FEELING I'M HAVING?**

   Is it a fleeting, temporary feeling? Perhaps you were reminded of someone, or you like your client's hair. Often these initial responses are just part of being human and are nothing to worry about. They aren't necessarily about the other person and don't need to be addressed with the client. What does matter is the extent you let yourself become distracted during the sessions, as well as your ability to refocus on the client's needs. Is the attraction enduring or intense? Do you fantasize about a client? Is there a client with whom you want to have sex? Do you experience certain kinds of patterns of attractions to clients? For example, you find you always like middle-aged businessmen, or for the past six months you have been attracted to every married female client. These attractions may indicate personal needs or countertransference issues which should be resolved in supervision. These are the situations which breed unethical behavior.

2. **DO I TREAT THIS CLIENT DIFFERENTLY IN SESSION THAN OTHER CLIENTS?**

   Breaches of ethics can occur with changes in behavior as subtle as flirting, lingering with your hand, or slipping past a normal boundary on a body part, or as blatant as engaging in sexual activity with the client. Practitioners rationalize their behavior by saying that the client initiated the behavior or propositioned the practitioner. In a therapeutic relationship, the practitioner is ultimately responsible for all interaction with the client, no matter who was the initiator. The practitioner is paid to know what behaviors and actions are beneficial or detrimental to a client, whether that concerns giving a particular treatment or hugging and kissing a client.

3. **IS THIS ATTRACTION SO STRONG THAT I WANT TO PURSUE A RELATIONSHIP?**

   The complexity of this question requires time to thoughtfully consider all issues. Generally, this is a boundary practitioners should not break, especially if they're in a pattern of wanting to date clients. However, there may be the rare instance that the attraction is so strong that a therapeutic relationship isn't feasible. First, you need to know if there are any laws in your state restricting practitioners in your field from dating former clients. If none exist, for ethical reasons it's useful to talk about the attraction to a trusted colleague or supervisor to assess the quality of the attraction and the underlying motivation.

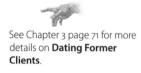

See Chapter 3 page 71 for more details on **Dating Former Clients**.

Assuming that you and the client are free to pursue a relationship and you decide to do so, know that you first need to discontinue the client-practitioner relationship. A significant lapse of time is recommended between the last session and the first social activity. Practitioners have been reported by clients for sexual abuse in situations where a date occurred immediately after a session. It is your responsibility to know the laws in your state regarding this issue.

Never ask a client for a date during a session when he is vulnerable and you're in the power position. Actually, in most professions, it's inappropriate to ever ask a client on a date. Just the act of asking is a betrayal of the client's trust that you'll remain therapeutically client-centered. He may feel shocked that you asked and want to end therapy. Be prepared that he may like you better as his practitioner and isn't interested in dating you. You, then, must decide if it's possible to continue as his practitioner. And, if you do continue, what will you do about the attraction and possible feelings of disappointment, rejection, anger, or sadness that you might experience? The attraction may be so strong that it interferes with your role as a practitioner, or you may just feel awkward continuing in that role.

Erections in the Treatment Setting

Is there any other bodily function that is so misunderstood, revered, or feared? While an erection is one of the most obvious indicators of physiological arousal, it doesn't necessarily mean that emotional or sexual desire is also present.

Men experience erections even when they aren't necessarily emotionally desirous of sex (e.g., when they're afraid or need to urinate). Touch, itself, on any part of the body can stimulate a physiological response that results in a partial or complete erection. Spontaneous erections in a therapeutic setting are often uncomfortable for practitioners and clients. The difficulty lies in that many practitioners are uncomfortable or fearful when a client has an erection response during a session.

Several realities shape female therapists' perceptions of erections. Many were raised with pervasive myths about erections: If you're with a man and he has an erection, a) you have caused it, and b) you're responsible for taking care of it. Additionally, having grown up in a culture rampant with sexual abuse and rape, erections are often associated with sexual violence. Intellectually, most women know this isn't true but the cultural message may be powerful enough to derail rationality.

If a male therapist notices a male client having an erection, several issues should be considered. A man isn't necessarily fearful of another man's erection unless he is being threatened or if it's perceived as a sexual come-on. Sometimes erections are even more disturbing to a male therapist if he responds by feeling aroused because then he may question his own orientation. Both male and female practitioners often either ignore erectile response or overreact, becoming passive or aggressive with the client in discussing the condition. Each of these responses puts the practitioner in a vulnerable position.

Ensure safety by obtaining sufficient information to discern the "intent" of the client's erection—whether it's merely a physiological response to touch or part of sexual desire. If a practitioner is verbally aggressive about the erection or hurts the client physically to quell the erection, the practitioner is abusing the client. Many practitioners learn in school to discourage erections by "pressing hard on certain points." There are more respectful, clear, and safe ways to deal with erections in men and arousal in women.

Arousal in Women

It is difficult to know when female clients are sexually aroused. Early signs of sexual arousal include changes to the clitoris, labia, and vaginal walls, but these aren't obvious to a practitioner. Other changes, such as nipple erection and skin flush, could be nonsexual reactions to cold, soft tissue manipulation (increased blood flow to the skin), and nerve enervation. As with males, client arousal doesn't mean sexual intent.

Practitioners whose female clients had an orgasmic response on the table usually say they had no clue that the client was aroused until she made verbal comments (e.g., direct communication, moaning) or displayed nonverbal behaviors (e.g., breathing changes, muscular rigidity, strange movements) that alerted the practitioner to the arousal.

Remember that, because of socialization, practitioners are less suspect, thus less alert to women who are sexually inappropriate within the context of a therapeutic relationship.

As well as being difficult to observe, female sexuality is often expressed much less directly than male sexuality. Be aware of female clients repeatedly exposing themselves during the treatment. One or two episodes may be an accident, poor boundaries, or a lapse in judgment. It may be helpful to distinguish the context surrounding the behavior. What were the client's verbal cues? Did the client watch to see your reaction? With a sexually inappropriate client, the number and intensity of behaviors usually escalate. Regardless of the reason, the practitioner needs to verbalize the physical boundary of draping at this time. A person with poor boundaries may seem like a well-adjusted individual, comfortable with nudity, while in actuality, her lack

> If you view all the things that happen to you, both good and bad, as opportunities, then you operate out of a higher level of consciousness.
>
> —Les Brown

of boundaries comes from a history of sexual abuse. You will probably never know. Taking a chance breaches the tenets of professional ethics.

Sometimes clients with an inappropriate attraction to the practitioner may sublimate or redirect those feelings by pumping the practitioner for personal information or giving gifts to the practitioner.[32] In this case, the client isn't aware of the attraction, which emphasizes the argument against accepting any gifts from clients. The client may also leave valuables and insist on seeing the practitioner when the valuables are retrieved. Some clients do know they're attracted to the practitioner and use the same techniques above to attract the attention of the practitioner. While all these examples of behaviors are inappropriate on some level, a more serious type of arousal expression during a treatment session is when a female client talks about her own sexuality or the practitioner's sexuality. This type of talk, combined with other verbal or nonverbal requests or innuendos, should not be ignored.

When To Address Erections and Arousal with Clients

When do practitioners need to talk to their clients about erections or arousal? The answer is simple: whenever the client or practitioner is uncomfortable. Once one party is uncomfortable, the session isn't going to be truly beneficial because the attention is diverted. There are several simple things to assess whenever an erection occurs:

- If a man has a partial or full erection, shows no signs of discomfort or embarrassment through verbal or nonverbal cues, and you're comfortable, it isn't necessary to talk about it at the time.
- If a man has a partial or full erection and acts uncomfortable via nonverbal cues (body tension, flushed face), and although he hasn't been inappropriate in any way during the treatment (and even if you feel comfortable), then it's wise to talk with him to assuage his discomfort.
- If a man has a partial or full erection and has displayed other verbal and nonverbal behaviors during the session that seem to indicate sexual intent, then you're ethically obligated to talk with him immediately (using the Intervention Model described in the next section).

This is also the case for sexual arousal in women. It is of ethical importance to immediately talk with the client if she indicates sexual intent in verbal or nonverbal behaviors.

Not every noise or movement a client makes is sexual or indicates arousal.

There is no recipe for dealing with the sexual arousal of a client. The action a practitioner takes depends on the client and circumstances. In any situation where a client indicates that arousal has occurred, the practitioner must determine, at that moment, the best way to handle the incident. When first aware of the situation, the practitioner must change what she is doing. The antidote to the parasympathetic response is activation of the sympathetic response. Actions, such as, changing tempo to a quicker pace and moderately increasing the pressure and depth of touch encourages sympathetic nervous system involvement. Move to a less risky area of the body, such as the upper extremity or the face and head. As long as the client doesn't indicate further sexual interest, give the client a minute or two to pass through this phase, since the arousal will likely subside, and she could continue without further arousal. In these cases, it's often more appropriate not to discuss the situation at that time. Whether it's discussed after the session depends on the situation and the practitioner's sense that it's fitting and necessary. Discussing it may simply mean informing the client that arousal can be a short-lived physiological response that may occur, and that, while it would never be acceptable to act on it, the incident wasn't interpreted by you as improper or unethical.

Both male and female practitioners need to be prepared for sexual arousal from both sexes and all sexual orientations. One proactive way to address the possibility of arousal and erection with clients is to include some basic written information in your client intake. If you model a healthy comfort level talking about all physiological changes a client might experience during a session, you have provided several things: an opening for the client to express concerns; an education for a client about how the body works; good boundaries; and a safe environment.

The Intervention Model

The Intervention Model is a communication model developed by Daphne Chellos[33] for practitioners to use when verbal or nonverbal communication from a client is unclear or when practitioners feel their boundaries are being violated. It was used, in part, in the previous section with clients crossing the line sexually. However, this model also applies when a client is having an emotional reaction or release during a session, such as crying or expressing anger. The goal is to empower you as you use these steps as a guide (combined with your intuition) to assess situations and make decisions. Let's explore the Intervention Model in more detail here.

> Important principles may, and must, be inflexible.
>
> —Abraham Lincoln

The Intervention Model is based on basic, sound communication skills. Many practitioners already possess these skills and will find this model quite familiar. However, most practitioners are generally unprepared to address sexual issues in a somatic setting even if they have had counseling experience, sex education training, and extensive professional training. Most don't practice discussing such complex, sensitive issues in the somatic setting. Role-playing situations in a school setting or with other practitioners is vital to prepare yourself so that you can feel confident when a questionable situation occurs.

The Intervention Model is a gender-free, orientation-free model. The same responses are utilized with both male and female clients. Sometimes this is a difficult concept to practice because people are socialized to communicate in different styles based on gender and other perceived differences.

Depending on the situation, you may need to go through all the steps or stop after step one. Typically, steps one and two follow in that order but steps three through eight might be addressed in a different order, and some steps may not be included at all. Learn them all and use your intuition and good judgment.

Figure 6.2 The Intervention Model

1. Stop the treatment using assertive behavior.
2. Describe the behavior(s).
3. Clarify the client's intent.
4. Educate the client.
5. Re-state your intent.
6. Continue or discontinue the session as appropriate.
7. Refer client to other professionals as appropriate.
8. Document the situation.

STOP THE TREATMENT USING ASSERTIVE BEHAVIOR

Assertive behavior means that you address the client with body language congruent with what you say verbally. Make eye contact if possible (by doing this, you're both reminded that you're dealing with a human being), stand in a relaxed, yet grounded, manner and use a firm voice. Do not shrink and get quiet (passive) or violate your client through yelling or touching inappropriately (aggressive).

Make sure the client is properly covered (i.e., redrape the body part being attended, adjust client's clothing/gown). This provides a literal boundary that reassures both client and practitioner. Additionally, if touch has contributed to a sexually aroused state, this ensures that you're stopping a potential cause of the stimulation.

Maintain safety. Store your belongings, including a cell phone, in an easily accessible place. If the client's behavior feels intimidating, don't stay too close to the client and position yourself so that you have easy access to your exit door. Leave immediately if the client actively threatens you and then call 911. If you're in a spa or clinic with others on site, go to the front desk. If you're in your private office or doing an in-home or hotel session, leave the premises—you can return later, accompanied by someone, to retrieve your equipment and supplies.

4. **DESCRIBE THE BEHAVIOR(S)**

Respond directly to the client's verbal or nonverbal communication by stating the obvious. This sounds so simple that it borders on the ridiculous, but is actually difficult to do. When we see a behavior, our first impulse is to interpret it rather than describe it. Describing a behavior lets the client know you're paying attention without judging the behavior. Examples of this kind of communication are:

- "I notice you're tightening your muscle and grimacing when I pass over this area."
- "I am aware that you made a comment about my appearance, then made a sexual joke, and now you have an erection."

5. **CLARIFY THE CLIENT'S INTENT**

Once you state the obvious, ask the client a direct question as a follow-up. Something simple like, "Tell me what's happening?" or "What are you experiencing?" allows the client to tell you what the behavior means. Some clients respond in a more straightforward manner about this than others depending on many factors, including their comfort level or their intent in receiving treatment.

Two cautionary reminders: resist answering for the client and wait for a clear answer. Often, when we are uncomfortable we tell someone what his experience is even if we asked him to tell us. Or we accept any answer, even if the response doesn't give us any information, so that we stop having to talk about it. Either way, if the practitioner doesn't clarify the client's intent, she can't accurately assess the situation and might put the client or herself in a difficult position.

6. **EDUCATE THE CLIENT**

Some clients experience unexpected, disturbing emotional and physiological responses during a session. When this happens and we become aware of their concern, we can share information. For instance, an educative statement for a client who has an erection and has expressed embarrassment is, "Sometimes clients become aroused as a physiological response to touch (or movement). It is a normal body response."

7. **RE-STATE YOUR INTENT**

This statement addresses and clarifies the therapeutic contract so that client and practitioner feel safe. After an education statement (as in step #4) you might add, "It is never my intent to create sexual arousal during a session. If it happens, and I am clear that your intent isn't for sexual inappropriateness either, then I'm comfortable in continuing the session if you are."

8. **CONTINUE OR DISCONTINUE THE SESSION AS APPROPRIATE**

You should terminate the session of any client who has sexual intent or is behaving inappropriately. Remember, you don't need to go through all the above steps to exercise this option!

Set conditions if necessary and have the client agree to them. Sometimes after going through all the above steps, a client's intent is still unclear to you. Perhaps she gave an answer that sounded good but felt incongruous and you're left uncertain. Let the client know that you'll continue this session but will stop if she behaves in any way that doesn't work for you.

9. **REFER CLIENT TO OTHER PROFESSIONALS AS APPROPRIATE**

This step is usually done after the session is complete. If it becomes obvious that a client could benefit by receiving other professional help such as a psychotherapist, counselor, or other medical practitioner, give this information to the client when he is fully dressed and alert.

10. **DOCUMENT THE SITUATION**

After the client leaves, document the occurrence and obtain supervision or peer support. Difficult communication with a client often evokes ethical questions and safety concerns. An objective person provides a reality check, or needed emotional support. Remember that client confidentiality must be honored unless you fear for the safety of yourself or someone else. Documenting the situation, and what you did to address the matter, is vital should a client decide to lodge a complaint against you. Demonstrate your commitment to ethics and professionalism by recording that you sought supervision to address the issue.

Intervention Model Practice

- Interview other professionals about their experiences with sexually inappropriate clients and discuss how those situations were handled or mishandled.
- Describe your reaction to a situation when a client exhibited sexual arousal or other behaviors in a session that made you uncomfortable. How do you wish you had handled it?
- With a colleague, practice the Intervention Model using the above experience or various scenarios such as: a flirtatious client, a client who makes questionable comments and touches you, a client who asks inappropriate questions, a sexually aroused client. Afterward discuss how you felt practicing the model and give each other specific feedback on your verbal and nonverbal responses. Identify what you might practice further to feel comfortable and confident. Role-playing is particularly important if you have a history of abuse, especially sexual abuse. Practicing can help you avoid going into a dissociated state and "freezing," which limits your ability to respond appropriately.

Sexual Misconduct and Sexual Harassment

Sexual misconduct and sexual harassment are similar in that each generally involves a person of greater power taking advantage of a person of lesser power. Michael Kimmel of SUNY Stonybrook, a sociologist and leader in men's studies[34] states:

> *Sexual harassment is particularly volatile because it often fuses two levels of power: the power of employers over employees and the power of men over women. It is the confusion of public and private, bringing together two arenas of men's power over women. Not only are men in positions of power in the workplace, but we are socialized to be the sexual initiators and to see sexual prowess as a confirmation of masculinity.*

His words about male-female sexual harassment apply just as well to sexual misconduct in the therapeutic relationship because the practitioner holds greater power in the dynamic between the practitioner and client. Over the last decade, more women have gained positions of power and we've witnessed a rise in harassment suits against them.

Sexual misconduct and harassment also are similar in that each often arises out of a lack of awareness of what kinds of behavior are offensive or even harmful. In other words, the intent to harass may be absent from the perpetrator's conduct. As a result, preventive measures for sexual misconduct and sexual harassment are quite similar: Both practitioners and consumers need to learn ways of prevention that safeguards those people with whom we work and those with whom we are involved in healthcare relationships.

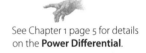

See Chapter 1 page 5 for details on the **Power Differential**.

Experience is a good teacher, but her fees are very high.

—W.R. Inge

Sexual Misconduct

The problem of sexual misconduct has been with us for millennia. The topic was addressed by the Greek physician Hippocrates in 400 B.C.E., which led to the Hippocratic Oath that members of the medical profession continue to use today. The key section, as it pertains to sexual misconduct, is: "Whatever houses I may visit, I will come for the benefit of the sick, remaining free of all intentional injustice, of all mischief and in particular of sexual relationships with both female and male persons."[35] Similar admonishments to doctors, warning them against inappropriate sexual behavior toward their clients, are found in European medical texts dating from the Middle Ages and Renaissance.

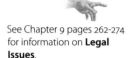

See Chapter 1 page 3 for details on the **Fiduciary Responsibility**.

Sexual misconduct isn't limited to sexual relations with a client. Sexual misconduct occurs when the fiduciary aspect of a therapeutic relationship is compromised. A continuum of behavior exists from sexual impropriety to sexual violation. Allegations of sexual misconduct create casualties on all sides: practitioners lose their licenses, practices, or reputations; clients are traumatized by inappropriate or abusive intentions or behavior, or behavior that they perceive as abusive; and healthcare professions are publicly humiliated or singled out for unflattering media attention. This impacts all somatic practitioners, whether you work in the service industry, health profession, or spa industry. Sexual misconduct complaints apply to employers, employees, practitioners, consumers, co-workers, teachers, and students. A comprehensive, even exhaustive, exploration of this and related topics is presented in the book *Sexual Abuse by Professionals: A Legal Guide.*[36]

See Chapter 9 pages 262-274 for information on **Legal Issues**.

Know your state's stance on sexualization of sessions. Many states prohibit sexualized intent, as well as sexual behavior. For instance, in North Carolina, the Rules & Regulations of the Board of Massage & Bodywork Therapy define sexual activity as:

> *any direct or indirect physical contact, or verbal communication, by any person or between persons which is intended to erotically stimulate either person, or which is likely to cause such stimulation and includes sexual intercourse, fellatio, cunnilingus, masturbation or anal intercourse. As used herein, masturbation means the manipulation of any body tissue with the intent to cause sexual arousal. Sexual activity can involve the use of any device or object and is not dependent on whether penetration, orgasm or ejaculation has occurred.*[37]

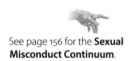

See page 156 for the **Sexual Misconduct Continuum**.

This type of inclusive definition attempts to protect the public not just from overt sexual behavior but also from covert sexualized intent which also violates clients. Touching non-erogenous regions of the body with sexualized intent is prohibited.

Statistics on the subject reveal that 70 percent of sexual misconduct complaints against healthcare practitioners are filed by female clients against male practitioners. Approximately 20 percent are from female clients complaining about female practitioners. Of the remaining 10 percent of complaints, roughly five percent are from male clients bringing allegations against female practitioners. Females, therefore, make up about 90 percent of the victims of sexual misconduct and 25 percent of the perpetrators. Many of those working in the field "have speculated that male victims of practitioners of either gender are underrepresented across the board because of particular male characteristics inhibiting both recognition and reporting [of abuse]."[38]

Examining the Roots of Sexual Misconduct

Sexual misconduct is a very complex problem, encompassing issues of sex, gender, power, and communication. Sexual misconduct is the result of the blatant disregard of ethics, boundaries, and genuine care for the client. Perpetrators of such behavior may do so because of psychopathology, ignorance, or a period of weakness brought on by unusual circumstances. Although most reported sexual misconduct is committed by males, female practitioners also commit acts of sexual misconduct.

Sociopaths prey on others to satisfy their own needs; they aren't inconvenienced by social, ethical, or legal considerations. Such a person could be involved in multiple cases of sexual misconduct or other inappropriate behavior throughout their lives. Sexual predators in the healthcare field are known to have had sexual contact with many of their clients throughout their careers, often with several individuals during the same time span. Reason, education, or peer-pressure have little or no effect on the sexual predator.

Most practitioners can't imagine themselves or their colleagues being sexually inappropriate with a client. Unfortunately, documented legal proceedings prove otherwise. For instance, consider the following cases taken from court transcripts.

A male massage therapist in the process of performing a full-body massage on a 20 year-old female client pulled down the client's bra and proceeded to massage her breasts and nipples. He asked her if she enjoyed his massaging her breasts and nipples to which she responded "no." He started to massage her legs and worked his way upward. Without her consent, he removed her underwear and massaged her vagina. The client attempted to turn over on her stomach to stop the therapist from massaging her vagina. The therapist penetrated her vaginally and anally with his finger while alternately massaging her back, shoulders, and buttocks. During the session, the client was covered from the waist up by a sheet. However, the massage therapist continually adjusted the sheet that was to cover her from the waist down so that it was "half on, half off." The massage therapist claimed that he touched the clients' breasts and genitals because she had not specifically indicated those body parts on his intake form on which he specifically asked, "What areas of your body would you prefer not to be worked on." The recommendation of the hearing was that his license to practice massage therapy be revoked and a $1,000 fine be imposed.[39]

Points to Ponder

Given your knowledge about power differentials, why do you think the client allowed the treatment to continue? Do the hearing recommendations seem sufficient considering the extent of the violation?

Ignorance is another root of sexual misconduct. Slowly, progress is being made through the increase of knowledge and education. Many individuals have no idea that casual sex with their clients or students is wrong. They didn't receive the education to lead them to an understanding of ethics, boundaries, and appropriate conduct with those in their care. These individuals may have engaged in sexual relationships with their teachers, supervisors, or healthcare providers in the past and are repeating learned behaviors. In other cases, these individuals were in environment(s) where this type of behavior was commonplace.

A patient, his wife, and daughter went to a chiropractor for treatments. The patient and his wife had difficulty in their marriage because of his wife's severe back injuries, which interfered with sexual activity. The chiropractor began having an affair with the wife during scheduled treatment sessions for which he issued bills and was paid. The chiropractor was sued for malpractice by the wife's husband.[40]

Points to Ponder

Besides the husband, who else might bring a case against the chiropractor? Should this practitioner have his license revoked like the massage therapist in the previous scenario?

It is possible the chiropractor realized that an affair with a client was unethical, but he chose to take the risk with the wife, never dreaming that the husband would file suit. Unethical behavior often leads to other unforeseen complications. In general, when given the proper education and training, practitioners learn that sexual relationships with clients are destructive and inappropriate, and in the future refrain from acting upon sexual urges.

Practitioners who find themselves in a period of weakness, brought on by unusual circumstances, may know what the right thing is to do but still have difficulty behaving appropriately. For example, an individual who has suddenly lost his spouse through an accidental death may be so distraught, confused, and vulnerable that rational behavior becomes nearly impossible. Many people have experienced times in their lives when rationality was gone and satisfying one's immediate needs was all that mattered. This isn't to excuse inappropriate behavior on the part of such practitioners, only to view it in context. These individuals may have inappropriate sexual contact with clients once or twice over their entire lifetime at these particular times of crisis. They need strong personal and professional support systems. If these practitioners receive the appropriate assistance at the time of crisis, they're less likely to inflict pain on others.

The Sexual Misconduct Continuum

As stated, the boundary violations that constitute sexual misconduct don't necessarily involve sexual intercourse between the practitioner and the client. The more common improprieties are: gestures or expressions that are seductive or sexually demeaning to a client; failure to ensure a client's privacy (e.g., improper draping, not providing a gown); sexual comments about a client's body or clothing; sexualized or sexually demeaning comments to a client; off-color jokes; strong interest in, or disapproval of, the client's sexual orientation; comments made during a treatment or consultation about sexual performance; conversation initiated by the practitioner about sexual problems, preferences, or fantasies of the practitioner or client; unnecessary examinations or treatments; the practitioner not obtaining informed consent to work on the breast or pelvic area; and inappropriate touching.

Remember that part of the power differential comes from the fact that clients often get to a deeply relaxed or altered frame of mind. In this more vulnerable and open place, a comment you might think is harmless joking is actually deeply upsetting to the client.

Sexual violations often involve actual sexual contact: encouraging the client to masturbate in the presence of the practitioner or masturbation by the practitioner while the client is present; intercourse; doing inappropriate work (e.g., touching breasts for any purpose other than therapeutic treatment; performing intra-anal coccygeal adjustments without gloves); or the most extreme case—rape. Regarding sexual contact or intercourse, it doesn't matter whether initiated by the client or the practitioner. It is ultimately the practitioner's responsibility. Because of the power differential of the therapeutic relationship, a client can't give clear, equal, authentic consent for any sexual contact; therefore, even if the client initiates or verbally says "yes," the practitioner is sexually violating the client.[41,42]

Analyzing Risk Factors

The following activity was adapted from a questionnaire developed by Ben Benjamin, PH.D. and Angelica Redleaf, D.C.[43] This questionnaire informs you about the clarity of your professional/sexual boundaries. If you answer these questions as honestly as you can, you get an accurate risk factor assessment. No one need see this but you.

Risk Factors Questionnaire

Place a check mark next to each statement that applies to you. After completing the questionnaire, add up all of your check marks in each of the three sections.

☐ I want a particular client to like me.
☐ I like it when my clients find me attractive, but I keep this to myself.
☐ I attend professional or social events where I knew a client would be present.
☐ I find myself cajoling, teasing, and joking a lot with clients.
☐ I feel lonely much of the time unless I'm working.
☐ I talk about my personal life to my clients.
☐ I notice that some of my clients are very dependent on me.
☐ I like it when my clients look up to me.
☐ I feel totally comfortable socializing with clients.
☐ Some clients feel more like friends.
   Total Section 1: _____

☐ I accept gifts/favors from a client without examining why the gift was given.
☐ A specific client often invites me to social events and I don't feel comfortable saying no.
☐ I like being alone in the office with specific clients.
☐ I invite clients to public or social events.
☐ I feel overly protective of some clients.
☐ I find it difficult to keep from talking about certain clients with people who are close to me.
☐ I talk a lot about myself with some clients, engaging in peer-like conversation.
☐ I invite clients to my home.
☐ I am surprised by how much I anticipate a particular client's visit.
☐ I frequently think about a particular client.
☐ I have trouble asking certain clients to pay my full fee.
☐ I find myself working weekends to accommodate a few clients whom I like.
☐ I feel under tremendous personal/professional pressure and I'm afraid I might burn out.
☐ I dress exceptionally well when I know a particular client has an appointment that day.
☐ I fantasize about what it would be like to have sex with some of my clients.
☐ I'm not charging one or more of the clients to whom I'm attracted.
☐ I have some of my clients take off more of their clothes than needed.
☐ I sometimes sneak looks as clients are undressing.
☐ I feel it's okay to date clients.
☐ I sometimes tell dirty jokes to my clients.
☐ I like doing work on those areas of clients' bodies that are close to their erogenous zones.
☐ I compliment clients when I think they look nice.
☐ I feel sexually aroused by one or more of my clients.
☐ I think that good-bye hugs last too long with one or more of my clients.
☐ Appointments with one or more clients regularly last longer than with others.
   Total Section 2: _____

❑ I've engaged in sexual contact with one or more of my clients.
❑ Sometimes I feel like I'm in over my head with a particular client.
❑ I sometimes drink or use recreational drugs with clients.
❑ I do more for a specific client than I would for any other client.
❑ I call a specific client a lot and go out of my way to meet with that client.
❑ I often tell my personal problems to clients, and allow them to comfort me.
❑ I enjoy exercising my power over some of my clients.
❑ If a client consents to sex, it's okay.
❑ I've touched clients in inappropriate ways at times.
❑ I've had sex with clients.
❑ I've had sex with clients in the office.
❑ I'm waiting to dismiss a particular client so that we can become romantically involved.

Total Section 3: _____

If you have one or more check marks in section 3, you're at the highest risk level. You are likely in danger of violating professional boundaries. Not only can this damage clients, but it could also damage your career. Asking for professional help from a psychotherapist or a consultant would be a good idea. You may also benefit from attending professional training in the area of personal and professional boundaries. Ignoring such a high risk level can result in serious consequences.

If you have more than three check marks in section 2, you have the potential to move into a higher risk category at any time, especially when stressed. If you have between four and eight check marks in section 2, you have entered a risk factor that is heading toward possible danger. You could use some help getting yourself on track concerning professional boundaries.

If you have more than five check marks in section 1, you could be overstepping your professional boundaries. You may not be in danger of crossing a sexual boundary, but you may be crossing other boundaries in your professional relationships.

Linking Client Impacts with Boundary Violations

Choose 10 Risk Factors from sections 2 and 3 above. Review the Impacts from Ethical Breaches chart (page 4). What damage do you think the client may experience from each of the risk factors?

> Figure 6.3 Sexual Misconduct Prevention Strategies

> - Do not seek emotional support from clients.
> - Limit personal self-disclosure.
> - Do not ask clients to do favors for you.
> - Avoid seeing clients after your normal hours.
> - Recognize and stop any problem behavior as soon as it occurs.
> - Be cautious when accepting gifts or tips.
> - Maintain your policies regarding fees.
> - Take immediate action to avert overtures from a sexually provocative client.
> - Establish a procedure to alert staff if there is a potential problem.

Sexual Harassment

Somatic practitioners often work in group practices or other healthcare offices. They must not only be aware of sexual misconduct in the treatment setting, they must be aware of sexual harassment in the work environment as well. Both sexual misconduct and sexual harassment create significant problems in a healthcare practice; each is a boundary violation occurring when one person's "safe space" is invaded by another.

Sexual harassment generally involves the behavior of a supervisor, manager, employer, or employee toward staff at the same or a lower level of power. An understanding of this issue is vital to all healthcare practitioners.

Sexual harassment is an issue arising in a workplace or an educational institution. It generally involves one person having power over another's employment, money, grades, or advancement, and abusing that power. Other instances of sexual harassment involve co-workers. There are two recognized forms of sexual harassment:

1. QUID PRO QUO: (Latin term meaning an equal exchange or substitution, "this for that"); a demand for sexual favors in exchange for job benefits;
2. HOSTILE WORK ENVIRONMENT: unwelcome acts such as physical or verbal conduct, or visually inappropriate displays, that make the individual's job difficult.

The U.S. Equal Employment Opportunity Commission (EEOC) defines sexual harassment as "unwelcome sexual advances, requests for sexual favors, and other verbal or physical conduct of a sexual nature" when:

- submission to such conduct is made a term or condition of an individual's employment, either implicitly or explicitly;
- submission to or rejection of such conduct is used as a basis for employment decisions affecting such individual;
- such conduct has the purpose or effect of unreasonably interfering with an individual's work performance or creating an intimidating, offensive, or hostile work environment.

Sexual harassment can be in the form of physical contact, such as touching, hugging, and stroking. Verbal sexual harassment includes inappropriate ways of addressing a person, use of sexually explicit language, or use of words, that refer to an individual's body parts. It can also be visual, such as displaying "girlie" or "hunk" calendars or other visually explicit material, regardless of whether that material is intended to offend. The intent of these actions is difficult to determine. A determination of intent isn't necessary to a finding of sexual harassment. Heavier penalties are usually exacted in cases where the intent to offend is established.

A finding of *quid pro quo* sexual harassment requires that a plaintiff prove that receiving job benefits or protection from job detriments was dependent upon his or her submission to a supervisor's unwelcome sexual demands.

Figure 6.4 Sexual Harassment Behaviors

- Physical Contact
- Touching
- Hugging
- Stroking
- Inappropriate Greetings
- Sexually Explicit Language
- Reference to Body Parts
- Displaying Visually Explicit Materials

A hostile work environment claim generally requires that a plaintiff prove a pattern of offensive behavior—unless the one incident was especially egregious. A single use of offensive language, or a single hug or bump in the hallway, isn't sufficient. A hostile work environment claim must prove two things: 1) subjectively, the individual had to regard the behavior as sexual harassment; and 2) another reasonable person would also regard this incident or behavior as sexual harassment.

The "reasonable person" measure has been modified in recent years in recognition of the fact that some material, speech, or behavior that is considered outrageous by most women is regarded as acceptable by many men. Instead of a "reasonable person," therefore, a "reasonable woman" standard has been substituted by the courts in some male-female harassment cases.

An institution's liability is established when the employer has had direct or legal notice of any of these types of sexual harassment and failed to take immediate and appropriate action. The major factors courts and enforcement agencies consider in determining liability are: the nature of the conduct; the frequency and openness of the conduct; and whether it could easily have been avoided by the victim.

Sexual harassment is perpetrated by the same gender as well as cross-gender. In a March 4, 1998, decision, the U.S. Supreme Court unanimously ruled that "federal law protects employees from being sexually harassed in the workplace by the same sex."[44]

Figure 6.5 Sexual Harassment Prevention Strategies

- Obtain training to facilitate an understanding of the power of roles.
- Gain an understanding of the impact of one's own sexuality and the sexuality of those with whom one interacts professionally.
- Learn appropriate ways of behaving around, and of communicating with, both genders.
- Discover what behaviors are considered unacceptable.
- Determine the types of situations that may lead to such transgressions.
- Ascertain the effects of abuse and harassment.
- Understand the potential legal and financial consequences of unacceptable behavior.

Further steps to take to help prevent sexual harassment by supervisors or co-workers are:
- Develop and post a policy against harassment.
- Teach employees what constitutes harassment.
- Improve morale and productivity.
- Address complaints before they develop into litigation.
- Establish an effective and confidential complaint process.

Breaking the Silence

Healthcare recipients previously kept silent about improper behavior. Today they're speaking out in record numbers. Until very recently, the complaint process has been little-known, little-used, and far from impartial. To quote the organizers of the Third International Conference on Sexual Exploitation by Health Professionals, Psychotherapists, and Clergy, "The tendency is to shoot the messenger, blame the victim, and coddle the man."[45] However, the number of complaints are expected to increase as clients become less afraid of complaining, as awareness of the complaint process rises, and as the process itself becomes fairer and less humiliating for the person filing charges.

In reality, clients' complaints serve as the major factor in monitoring the behavior and regulation of practitioners. Women, especially, are increasingly sensitive to inappropriate behavior on the part of either male or female practitioners. In the treatment setting, as in greater society, they have taken the lead in the fight against abuse, misconduct, and harassment.

Marshaling evidence to prove sexual misconduct malpractice is difficult because the actions often occur behind closed doors and proof becomes a matter of the word of the victim against that of the alleged perpetrator. Tangible evidence of the boundary violation can include cards, letters, diaries, journals, gifts, receipts for meals, phone records, voice mails, photos, videotapes, appointment books, and self-disclosures by the victim to friends and relatives.

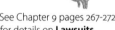

See Chapter 9 pages 267-272 for details on **Lawsuits**.

Widespread education about ethical behavior is necessary to prevent the next generation of health practitioners from compromising their clients' welfare and the public trust. That training already has begun in some schools. As for the current practitioners whose education included no substantive training in sexuality, ethics, communication, and other important skills—it's never too late to learn.

The healthcare market is an increasingly consumer-driven market. Practitioners who develop a strong sense of awareness of their own attitudes and behavior cultivate a wide range of skills in interpersonal communication, and adopt office procedures with their clients (especially their female clients) in mind, are far more likely to become or remain successful—as well as to prevent unnecessary difficulties for themselves and their clients.

Analyzing Sexual Misconduct

Consider the following scenario:

A new client of yours tells you that she received a very uncomfortable session from a female practitioner in town. She said the woman's fingers kept touching her pubic area and the practitioner's body contacted the client in ways that felt intrusive.
- What do you do?
- How would this scenario differ if the practitioner was a male?
- How would this scenario differ if the client was a male?

▍ Desexualizing the Touch Experience

Good intentions and the number of years in practice don't guarantee appropriate professional behavior regarding sex, touch, and intimacy. The ethically safe touch experience doesn't just happen; it must be created, structured, and sustained. Structuring safety means at all times proactively demonstrating absolute professionalism in all aspects of practice, particularly around the connections between sex and touch. The following suggestions apply to practitioners of both genders.

Figure 6.6 Tips to Desexualize Touch

Preparation, Language, Behavior	• Observe and know yourself. • Establish a pre-treatment thinking process. • Describe your techniques. • Maintain a professional appearance and demeanor. • Participate in ongoing supervision. • Commit to continued education.
Office Space	• Choose an appropriate office location. • Establish a professional space. • Set up a space that feels like an office when doing home or hotel visits.
Treatment Interactions	• Provide Informed Consent. • Allow privacy. • Always use proper draping techniques. • Use respectful communication. • Be mindful of body contact during the session. • Prevent straying strokes or movements.
Practice Management	• Keep accurate records. • Inform your clients of their rights. • Treat all clients equally. • Effectively respond to inappropriate inquiries.
Marketing Materials	• Maintain a professional image. • Choose an appropriate business name. • Set up separate business and personal email accounts. • Be careful with the links you include on your website.

Preparation, Language, and Behavior

OBSERVE AND KNOW YOURSELF. Monitor your inner experience, as well as your language and behavior. Consider how you come across and the messages you transmit to others, especially clients. Take time to think about your work environment and your approach with clients. Ask yourself, "Is there anything about me or my work space, or that I say or do, that is likely to be sexualized?" or "Would I act this way if I wasn't attracted to the client?"

ESTABLISH A PRE-TREATMENT THINKING PROCESS. Ask yourself the following questions before working with a client: Is this course of treatment necessary? Am I the right person to do this? Should someone else be in the room?

DESCRIBE YOUR TECHNIQUES. Strive for precise ways to communicate about your work. Realize that what you say might be interpreted differently from what you mean and avoid language that can be sexualized. For instance, acupuncturists might want to refrain from using a phrase such as "sticking in a needle" and instead say something with a less emotional charge like "gently apply a needle." Massage therapists might avoid the term "full body massage" which can be suggestive or misleading. Instead, use terminology which more accurately describes the therapeutic aspect of your work. The term "out calls" has long been associated with prostitution and escort services so consider using the phrase "in-home" or "on site treatment" when talking about appointments in a private residence or hotel setting.

MAINTAIN A PROFESSIONAL APPEARANCE AND DEMEANOR. Your appearance is an outward representation of your professional standards. Make sure that your image projects competence and doesn't sexualize you. Dress appropriately for the work environment, maintain good hygiene, keep jewelry to a minimum, don't wear heavy perfume or cologne, and avoid provocative or revealing attire. Some examples of inappropriate clothing are: tank tops (especially for women); short shorts; shirts that show cleavage or nipples; shirts that expose the midriff; shirts that have questionable statements or provocative images. Remember, your attire isn't meant to be a distraction or a loud statement.

PARTICIPATE IN ONGOING SUPERVISION. Seek help immediately from a supervisor, colleague, or other professional if you find yourself overly attracted to a client or are in a vulnerable situation.

COMMIT TO CONTINUED EDUCATION. Your business requires that you maintain healthy client/practitioner interactions. Invest is lifelong learning, particularly in the areas of ethics, boundaries, and communications skills.

> The value of an idea lies in the using of it.
> —Thomas A. Edison

Office Space

CHOOSE AN APPROPRIATE OFFICE LOCATION. Practitioners often choose an office location based on what's close to where they live or where they can find a good deal. More importantly, choose a location where you and your clients feel safe. Check out the location at different times of the day, especially if you plan on being open in the evenings or weekends. A busy weekday locale with lots of foot traffic might be dark and deserted on evenings and weekends when you plan on working.

ESTABLISH A PROFESSIONAL SPACE. Sight, sound, smell, touch, and imagination all have the potential to arouse. Often times, practitioners attempt to set up a very relaxing space with dim lights, candles, and soft music. These can be wonderful, but they can also send confusing messages—particularly to new clients or people who are in a vulnerable state in terms of their romantic relationships. Ideally, start with the room fairly well-lit and ask clients if they want the light dimmed, or offer them an eye pillow. Choose music that is soothing, without being sensual or romantic. You can never know what scent might trigger a sexual response in clients, but in general, it's wise to be judicious with scents, as many people have allergies and sensitivities to fragrances. Create a comfortable, yet professional treatment room. Use high-quality equipment and supplies. Keep extra linens handy for additional draping needs. Consider hanging anatomical charts and other posters that are health related. Limit your displays of personal photos and keepsakes.

SET UP A SPACE THAT FEELS LIKE AN OFFICE WHEN DOING HOME OR HOTEL VISITS. Consider investing in a hard case on rollers that holds your supplies. When you set up the working space, also arrange your supplies on top of the case. This helps to make the space look a bit more office-like. Avoid working in a bedroom unless you're doing a session at a hotel, or if your client is injured or ill.

Treatment Interactions

PROVIDE INFORMED CONSENT. Before the first treatment begins, always inform the client about what you intend to do for the session protocol so she knows what to expect. Take her into the treatment space and discuss the session scenario. If doing hands-on work, explain whether you begin prone or supine, the anticipated sequence of where you'll work, how she'll be draped, and any other pertinent details. Repeat this process whenever there's a

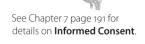

See Chapter 7 page 191 for details on **Informed Consent**.

major change in the session procedure or the areas you work on. Invite the client to have a third party present, particularly during sensitive procedures (such as working on an injury in the breast area), when working on minors, or if the client has any history of abuse.

ALLOW PRIVACY. Regardless of how well you know the person, always allow him complete privacy while changing. Some clients begin undressing before you have a chance to leave the room. In these instances ask them to wait and leave promptly. Remember, they aren't responsible for setting professional boundaries, you are.

ALWAYS USE PROPER DRAPING TECHNIQUES. If your treatment requires clients to partially or fully disrobe, make sure they're properly draped. While clients have clear choice about what to wear under the draping linen so they're comfortable (e.g., underclothes, shorts, swimwear), proper draping isn't optional. If a client insists on forgoing the draping linen, explain that you're more comfortable when draping is used, and that in the interest of your professionalism, draping techniques are used with all clients. Offer to adjust the room temperature, turn on a fan, or uncover her feet if she claims to feel too warm. Ensure that draping is secure and doesn't allow partial exposure of areas intended to be draped.

USE RESPECTFUL COMMUNICATION. All practitioners need to be thoughtful when talking about a client's body. Anatomical terms are far less suggestive and less offensive than slang words. For example, use clinical terminology such as "gluteal area" versus "butt" and "inguinal area" or "groin" instead of "crotch." Phrases such as "move your legs apart" or "open your legs" might seem innocuous but could be emotionally triggering for a client. Saying instead, "move your feet apart" is more emotionally neutral. If you notice a physical symptom during a session that's a health concern, it's essential to tell your client. Otherwise refrain from commenting on weight gain or loss or other physical appearance issues. When you make such comments, it fosters the notion that you're observing the client's body in a judgmental way. Also, compliments can be misinterpreted as flirtation. If a client thinks you're flirting, and he happens to become sexually aroused during the treatment, he may become confused about your intentions and respond inappropriately. Additionally, be aware of cultural language and how you use colloquialisms. For instance, in some locales calling people "honey" is commonplace and can be endearing; even so, some may find the expression demeaning or too intimate.

BE MINDFUL OF BODY CONTACT DURING THE SESSION. Beyond using proper body mechanics, pay attention to how you brace, support, and lean. Be conscious of where your body may contact the client's body during your strokes, manipulation, stretches, and other techniques. Avoid contacting the client with areas other than your extremities. Maintain a professional posture and stance throughout the session. Even accidentally allowing your genital region or breast to touch or brush against a client can be quite unnerving. Consider the following example of how a client can perceive an action as a subtle sexual contact: A chiropractor performs a manipulation on a client's back. While standing at the client's head, the practitioner unconsciously leans over allowing her pelvis to come in contact with the top of the client's head.

PREVENT STRAYING STROKES OR MOVEMENTS. When working areas such as the medial thigh, ischial tuberosity, the sacrum, or the subclavicular/pectoral area, strokes must not stray, even accidentally. The slightest "slip" in these areas is invasive and inappropriate, and could give the client the wrong message about your intentions.

Practice Management

KEEP ACCURATE RECORDS. Document whenever a client does anything questionable (e.g., flirts, sends inappropriate correspondence, gives you improper gifts). Write a summary of the impropriety as though it were to be read in court or before a board. Include the basic details, how you handled it, and the names, dates, and telephone numbers of other professionals with whom you discussed this (such as a peer supervision group).

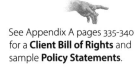

See Appendix A pages 335-340 for a **Client Bill of Rights** and sample **Policy Statements**.

INFORM YOUR CLIENTS OF THEIR RIGHTS. Develop and post a Policy Statement. Address client complaints and dissatisfaction promptly, before they develop into litigation.

TREAT ALL CLIENTS EQUALLY. All clients should be given the same consideration regardless of age, gender, or attractiveness. Be particularly careful of extending special considerations or expressions of endearment that you wouldn't ordinarily give to anyone else. For example, a physical therapist was treating a client who disclosed personal information about a recent death of a loved one. At the conclusion of a treatment session, touched by the client's disclosure, the therapist gently kissed the client's forehead. While the kiss was well-meaning, the gesture could easily be misinterpreted and the therapist could be charged with sexual misconduct.

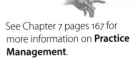

See Chapter 7 pages 167 for more information on **Practice Management**.

EFFECTIVELY RESPOND TO INAPPROPRIATE INQUIRIES. Be prepared with a script to respond to someone contacting you for sexual services via telephone or email. Do not wait until new clients arrive for their appointments to discover if they're ethically appropriate. If a receptionist takes your calls, or if you use an online scheduler, be sure to call the clients prior to their sessions. Determine their intentions and goals for the treatment when you first talk with them to set up the appointment (either on the phone or in person). Assess them by their demeanor, language, and approach as to whether they're seeking non-sexual treatment. Ask questions such as, "Why are you seeking this course of treatment?" and "What are your goals for this session?" If they remain vague and obscure, inform them directly that the treatment you offer is "therapeutic and non-sexual." Beyond determining that they aren't seeking sexual services, it's wise to ensure your own ethical and physical safety. This is especially critical in the massage and bodywork professions, particularly when doing a home or hotel visit for a new, unknown client. For instance, if you have concerns for your safety, in the client's presence, place a telephone call to a friend (or the concierge if at a hotel) and tell that person where you are, when you expect to be done, and that you'll call back when the session is over.

Marketing Materials

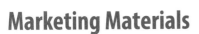

MAINTAIN A PROFESSIONAL IMAGE. Marketing materials (e.g., brochures, business cards, website, business name, email address) need to be professional and project the desired image. Use appropriate language and terminology. Avoid phrases like "full-body massage." Even words such as "release" can be taken out of context. Be sure your photos and artwork aren't provocative: view pictures from all angles because sometimes images look fine from one direction, but suggestive from others. Ideally, have your picture taken by a professional photographer, but refrain from using "glamour" shots.

CHOOSE AN APPROPRIATE BUSINESS NAME. Many practitioners use their personal name as their company name. This is a fine option and a business name that says "Terry Smith, L.M.T." sounds much more professional than "Massage by Terry." Use caution if you decide to have a separate business identity: avoid anything gimmicky or that could have a double meaning. Also verify that your business name doesn't mean something derogatory in another language.

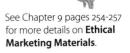

See Chapter 9 pages 254-257 for more details on **Ethical Marketing Materials**.

SET UP SEPARATE BUSINESS AND PERSONAL EMAIL ACCOUNTS. Either use your name, company name, or the type of work you do as the first part of your email address. There are too many examples of practitioners with business emails like rockerchick@example.com or angelhands@example.com. In a marketing class where students critiqued each other's email addresses, one woman's email was healinghands69@example.com. As soon as she said it out loud there was a lot of snickering in the room. She didn't get it. The year 1969 was very important to her. She failed to realize how the number 69 has a sexual connotation and that using that email address for a business could send the wrong message. Ideally, you have a website and an email address that match (e.g., TerrySmith@DesertWindsMassageTherapy.com).

BE CAREFUL WITH THE LINKS YOU INCLUDE ON YOUR WEBSITE. In addition to links becoming inactive, sometimes a link that originally went to one site all of a sudden takes you to a totally different site. This can be a purposeful act of misdirection or just something that went haywire. So, in addition to periodically checking the links you list on your site, make sure that you check your own internal links.

Conclusion

Sexuality is a natural part of the human experience. By recognizing this fact, you can consciously choose to create a professional treatment space, to maintain clear boundaries, and to deal ethically and compassionately with unintended sexual responses. You can also protect yourself and your clients from sexually inappropriate or damaging behavior. Through an awareness of the physical, social, and cultural dynamics, and knowledge of behavioral strategies, you can enhance your effectiveness as a safe, healing presence in the treatment setting.

7
Practice Management

"You can't build a reputation on what you're going to do."
—Henry Ford

Professionalism
- Intentional Practice
- The At-Risk Practitioner

Scope of Practice
- Key Factor One: The Law
- Key Factor Two: Educational Training
- Key Factor Three: Competency
- Key Factor Four: Self-Accountability

Standards of Practice

Client/Practitioner Expectations
- Procedures
- Draping
- Communication
- Attitudes
- Interaction
- Etiquette
- Illness

Time Management
- Start and End on Time
- Cancellations

Confidentiality
- Maintaining Confidentiality
- Limits of Ethical Confidentiality
- Actions That Minimize Confidentiality Problems
- Documentation

Health Insurance Portability and Accountability Act
- HIPAA Compliance

Informed Consent
- The Well-Informed Client

Working with Minors
- Special Considerations
- Infants and Children
- Teenagers

Declining Potential New Clients
- A Full Practice
- Inability to Help
- Countertransference

Referring Out

Dismissing A Client
- Discomfort
- Transference and Countertransference
- Lack of Results
- Completion

Client Policy Statements
- Type of Service
- Training and Experience
- Appointments
- Finances
- Client/Practitioner Expectations
- Personal Relationships
- Confidentiality
- Recourse Policy

Key Terms

Abandonment
Assessment
Benchmarking
Certification
Competency
Confidentiality
Countertransference
Demeanor
Diagnosis

Etiquette
Health Insurance Portability and Accountability Act (HIPAA)
Informed Consent
Licensure
National Provider Identifier (NPI)
Policy
Professionalism
Protected Health Information (PHI)

Registration
Scope of Practice
Self-Accountability
Standards of Practice
Therapeutic Constellation
Title Protection
Transference
Work Ethic

You set the tone for an ethically run practice by developing and implementing business and practice management systems. How you manage your business impacts how your clients feel about you and your practice. You may do wonderful work and be a caring and compassionate person, but your clients won't hold the same level of trust in you and your abilities if the foundation of your business is poorly considered. Ethical practice management involves the art and skill of managing daily working affairs with others from a base of honesty, integrity, and forthrightness. In this chapter we explore attitudes, policies, and procedures relating to your conduct with clients; maintaining client records; honoring confidentiality; working within the appropriate scope of practice; and accurately representing abilities. The business management issues that relate to the topics of finances, marketing, negotiating contracts, legalities, employees, insurance claims, and ethical issues relating to specific practice environments are covered in Chapters 8 and 9.

Professionalism

The root of the word professional is "profess" which means to declare, claim or openly affirm a belief or an opinion. *Webster's Dictionary*[1] defines a professional as a person who conforms to the standards of a profession; has or shows great skill; engages in a given activity as a source of livelihood; follows a learned profession. The term *professionalism* encompasses the behaviors and qualities that mark an individual as a reliable, competent, trustworthy, and polished professional person. Professionalism stems from your attitudes and is manifested through your technical competency, your communication skills, your ability to manage boundaries, your respect for yourself and clients, and your business practices.

High standards of action with clients result in both ethical and professional behavior. Obviously, ethical violations are unprofessional. However, not all unprofessional behavior is unethical. For example, wearing torn workout clothes when working with a client is unprofessional but not unethical, and having a messy waiting room with visible dust bunnies is unprofessional but certainly not unethical.

Figure 7.1 What is a Professional?

- Gives high quality performance
- Is predictable and consistent
- Is self-motivated
- Is self-reliant and takes responsibility
- Works well under pressure
- Is always willing to learn
- Understands her interconnectedness with humanity

by Jerry Buley, PH.D.[2]

In their book *Communication & Ethics for Bodywork Practitioners*[3], Patricia M. Holland and Sandra K. Anderson describe someone with a professional work ethic as one motivated to "arrive at his job on time every day, do the best work he can do at all times, work until his job is done, not take excessive amounts of time off, and cooperate with his colleagues and supervisors." They go on to say that employers are looking for "employees with good work ethics, appropriate social behavior, and self-discipline." Your attitude about professionalism and work ethic can help or hinder your ability to secure and maintain an employment position or private practice, and most importantly, secure and maintain clientele. You start by evaluating and meeting client expectations of personal etiquette and behavior. Most people feel comfortable in a clean and neat office that is appropriately equipped for the type of work done, with a clean and conservatively dressed practitioner who acts respectfully and sets professional boundaries. The personal appearance of a practitioner may vary widely, depending on the work environment and his own personality, but inevitably clients feel more comfortable with practitioners who are like them. Consider your target clientele in terms of what they look like and how they act, and be sure that your attitude, appearance, and behavior match their expectations.

What Does a Professional Look Like?

- Think about someone you regard as being very professional. Identify the ways that person manifests professionalism. Describe how you feel when you're with this person.
- Describe yourself in terms of professionalism.
- Describe how you imagine others see you in terms of professionalism.
- List the changes you would like to make in terms of demonstrating professionalism.

The basis for true professionalism lies in integrity. Someone may talk, walk, and look the part, but if that person doesn't come from a base of integrity, the façade wears thin quickly, ultimately resulting in the loss of clientele. The dictionary[4] defines integrity as the quality or state of being complete; unbroken condition; wholeness; honesty; and sincerity. Integrity is an essential quality for a true healing professional. People who possess integrity behave ethically, honor confidences, and keep their word. Integrity can be divided into three major levels: the first level is keeping one's agreements; the second is being true to one's principles; and the highest level is being true to oneself.

It is rare to find somatic practitioners who value professionalism without the integrity behind it. More often, they love what they do and are genuinely concerned about the wellbeing of their clients, yet may neglect to develop a professional demeanor. A truly effective practitioner combines outward professionalism with internal integrity.

Intentional Practice

What is an intentional practice? Having an ethical and professional practice doesn't just happen automatically, even for the practitioner with integrity. A professional practice is created and maintained by cultivating professional knowledge and behavior, and by proper planning.

Cultivating professional knowledge most obviously includes learning and practicing technical skills with an in-depth understanding of the human body, but it also includes an understanding of human nature, sexuality, and the risk factors involved in somatic relationships. Cultivating professional behavior includes establishing and maintaining healthy boundaries, as well as following policies and procedures (yours or those set by your employer). The ability to self-monitor is crucial, as inappropriate behavior runs the continuum of subtle to obvious and minimal to criminal. Subtle boundaries are crossed much more frequently than the overt, and it takes an intentional practitioner to know the difference and make immediate corrections to preserve professionalism at all times.

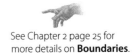

See Chapter 2 page 25 for more details on **Boundaries**.

Proper planning can help the intentional practitioner be prepared. For example, planning a session structure before the treatment begins, and having contingency plans if something goes awry, allows the practitioner to avoid potential boundary crossings or inappropriate behavior that often result from the surprise of the moment. When variations are thought through ahead of time, the practitioner can simply move to plan B with little effort or anxiety.

Intentional practice becomes paramount when touch is introduced. Understanding the difference between intentional and accidental touch, and behaving accordingly, is of utmost importance to a professional practice. While much of touch therapy is intentional, accidental touch does occur. Avoiding client discomfort or further at-risk behavior requires presence and proper planning, and knowing what to do when it does occur. Intentional practitioners make it their business to know the difference, and take the proper steps to plan for successful and professional interactions. The topics in this chapter can be used as that professional foundation.

The At-Risk Practitioner

See Chapter 9 page 270 for **High Risk Client Characteristics**.

The consequences of not being an Intentional Practitioner can be more severe than just having a struggling practice. Not being intentional puts you, your practice, your place of employment, and your clients at risk. The unintentional practitioner risks being sued, acquiring a damaging reputation (both yours and that of the whole profession), losing clients, losing your job, and potentially losing your license. Be aware of the characteristics of at-risk practitioners, and work intentionally to avoid them.

Figure 7.2 The At-Risk Practitioner

- Under Major Stress
- Insufficient Knowledge
- Poor Organization
- Inappropriate Boundaries
- Working Beyond Scope

- Insufficient Documentation
- Not Following Policies & Procedures
- Lack of Contingency Plans

Scope of Practice

More than 2,500 years ago Hippocrates proclaimed this primary warning to physicians: Do no harm.[5] This decree is the basis for the enduring responsibility of all helping professions to define, clarify and regulate what they do. Scope of Practice (Scope) regulations are an extension of this mission. Many of the hands-on professions are still developing consistent standards, mainly due to varying educational requirements and outdated regulations. Most professions' Scope evolves over time. For instance, in the fairly recent past, physical therapists needed a prescription from a medical doctor to provide services; now, in many states, they don't. All things considered, it may be difficult for individual practitioners to discern the parameters of their scope of practice. This section defines Scope and introduces the four key factors which shape and change it.

Many practitioners enter a wellness career because of their experience with the results of that particular modality. Their enthusiasm often leads to the misconception (and often arrogance) that this particular technique helps almost anything. Exactly what is Scope and who determines its parameters? What determines whether a practitioner is functioning within her Scope? Is a practitioner qualified to teach a client to do stretches at home, perform passive stretches on a client during a treatment, or sell nutritional supplements in the waiting room?

Sandy Fritz, author of *Mosby's Fundamentals of Therapeutic Massage*, defines Scope as, "The where, when, and how a professional may provide their service or function as a professional."[6] As succinct and simple as this sounds, the *where, when,* and *how* can be quite complicated, and they vary greatly throughout geographic regions. Despite its broad diversity, however, Scope is consistently influenced by four key factors: the law, educational training, competency, and personal accountability. Together, these factors circumscribe and ultimately define one's Scope.

Figure 7.3 Key Scope of Practice Factors

- The Law
- Educational Training
- Competency
- Self-Accountability

Key Factor One: The Law

The law is a pivotal factor in determining Scope, yet it's often the most difficult to decipher. Four levels of government make laws that affect practitioners: federal, state, county, and local municipalities (city and town). The federal government, besides imposing taxes, authorizes the accreditation of schools and regulates financial aid. The subordinate governing bodies (state, county, and municipal) exert a more tangible influence on Scope, offering four regulatory methods known as *licensure, certification, registration*, and *title protection*. Each method has its particular requirements and provisions, and each state has its preferred method of regulation. Licensure, certification, and registration typically have a mechanism for revoking professional practice status from individuals who engage in prohibited activities, whereas title protection rarely has such a mechanism.

> Laws should be interpreted in a liberal sense so that their intention may be preserved.
>
> —Marcus Tullius Cicero

Figure 7.4 Regulatory Methods

Licensure	Certification	Registration	Title Protection
required by law to practice	voluntary, non-governmental	governmental tracking/recordkeeping	voluntary, only required to use title
high consumer protection	high consumer protection	minimal consumer protection	no consumer protection
code of ethics and professional conduct requirements	code of ethics and professional conduct requirements	no restrictions	no restrictions
educational and exam requirements	educational and exam requirements	non-practice related requirements	minimal requirements

---

LICENSURE is the most restrictive form of regulation, and it provides the greatest level of public protection. Licensing programs typically involve the completion of a prescribed educational program and passing an examination that measures a minimal level of competency. Licensure requires practitioners to obtain a license to perform their services; unlicensed persons who practice, break the law. Holding a license generally requires the licensee to adhere to a code of ethics or professional conduct. If this code is violated, the license can be revoked or other disciplinary actions taken. Some municipalities require a business or occupational license in addition to a license to practice a specific trade. Legal names and professional titles cited in the law are numerous and varied. License titles aren't necessarily the same as professional certification titles.

CERTIFICATION offers a level of consumer protection similar to licensure, but the entry requirements are generally lower. Certifying bodies are frequently non-governmental agencies that establish the training requirements, and own and administer the examination. Certification, from a governmental view, is a voluntary option which offers the use of vocational titles to distinguish professional services from adult entertainment. Other certification documents show that you have passed specific professional tests, such as those from the National Certification Board for Therapeutic Massage and Bodyworkers (NCBTMB) or the National Certification Commission for Acupuncture and Oriental Medicine (NCCAOM). In some states, certification is used as the designation for practitioners rather than licensure, and in those places certification is made conditional upon the individual practitioner obtaining and maintaining the relevant private credential. These types of programs usually entail title protection and ensure that only those who are deemed competent may practice.

REGISTRATION is the means by which a government agency keeps track of practitioners by informational recordkeeping. Registration can serve to protect the public, although the entry requirements are usually minimal and non-practice related, such as proof of insurance coverage or the use of certain client forms. These types of programs can entail title protection and practice exclusivity. In Canada and some states in the United States, practitioners must be registered to legally use their professional title.

TITLE PROTECTION represents one of the lowest levels of regulation. Only those who satisfy certain requirements may use the relevant prescribed title. Practitioners aren't required to register or notify the state. Thus, anyone may engage in the particular practice, but only those who satisfy the prescribed requirements may use the specific title.

Credentialing can be complicated and confusing, and thus many competent, conscientious practitioners are unclear about the regulatory laws that apply to them. For example, although a practitioner was licensed many years ago, she may not have received notification of updated revisions. Even recently licensed practitioners with current awareness of applicable laws may find it difficult to understand the vague and tedious terminology. A myriad of inconsistencies further complicates matters including the delivery of the information. Some governing agencies issue ponderous amounts of information that attempt to define everything from the wording used in advertising to legal hours of operation; others offer little clarification.

There are a few states that have specific health freedom laws. These states allow greater freedom to the practitioner, especially the unlicensed practitioner. For instance, the state of California passed a law that says any individual can choose anyone to be his health practitioner. The caveat is that the practitioner must disclose her education, or lack thereof, to each client. This puts the responsibility of one's health on one's own shoulders. This offers great freedom for the receiver of the health services, as well as great responsibility. The same can be said for the practitioner—great freedom and great responsibility. In states with basically no scope of practice for any practitioner, we only hope that each practitioner adheres to very strong professional ethics.

Procedures, Techniques, and Other Regulations

The law can permit or forbid any number of activities, so it's wise for practitioners to consult laws and regulations in their state, province, or locality regarding Scope. Some of these laws are straightforward and others vague. Many seem frivolous. These laws typically restrict practitioners from performing services or procedures that require a different license (e.g., M.D.) or limit activities which could be linked with sex or sexual enterprise.

Assessment and Diagnosis

For somatic practitioners who aren't considered primary care providers (PCPs), the areas of *assessment* and *diagnosis* can be of concern. While diagnosis is generally restricted to the

Scope of physicians and other PCPs, assessment is an integral part of most practitioners' work. Many people confuse the concepts of assessment and diagnosis, and, for that reason, they shy away from learning about them. Understanding the difference, however, is important for ethical practice since assessment skills are a critical component of wellness practices. Whitney Lowe, L.M.T.[7], and Clifford Martin, M.D., provide the following definitions:

ASSESSMENT is a systematic method or approach to gathering information about a client's condition and symptoms. The information gathered in the assessment is then used to make informed decisions about, if, and how treatments should proceed. Information can be subjective (provided by the client) and objective (directly observed by the practitioner). Subjective sources include information provided in written or verbal form by the client regarding her symptoms. Objective information comes from the practitioner's direct observation, usually in the form of physical examination and observation before, during, or after treatment sessions. Since assessment is information gathering, you can't provide any kind of treatment without performing some level of assessment. For instance, when your hands feel a tight area in your client's muscle tissue, you naturally focus your attention on reducing the tension in that area. In this case, you performed an assessment through palpation and chose a particular course of action as a result of your assessment of the client's tissue state. Gathering information about a client's condition to determine if you should proceed with a given treatment is assessment, not diagnosis.

DIAGNOSIS, on the other hand, is the identification of the underlying cause, etiology, pathology, or nature of a set of signs or symptoms. Diagnosis relies on assessment, often including further information such as advanced physical exam findings, laboratory evaluation, and radiology results. The ability to diagnosis is limited to physicians and certain other PCPs, and it carries with it a high level of medical legal responsibility. If the patient has a specific diagnosis that underlies his symptoms, that information can be used in the assessment done by a somatic practitioner to inform treatment decisions.

> A client visits a somatic practitioner complaining of neck pain accompanied by bouts of dizziness. During the intake and assessment phase, the practitioner realizes that he understands neither the cause of the client's neck pain nor the dizziness associated with it. Nevertheless, the practitioner has been trained in a variety of techniques and feels competent in proceeding with treatment. This action is outside of his scope of practice because he doesn't have the training to diagnose what is actually occurring. These symptoms could indicate a brain tumor, pressure on the intervertebral artery, cancer, or disc injury. While the treatment may not immediately harm the client, if the client feels better after the treatment, he might not seek the establishment of an accurate diagnosis and therefore delay appropriate treatment.
>
> **Points to Ponder**
>
> If this was your client, would you treat the client? Would you refer your client to another healthcare practitioner? Think about how you would discuss such a referral, without suggesting the possible indications (without diagnosing).

Educating vs Prescribing

Two common areas where the scope of practice for many somatic practitioners is limited are stretches/exercises and nutritional supplements. Some states don't allow practitioners to even recommend specific stretching routines to clients unless the practitioners also have a specialty certification (e.g., personal training). Most somatic scopes of practice don't include actions such as telling a client to take specific nutritional supplements products, how much to take, or the frequency. They don't include putting a client on a particular diet or setting up a rigid rehabilitation exercise plan for the client.

This can be a challenge. As we know, clients usually want us to "tell" them what to do. If we demonstrate a stretch and recommend that the client do this stretch, the client often says, "How often? How many times a day? For how long should I be doing this?" In some states, only fitness professionals or physical therapists can give this type of information.

However, the Scope in most locales doesn't restrict the practitioner from educating clients about health. Somatic practitioners who aren't considered PCPs can't "tell" a client that she has a condition such as vitamin deficiency, nor can they "tell" the client how much of a particular Vitamin to take as this would be "prescribing." Only certain licensed professionals (e.g., a licensed physician or a licensed dietitian) are allowed to do this. Practitioners who choose to expand their practices to include offering nutritional consultations or selling supplements, must take responsibility to find out if the laws and scope of practice for these other licensed professionals are stated in such a way that the nutrition consultations the practitioner plans to provide step over the line into the scopes of practice of those other licensed professionals.

For example, if a bodywork practitioner lives in a state where the scope of practice for a licensed dietitian/nutritionist includes "providing nutrition counseling in health and disease," the practitioner couldn't advertise that he offers nutrition counseling, nor could he offer nutrition counseling in conjunction with his bodywork practice without breaking the law. Distinguishing between "nutrition counseling" and "nutrition consulting" is quite challenging, but makes the difference between practicing outside one's scope of practice and practicing inside one's scope. The language of the practitioner must clearly remain educational, not slipping into potentially diagnosing or prescribing. This can be a very slippery slope.

> During a bodywork session, the client tells the practitioner that she knows Vitamin C is really good to take in the winter. She heard that it helps people avoid getting colds and the flu.
>
> She asks the practitioner, "Do you take Vitamin C?"
>
> The practitioner responds, "Yes. I learned that Vitamin C boosts the immune system."
>
> "How much Vitamin C are you supposed to take each day?" asks the client.
>
> The practitioner's response is, "Vitamin C is water soluble, which means the body will eliminate whatever it doesn't use within about 2 or 3 hours. Taking some of the vitamin throughout the day allows the body to have more usable C than taking a large dosage once a day."
>
> Again, the client asks, "But how much should I take in a day?"
>
> Since the client has asked this a second time, the practitioner clearly states, "I can't tell you how much you should take because each body is different. However, I can email you a link to some educational websites, and you might want to do some additional research on your own or talk with your primary healthcare provider."

Points to Ponder

Would it be okay for this practitioner to tell the client how much Vitamin C she takes each day? Why or why not?

In the above scenario, the practitioner has educated the client about Vitamin C, offered additional information to the client, but hasn't slipped into the easy role of "prescribing" dosages or frequency.

Technique Restrictions

On occasion, a Scope rule may also refer to rarely heard-of procedures. An example is the term "heliotherapy." New Jersey law permits massage practitioners to do this procedure, and Rhode Island law prohibits it, further specifying that it can only be performed by physical therapists. *Taber's Cyclopedic Medical Dictionary*[8] defines heliotherapy as, "Exposure to sunlight for therapeutic purposes." One is left to wonder if that means using heat lamps, tanning lights, or working on a client outdoors or under a skylight with the sun shining in.

Each profession has certain prohibitions against treating certain parts of a client's body. For example in most places in the United States where there is licensure, massage/bodywork therapists aren't permitted to work directly on breast tissue. In some states, breast massage is permitted as long as there is informed consent. In other countries, such as Canada, it's an integral part of the training and the therapy.

Sexual Enterprise

Government officials (particularly in the United States) enacted laws and regulations in the attempt to hinder sexual enterprise. Examples include limiting hours of operation, placing physical restrictions (e.g., treatment room doors to remain unlocked, treatment rooms must have a window), not allowing practitioners to work out of their homes or do out-calls, requiring annual fingerprinting, and making cross-gender treatments illegal.

These examples demonstrate that state regulation is hardly a cure-all to a profession's problems. While state regulation is often perceived as the remedy to the problems caused by a hodge-podge of local laws, state laws can be as irrelevant and outdated. Such spurious restrictions tend to anger legitimate practitioners. If practitioners want to influence the laws that govern them, they must do more than vote in elections. They must know their laws and become active in changing them.

> Wisdom too often never comes, and so one ought not to reject it merely because it comes late.
>
> —Felix Frankfurter

Unregulated Professions

Many professions have surfaced that aren't regulated by state boards, such as holistic health coaches and nutrition consultants. If a state doesn't have laws that specifically regulate a field, then most likely a clearly designated scope of practice doesn't exist.

Often, somatic practitioners choose to engage in dual professions. Practicing two professions, one that is licensed or credentialed and the other that isn't, has legal and ethical ramifications. Legally, the practitioner is required to perform within the scope of practice of the licensed profession. Ethically, it's a session-by-session decision regarding what information is provided and the language in which this information is stated. This carries with it a sense of freedom, as well as an imposing responsibility.

It is the practitioner's responsibility to check state and local laws, verifying that the services she offers in an unregulated profession doesn't fall within the scope of practice of another regulated profession. For instance, nutrition consultants need to ensure that they aren't practicing as a dietitian or a nutritionist, as these are generally licensed, regulated professions in most states. The scope of practice for the dietitian states what services the licensed professional in that field can provide. The nutrition consultant can't provide those services.

1. Jerry is a distributor for a line of vitamin and mineral supplements. He believes in this product line and takes many of the supplements himself. It is because he has done research and learned the high quality of this product line that he has chosen to sell these in his office. When a client arrives and begins looking at the bottles of supplements, the practitioner offers the client a brochure about the product line. There is no sales pitch or pressure—just informational data is provided. Should the client choose to purchase any of these products, great! If not, fine.

2. Tom is a distributor for a line of vitamin and mineral supplements because he learned that this was a terrific passive revenue source. He had attended a convention where this line of products was advertised and the representative gave him an amazing sales talk about how much money could be made by selling these supplements. The practitioner's business had been down the past year and he was looking for ways to increase his income. The products were beautifully packaged, priced a bit on the high end, and were endorsed by a really cool movie star!

   When a client arrives and begins looking at the various bottles of supplements, the practitioner notices and approaches the client with an enthusiastic, "These are the vitamins that I take. They are a very high quality and the company that manufactures them is known worldwide. They're priced a bit higher than other brands you might find at a superstore or the local health food store, but well worth it! I feel so much better, I haven't gotten sick since I started taking them, and wait until you read the testimonials from the famous people who take these! You should take them for a while and see how great they can make you feel."

Points to Ponder

How does Tom's response differ from Jerry's? Did either lie to the client? Did either break the law? Which one is practicing the most appropriate professional ethics?

For the nutrition consultant who is educating the client about a supplement, the client will inevitably ask, "How much of that should I take? Should I take it every day? For how long?" The unlicensed nutrition consultant isn't qualified to prescribe this supplement, and answering these questions can definitely be considered as prescribing. So, what is the appropriate response?

Figure 7.5 Ethical Client Education Checklist

- Make referrals to your published resources of clinical studies.
- State facts in a generic manner.
- Make "I" statements about "What I would do if I were you."

Using statements, like the following, allows the practitioner to remain ethical, even when practicing in unregulated territory.

1. **MAKE REFERRALS TO YOUR PUBLISHED RESOURCES OF CLINICAL STUDIES**
   According to Dr. Elson Haas in his book, *Staying Healthy with Nutrition*, there have been clinical studies that show X amount of this supplement improves the immune response.

2. **STATE FACTS IN A GENERIC MANNER**
   The American Dietetic Association states that X amount of this vitamin is the daily recommended dose.

3. **MAKE "I" STATEMENTS ABOUT "WHAT I WOULD DO IF I WERE YOU"**
   - If this was for me, I would take X amount of that supplement several times throughout the day.
   - When my neck gets stiff, I do these stretches every few hours, especially when I sit at the computer for any length of time.
   - If I were running every morning, I would do these stretches to keep my legs from getting too tight.

Empowering a client is the goal of every practitioner. Telling a client what to do doesn't empower the client; educating the client, offering ideas and recommendations, and then allowing the client to make the final decision does empower.

Getting Involved

Ethical practitioners are concerned about the quality of the overall profession. This quality is affected by both good and bad laws. Therefore, it's important for practitioners to work in their communities to increase the understanding and acceptance of their services as a valuable wellness modality. It is equally important to abide by all laws governing their practice and work for the repeal or revision of detrimental or specious laws. In brief, practitioners must get civically involved. Individually and collectively, practitioners make a difference by helping shape and change the laws that govern them. Here is where to start if you want to find out about your laws, clarify the meaning of a law, or if you disagree with a law and want to change it:

- If you have state licensure, call the state office that issues your license. If you don't have state licensure but have municipal regulations, call your city or town hall and ask for the department that issues licenses for your profession.
- Ask for the person who answers specific questions about practice laws. Find out if a professional board exists. Ideally, a governing body has an appointed advisory board consisting of both licensed, experienced practitioners and lay persons. A board serves to oversee the relevance and implementation of the laws.
- Ask for a copy of applicable laws to be sent to you. Read these laws.
- If a board doesn't exist, ask what must be done to create one.
- In the event that a bill must be passed to create a regulatory board, contact your local senators and representatives. Be prepared because they're likely to ask you for specific, documented ideas. Find ideas of what you want by researching other states' laws.
- If no laws govern where you practice, contact your professional organization's local chapter for information on action that has been taken toward legislation.

> Never doubt that a small group of committed people can change the world. Indeed, it's very often the only thing that does.
>
> —Margaret Meade

Key Factor Two: Educational Training

One definition of Scope is "the knowledge base and practice parameters of a profession."[9] Use of the term "practice parameters" implies there's a collective Scope for a profession. However, defining these practice parameters isn't always an easy task. The phrase "knowledge base" suggests that there's a common framework of fundamental information provided by the educational training process in a particular field.

Training in many of the somatic modalities is unlike training in the branches of chiropractic, acupuncture, and physical therapy. In these latter standardized professions, basic training programs throughout the country are fairly consistent in what they teach the students to know and do. Educational offerings in massage and bodywork training programs are as diverse and inconsistent as the local laws that govern them; it's difficult to define a comprehensive, consistent, common knowledge base.

Ultimately, if local licensing laws exist where you practice, they govern your Scope and determine what you can and can't do. Even if laws exist, many of them are very general and make no mention of specific modalities. So, while the laws serve as a guide, two practitioners governed by the same laws may have significant differences in their scopes of practice based on their education and unique knowledge base. Beyond the law's watchful eye, educational training individualizes Scope and it becomes a personal issue rather than a collective one. Ethical practitioners must be mindful about the limitations of their training, regardless of what they're lawfully permitted to do.

Key Factor Three: Competency

Ability and proficiency influence Scope, as well as educational training and laws. This brings forth the questions, "What determines competency?" and "Who is the ultimate judge of competency?" In many localities, the law states that competency is presumed once the required number of hours of formal education is complete. Growing numbers of city and state laws require practitioners to pass a written exam as a method to verify competency requirements. Unfortunately, written exams vary in degree of difficulty and efficacy, which is why many licensing boards defer to tests developed by independent organizations or national certification boards such as the Federation of State Massage Therapy Boards (FSMTB), the National Certification Board for Therapeutic Massage and Bodywork (NCBTMB), and the National Certification Commission for Acupuncture and Oriental Medicine (NCCAOM).

http://www.fsmtb.org/
http://www.ncbtmb.org/
http://www.nccaom.org/

Beyond basic training, offerings for advanced studies abound. Once again, the ethical concern of competency brings more questions. Does a practitioner need credentials from a week-long course, or does it suffice to attend a two-hour seminar to become adept in a new method? Is watching a video on the subject, or reading a book, adequate to claim proper training and competency? How much and what type of training is adequate?

A client comes to a practitioner complaining of fatigue and achiness throughout his body. With little more than a weekend's training in nutrition, the practitioner recommends dietary supplements and a change in diet for the client. The client's condition deteriorates over the next few weeks and he ends up in the hospital.

Points to Ponder

Should this practitioner have advised the client at all? If so, what should the practitioner advise in this case?

Patricia J. Benjamin, PH.D., former national director of education for the American Massage Therapy Association (AMTA), warns against "paper tiger" credentials: credentials, titles, or certifications which may sound impressive but which lack teeth. She says:

> A disturbing number of practitioners are claiming credentials in various disciplines or specialties only after an introductory workshop or a few hours on the subject. If a credential is to mean something of value, it must represent meeting a certain standard of quality or the significant mastery of a particular area, and not just a passing familiarity.[10]

In an evolving profession, determining competence requires self-accountability on the practitioner's part. In addition to meeting all legal and educational requirements, the ethical practitioner must seriously evaluate her training, experience, and confidence before offering treatment to clients as a professional.

Key Factor Four: Self-Accountability

Scope of practice is a very individual thing. Self-accountability is the most decisive factor that keeps you functioning within your individual Scope. When you're self-accountable, you're answerable to, and responsible for, what you say and do, even when there's no external authority present. Unless you have internalized the laws and guidelines that define the limits of your practice, you're at a high risk of violating your professional scope of practice and ethical responsibilities.

See Chapter 1 pages 17-19 for details on **Self-Accountability**.

In the seclusion of your private practice, and behind the closed doors of your treatment rooms, you're often left with no one but yourself to hold you accountable, and you could transgress the scope of your practice without anyone ever knowing. Governing laws, education and training, and competency influence your Scope only when you obey the laws, carry out what you have learned and been trained to do, and perform your work competently. No matter what code of ethics you outwardly subscribe to, and regardless of your proclaimed litany of beliefs, it's self-accountability that creates and sustains your personal and professional ethics and keeps you functioning within the parameters of your Scope. Self-accountability enforces scope of practice.

Personalize Your Scope

Governing laws in your locality, an individually acquired knowledge base, and a capacity to apply and practice responsibly and well are what personalize the Scope.

Figure 7.6 **Personalizing Scope Checklist**

1. Update Your Resume.
2. Define Your Personal Strengths.
3. Review Local Licensing Laws.
4. Retire Old Techniques and Modalities.
5. Network with Other Professionals.
6. Represent Yourself Honestly.
7. Be attentive to High Risk Areas.

These steps assist in clarifying and personalizing your Scope:

1. **UPDATE YOUR RESUME**

   This is a very effective way to outline what you know about the breadth and width of your acquired knowledge base. List education, training, and work experience, including what you did before you became a practitioner. Everything you know, and have done, contributes to who you are as a person. In some cases, the work may actually enrich your Scope. For example, a practitioner who was a physical therapist before becoming a massage therapist has a knowledge base and experience that makes her personal Scope different from a chiropractor who becomes an acupuncturist. She would most likely have very different approaches to working with a client who sees her for low back pain.

2. **DEFINE YOUR PERSONAL STRENGTHS**
   List techniques, procedures, and modalities that you do regularly and in which you feel competent.

3. **REVIEW YOUR LOCAL LICENSING LAWS**
   Become familiar with what is permitted and prohibited by the law and stay current with legislative changes that affect you. Function honestly within your legal limits.

4. **RETIRE THE TECHNIQUES AND MODALITIES YOU KNOW BUT SELDOM DO**
   As in all skills, "Practice makes permanent" (not necessarily perfect) and, "Use it, or lose it." If, for example, you haven't performed foot reflexology since your course in school three years ago, serve the client who requests a reflexology treatment by referring him to a colleague who does it regularly. Do not list reflexology on your business card. If your list reminds you of aspirations you have long forgotten, decide if you want to pursue them at this time.

5. **NETWORK WITH OTHER PROFESSIONALS**
   Talk with them about their Scopes and see how yours is different from theirs. The contrast helps you better identify your own parameters, strengths, and limitations. Also, knowing what others do and their specialties offers you referral options for clients whose needs exceed your abilities.

6. **REPRESENT YOURSELF HONESTLY**
   Be realistic about what you were officially and properly trained in, versus information you acquired in your travels through life. Being self-taught is a valuable attribute, but there are substantial differences between working in a field or researching it for years and watching one or two videos on a subject.

7. **BE ATTENTIVE TO HIGH RISK AREAS**
   These situations tempt you to go beyond your qualifications. Prepare responses for these situations such as, "That isn't within my scope of practice; I can refer you to someone for that."

 Defining Your Scope

LAW
- Discuss the advantages and disadvantages of licensure, certification, registration, and title protection with a colleague or partner. Summarize this discussion in your journal.
- Review your state (or city) laws and regulations. Identify any items of concern.

TRAINING
- Describe the activities and modalities that are within your Scope.
- Describe the ways in which your Scope might be different than your colleagues' Scopes.

COMPETENCY
- Describe the characteristics that determine competency and list ways to objectively identify competency.
- List factors that could contribute to different Scopes for colleagues in the same field.

SELF-ACCOUNTABILITY
- Identify areas and activities that technically fall within your Scope but might be questionable for you to do.
- Determine the areas or circumstances that are high risk and might tempt you to go beyond your qualifications.
- Identify past actions or circumstances that you would prefer no one knew.

Standards of Practice

Scope of Practice mainly covers the limits of a practitioner's service, whereas Standards of Practice describe the underlying principles of a given field, the expectations of professional conduct, and the quality of care provided to clients. Standards of Practice often elaborate upon the items in a Code of Ethics. The contents of Standards of Practice, Scope of Practice, and Codes of Ethics frequently overlap.

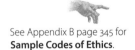

See Appendix B page 345 for **Sample Codes of Ethics**.

The broad categories covered in Standards of Practice are: professionalism, competence, professional excellence; legal and ethical requirements; protecting the public and profession; responsibility to the client; confidentiality; business practices; professional relationships, roles, and boundaries; prevention of sexual misconduct; professional conduct; educating the public; research; fees; accurate representation of Scope; professional appearance; continued education; courtesy; and integrity. Some Standards of Practice list a broad statement for each category, while others elaborate in great detail. The specific requirements vary greatly in the different professions. Check with professional associations (most associations post this information on their websites) to find the most current standards. The following list contains common statements in most Standards of Practice:

- Conduct practice in a professional manner.
- Dress appropriately.
- Respect the rights and dignity of all clients.
- Provide accurate information to the client about the profession and services provided.
- Maintain high standards and give highest regard to the clients' welfare.
- Communicate clearly using appropriate terminology.
- Provide services within the profession's Scope of Practice and in accordance with the laws.
- Abide by the profession's Code of Ethics.
- Accurately represent your level of competence, education, training, and experience.
- Make judgments that are commensurate with qualifications and accept responsibility for the exercise of sound judgment.
- Perform appropriate assessment.
- Refer to other practitioners when appropriate.
- Seek professional advice when needed.
- Act with due regard for the needs, special competencies, and obligations of colleagues.
- Refrain from falsely impugning the reputation of any colleague.
- Remain in good standing with professional associations.
- Maintain accurate records and store them properly.
- Protect clients' confidentiality.
- Provide a safe physical environment.
- Maintain adequate and customary insurance.
- Promote business in an honest and dignified manner.
- Recognize the psychological principles involved in working with clients.
- Avoid dual relationships that could exploit or harm clients, employees, or co-workers.
- Refrain from practicing when your judgment or competence is impaired by intake of drugs or alcohol, or by a physical or mental incapacity.
- Refrain from participating in sexual conduct, sexual activities, or sexualizing behavior with clients.
- Maintain and promote high standards of practice, education, and research.
- Seek remuneration for services that is deserved and reasonable.
- Protect the public and profession from unethical, incompetent, or illegal acts.
- Report to the proper authorities any other practitioner's alleged violations of the law, Code of Ethics, Scope, or Standards of Practice.
- Participate in activities that contribute to the health and wellbeing of the public.

Analyze your Profession's Standards of Practice

Review your state/province/national Standards of Practice and identify the following: items that you highly value; statements that are vague; standards that you don't agree with; additions you would like to include.

Client/Practitioner Expectations

Creating a practice with integrity is made much easier by clearly expressing your expectations. Topics to consider are procedures, draping, communication guidelines, attitude, interaction level outside of the actual treatment, illness, and etiquette expectations.

Procedures

Ease the anxiety some people feel about seeing a practitioner for the first time by giving new clients a description of what occurs during the first and subsequent sessions. Address these questions: Do you start with an intake interview and a history? If so, how much time is allotted and does this take away from the "hands-on" portion of the session? Does the length of sessions vary? Will the client need to disrobe or wear specific clothing? What safety measures are observed? What happens if something occurs that makes the client uncomfortable? Should a client refrain from eating prior to sessions? Do you allow interruptions (e.g., telephone calls)? If so, how are they handled? Are there any unusual reactions the client might experience during or after the first (or subsequent) session?

Draping

Appropriate draping is crucial if clients need to remove some or all of their clothing to receive your treatment. Draping, or covering a client, fosters a sense of safety and emphasizes your professionalism. Instruct clients about your standard procedure: tell them to undress to their level of comfort; direct them as to which articles of clothing to leave on; or ask them to put on a smock. Tell them how to position and cover themselves on the table (e.g., lie on the table and cover yourself with the top sheet or towel). Inform clients that you leave the room while they change in private and you knock before entering.

Draping concerns aren't limited to the initial covering of the client: they also include draping for privacy throughout the session. Sometimes it's necessary to add more draping in the course of the treatment if your work entails some type of movement, positioning, or work that exposes another part of the body. Also it's best to only uncover the area that is directly receiving work and never work under the drape.

Communication

Understanding the communication expectations of your clients and choosing appropriate language and terminology is very important. Therapeutic outcomes and client retention improve as expectations are met and trust grows. The clearer you communicate in the beginning of the therapeutic relationship about your own style and expectations, the sooner the client can be at ease. Consider the depth of information you require during your client intake, and be sure you can articulate the reasons for your requirements. Both you and the client should be comfortable with the levels of self-disclosure. Also, keep in mind that confidence is instilled by your ability to remain professional.

Attitudes

Your attitudes toward your work and toward people greatly impact the therapeutic outcome. Ethical healthcare professionals demonstrate respect for all clients regardless of their age, gender, race, national origin, sexual orientation, religion, socio-economic status, body type, political affiliation, state of health, and personal habits. Unfortunately, not everyone has reached this point of maturity. Nina McIntosh states the following in her book, *The Educated Heart*:

> *We owe clients our care and attention. We may not connect with a person right away, but if we cannot imagine ever having a caring attitude toward a particular client, we shouldn't work with him/her. We need to be on the alert for anything that interferes with our abilities to touch a client in a respectful, non-judgmental way. We are not just touching bodies—we're touching spirits"*[11]

Interaction

Clarify the level of your availability to clients: your hours (including parameters for extended hours); location (e.g., do you also work with clients at their business or home?); how quickly you return telephone calls and e-mail; and the time allotted before and after sessions to answer questions or offer support.

Follow-up tends to be a weak area in most practices. While it's a good idea to place appointment reminder calls, first find out if your clients want you to do it, when they want it, and where they want to receive the calls. Some practitioners call new clients within 48 hours after their first session just to check in. Others also like to call clients who have experienced a major shift or event during the session. Regardless of the type and frequency of follow-up, always discuss the policy first with your clients.

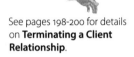

See pages 198-200 for details on **Terminating a Client Relationship**.

Etiquette

Etiquette is a code of behavior that delineates expectations. Professional etiquette concerns behaviors that fall under the heading of good manners: cancellation notification and being punctual; hygiene (e.g., bathing prior to a session and refraining from wearing strong perfume); and personal habits such as smoking on the premises or arriving in an altered state.

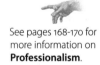

See pages 168-170 for more information on **Professionalism**.

Illness

An ethical question arises whenever a practitioner is at risk of infecting a client. If a practitioner has a condition that is clearly infectious, the decision to cancel an appointment is easily made. More difficult is the case of the common cold. When a practitioner has a cold, or symptoms which may indicate the onset of a cold, there's a tendency to ignore the situation or dismiss it as inconsequential. This avoidance of clear decision-making can be exacerbated if the practitioner is experiencing financial pressure. Nevertheless, the practitioner's responsibility to the client should take precedence ("Do no harm"). The practitioner is obligated to notify the client prior to the appointment to discuss it.

This becomes even more important if the client is immunologically compromised. Two of the most common clients in this category are those receiving cancer treatment, especially chemotherapy, and those with HIV; these clients are most susceptible to all infections. Their cases are clear-cut but only if the practitioner is aware of the client's condition. If there's ever any question of compromising a client's health, the ethical action is to call and cancel the session or offer the client the option of canceling the session.

The same expectations apply to clients. You should clearly communicate the expectation that if a client is sick and may be infectious, he should either postpone his appointment or at least call you to discuss the situation.

Figure 7.7 **Client/Practitioner Expectations**

- Procedures
- Draping
- Communication guidelines
- Attitude

- Level of interaction outside of the actual treatment
- Etiquette
- Illness

Time Management

Successful practitioners make time management a priority. Create appropriate time frames for your appointments that help you stay on time. Establishing a time frame for your interactions with a client creates a boundary. The structure and expectation about treatment time and your availability is determined by the specific situation. Clarification is particularly important at the beginning of the treatment process since different disciplines (as well as individual practitioners) have varying time policies, and clients may easily make inaccurate assumptions about yours.

Punctuality on the part of the practitioner connotes respect for both parties. While being late under certain circumstances is understandable, tardiness is usually perceived as annoying and disrespectful. Be sure to communicate the length of initial and follow-up appointments to your clients, and set clear guidelines for scheduling changes, lateness, cancellations, and emergencies.

Start and End on Time

Starting and ending a session on time establishes a clear boundary. Practitioners who run professional practices are generally on time. Every practitioner may be late occasionally but if the practitioner consistently runs a little late, this is a significant signal that he has difficulty with the boundaries of time and has possibly set up his schedule without enough space to respect the client's time. For instance, if a practitioner needs 45 minutes of actual treatment time for each appointment and schedules clients at 45 minute intervals, there's no leeway for the unexpected. If this practitioner finds it difficult to keep this schedule and run on time, it makes sense to change the interval to an hour. Schedule appointments with 10 or 15 minutes of leeway to make calls between sessions, take notes, enjoy a snack, stretch, or accommodate clients who need a little extra time to get ready.

Another type of time problem occurs when a practitioner keeps a client significantly beyond the ending time of the appointment without asking the client's permission. The client may have other commitments after the appointment with this practitioner. Blatant disregard for the client's time is as much a boundary violation as any other.

The concept of time varies for different cultures. In certain cultures time isn't very important or it may even be a non-issue. Time is often a precious commodity in Western culture and usually holds great significance to clients. If the boundary of time is consistently violated a client may draw several conclusions: the practitioner doesn't care; the practitioner is too busy to really listen; the practitioner is unprofessional; the practitioner is inattentive; the practitioner is irresponsible; the practitioner is overwhelmed; the practitioner has poor time management skills; or the practitioner has no respect for time.

Cancellations

Cancellations can be disconcerting for both parties, particularly if they happen frequently and at the last minute. A clear cancellation policy reduces this problem. Some practitioners require a 24-hour cancellation notice or the client is billed (either in part or full) for the session. Other practitioners whose practices consist of last-minute or walk-in clientele often only require a four-hour or eight-hour cancellation policy. Along with this policy, some practitioners stipulate that the client is not billed if the appointment slot is filled. A simple statement often suffices, such as; "If cancellation is necessary, please give 24-hour notice or you're charged for the appointment unless it can be filled. Emergency cancellations are determined at the practitioner's discretion."

Turnabout is fair play. Consider including a statement like this: "If I need to cancel an appointment, I do so within 24 hours whenever possible. If an emergency arises and I can't keep an appointment, I provide a 50 percent discount with a client's next session. For non-emergency cancellations of less than 24 hours, your next session is at no charge."

▌ Confidentiality

Confidentiality can be defined as the practitioner's guarantee to the client that what occurs in the therapeutic setting remains private and protected. First and foremost, the issue of confidentiality concerns the client's rights to privacy and safety. These rights belong equally to every client you see regardless of age, status, or relationship to you or another client. These same rights apply to both verbal and written interactions you have with anyone other than the client.

As a model for confidentiality in the somatic professions, we turn to the profession of psychotherapy where these issues have been examined and developed over many years.[12] The ethical guidelines of most helping professions include a statement about confidentiality (with the goal of helping practitioners make ethical decisions regarding confidentiality). Nevertheless, these ethical statements often fall short of satisfactorily defining the parameters of the client's right to confidentiality. As with other ethical questions throughout the book, practitioners may find it challenging to apply confidentiality guidelines in complex situations.

Most people are clear about major confidentiality breaches, such as sharing important personal information about a client with a third party, yet subtle situations occur where boundaries are easy to cross. Consider the following scenarios:

> The closer and more confidential our relationship with someone, the less we are entitled to ask about what we are not voluntarily told.
>
> —Louis Kronenberger

1. A well-known politician comes to you for treatment. Do you think twice about sharing this exciting news with your friends?
2. Your best friend sends his wife to you for a session. Do you stop and consider if it's appropriate to answer his questions about her session?
3. You schedule a session with a 13-year-old boy who will be accompanied by his mother. Prior to the session do you think about whether to work with the boy alone or with the mother present?

Points to Ponder

If you answered "yes" to any of the questions posed in these scenarios, you have already begun to deal ethically with the issue of confidentiality in your work. Do you think you would maintain confidentiality and trust in these or similar situations?

Maintaining Confidentiality

Confidentiality guidelines for somatic professions generally state that information shared between client and practitioner during a session remains private. These guidelines are usually further interpreted to mean that client names, details of treatment, and information shared by clients during sessions are not discussed by the practitioner with anyone else.

Behind confidentiality issues are two assumptions: that an important and personal relationship exists between client and practitioner, and that trust is an essential element in this relationship. The client who knows that his right to privacy is honored is more likely to develop the trust necessary for a successful, healthy outcome of the therapeutic encounter. For example, it may be very tempting to tell your friends about the well-known politician/athlete/musician/film star who is your client, or to do a little name-dropping at a social function. You might even be tempted to use this client's name or title in your advertising (e.g., "acupuncturist to the mayor!") All of these actions, however, cross the ethical boundary of confidentiality. The mayor, like every client, has the right to privacy about her sessions with you.

If the mayor chooses to tell others that she knows your work, you have gained a valuable referral. You, however, are still bound by the ethics of confidentiality. Her reference to you doesn't give you permission to discuss her case with others. If you break this ethical policy, even in casual conversation, it looks as though you're trading on a well-known name and you always run the chance that what you have said could get back to your client. If the situation turns out negatively, you may lose not only the client but professional respect as well. If you work with celebrities or public figures and you want to let others know, obtain disclosure permission (preferably in writing) from the client.

All your clients deserve the same confidential treatment you would give the mayor. In the introductory scenarios, the spouse asking about his wife is, hopefully unknowingly, asking you to cross an ethical boundary. And though a number of your friends may know you treat each of them, you aren't implicitly authorized to say anything about another's session. You can avoid unethical behavior by saying in a light-hearted manner, "You know it's against my policies to discuss anything that happens in a session with anyone. I'm sure [Terry] would enjoy talking with you about her session." Finally, if you trade sessions, or otherwise treat a fellow health professional, he too benefits more from your work together if you maintain his privacy and safety.

Limits of Ethical Confidentiality

The limits of confidentiality can be an area of confusion and misinformation on the part of both practitioners and clients. Not all healthcare relationships are held to be "privileged" relationships. Unlike a psychotherapist, medical or psychological information about the client isn't necessarily legally held in confidence by the practitioner. Therefore it's vital that a well-researched and clear policy statement regarding confidentiality be presented and the practitioner discloses any exceptions to absolute confidentiality.

Two major considerations underlie the limits of professional confidentiality: the practitioner's obligations to the law, and the practitioner's obligations to others.

In regards to your obligations to the law: the legal system may have the right to subpoena your client lists or even your client records. Client files contain information so that you can properly work with any given client. Although you want your files to contain accurate and thorough information, your actual treatment records should only include information as it relates to the treatment and not superfluous notes (e.g., refrain from inscribing details about a client's eccentricities or personal relationships).

Some reasons for breaking confidentiality include: there's a clear and imminent danger to the client or another individual; a client discloses an intention to commit a crime; you suspect abuse or neglect of a child, an elderly person, or an incapacitated individual.

Confidentiality and its limits don't exist in black and white terms. When making ethical decisions, practitioners choose among various levels of thinking and functioning. From one vantage, abiding by the law may seem clear-cut; from another vantage, doing what is best for your client may mean questioning the law; from still another vantage, protecting a third party may mean breaking the client's trust. The practitioner must combine knowledge of the situation with a clear understanding of the ethics involved, and temper these with wisdom and experience.

Practitioners may also reveal details of therapy encounters to their supervisors or supervision groups. In these discussions the names of clients are withheld although other pertinent information and treatment particulars may be shared.

Actions That Minimize Confidentiality Problems

When you tell your clients up front about the limits to the confidentiality of your work together, they're much better able to give informed consent regarding treatment from you. Therefore, early in your professional relationships let your clients know that you hold your work together as confidential, and that you may discuss your work with your supervisor, and that legal or ethical obligations may require you to break confidentiality in extreme circumstances.

The practitioner should avoid making unilateral decisions about breaking confidentiality. Even in some of the legal instances described above, if you must make the decision to break confidentiality, you should discuss your decision with the client beforehand. In this way, while the client may not agree with your decision, she is informed of your reasons.

When you want permission to discuss the professional relationship elsewhere, you should have a specific reason for doing so. This reason should be discussed with the client, and the client needs to give specific written consent. For example, you may wish to correspond about the client with another healthcare provider, or to use details about the client's condition, treatment, and outcome in an article or presentation. The client's permission should specify exactly what details, such as name, dates of visit, and treatment records he is authorizing you to share, as well as any specific limitations on where, when, and how you may share the information.

In general, as soon as you perceive a potential problem surrounding confidentiality, the situation should be discussed with the client. When the 13-year-old boy and his mother are in your treatment room together, whatever one shares, the other hears and confidentiality between the two of them is implicitly set aside. At the first session these clients should be informed about whether you'll work or speak with either of them privately; if so, specify whether you keep what one says to you confidential from the other and what limits you may put on this confidentiality. In this way, both son and mother utilize the therapeutic encounter more successfully.

See pages 193-195 for more information on **Working with Minors**.

Documentation

Confidentiality certainly involves not sharing client information, and also involves the safe-keeping of client records.

The documentation of client sessions (also known as charting) is a vital activity in all wellness practices. Charting is an important way to document and monitor client progress and outcomes. The most accurate charts are those in which notes are taken in a timely manner, preferably during or just after the session. Charts should only include information related to the client's condition and treatment, not unrelated personal information. If what a client had for breakfast directly affects his condition or treatment plan, include it; if not, leave it out. Accuracy is important, so if you have to change anything in a chart after the fact, be sure to initial and date the change.

Intake forms, charts, treatment plans, payment information, and any other documented client information are considered private and must be protected. As we will see in the next section, health records are protected under law.

Breaking Confidence

- Describe situations where it could be easy to inadvertently break confidentiality.
- Identify circumstances when it's okay or even necessary to break confidentiality.
- Specify actions to minimize confidentiality problems.

Health Insurance Portability and Accountability Act

HIPAA Privacy Rule

http://www.hhs.gov/ocr/privacy/

Significant changes have been made regarding how healthcare practitioners protect their clients' privacy. The right to privacy is mentioned in many places in American law (and probably many other countries). The Fourth Amendment to the U.S. Constitution in particular guarantees that "the right of the people to be secure in their persons, houses, papers, and effects, against unreasonable searches and seizures shall not be violated."

In 1996, the U.S. Congress passed the Medical Records Confidentiality Act in an effort to establish uniform privacy protection for personally identifiable health information. On one hand, clients gained access to any health information about themselves and it gave people a chance to correct this information. In 1998, the Children's Online Privacy Protection Act was enacted to safeguard children online.

A far more comprehensive strategy was passed in 1996 known as the *Health Insurance Portability and Accountability Act*, or **HIPAA**, and healthcare providers (and other agents) were mandated to comply with its requirements as of April 2003.

Figure 7.8 **The Four Facets of** HIPAA

1. **ELECTRONIC HEALTH TRANSACTIONS STANDARDS**
   When billing insurance, practitioners are required to use the Standard Code Sets of the International Classification of Disease (ICD) codes and the Current Procedural Terminology (CPT) codes.

2. **UNIQUE IDENTIFIERS FOR PROVIDERS, EMPLOYERS, HEALTH PLANS, AND CLIENTS**
   Each practitioner who transmits electronically is assigned a National Provider Identifier (NPI).

3. **SECURITY OF HEALTH INFORMATION & ELECTRONIC SIGNATURE STANDARDS**
   All practitioners must provide uniform levels of protection of all health information that is stored or transmitted electronically. This includes your computer, along with any faxes and email messages sent. An electronic signature is required for all HIPAA transactions.

4. **PRIVACY AND CONFIDENTIALITY**
   Limits the non-consensual use and release of private health information; gives clients new rights to access their medical records and to know who else has accessed them; restricts most disclosure of health information to the minimum needed for the intended purpose; institutes criminal and civil sanctions for improper use or disclosure; and establishes new requirements for access to records by researchers and others.

HIPAA has three major purposes: (1) to protect and enhance the rights of consumers by providing them access to their health information and controlling the inappropriate use of that information; (2) to improve the quality of health care in the United States by restoring trust in the healthcare system among consumers, healthcare professionals, and the multitude of organizations and individuals committed to the delivery of care; and (3) to improve the efficiency and effectiveness of health care delivery by creating a national framework for health privacy protection that builds on efforts by states, health systems, individual organizations, and individuals.

HIPAA Compliance

Who are the covered entities under HIPAA? Section 1172(a)(1) describes "health plans, health care clearinghouses, and healthcare providers who transmit any health information in electronic form in connection with a transaction referred to in section 1173(a)(1) of the Act." **If you have read this far and are thinking that because you don't use electronic claims submission (ECS) you're exempt, think again**. If all your information is kept on paper, you don't have to comply on the surface; however, if you plan to fax, e-mail, or in any other way electronically send information, you're responsible. Nor are you exempt if you bill insurance and any of the other entities (e.g., a health care plan) electronically submits your typed claim form. In any event, plan on complying with HIPAA. As an ethical practitioner, you have a duty to protect your clients' privacy.

Get your assigned **National Provider Identifier**

https://nppes.cms.hhs.gov/ NPPES/Welcome.do

Following the HIPAA guidelines actually makes good business sense, and the requirements are fairly easy to implement. Consumers are used to receiving privacy policy statements from other healthcare providers. Your clients might find it disconcerting if you don't follow suit. Note that even if you don't need to be HIPAA compliant for your own practice, you still need to be compliant if you work with other covered entities. Thus, if a PCP refers a client to you or you send a client's progress report to her doctor, then you're considered a Business Associate: persons, companies, or entities hired by the practitioner to perform duties, requiring access, the use of, or disclosure of a client's Protected Health Information (PHI). Also, be aware that state regulations might be more stringent than the federal requirements.

Failure to heed the HIPAA regulations can result in civil and criminal penalties, starting at $100 per person per violation, not exceeding $25,000 per year per person. The penalties get worse for knowingly violating HIPAA, especially if the offense is "under false pretenses" where there is a potential fine of up to $100,000 and/or imprisonment up to five years. If the offense is with intent to sell a client's information the penalty is up to $250,000 and 10 years imprisonment.

In her blog, Tara the SpeechyKeenSLP, discusses the use of the Double Lock Rule(DLR)[13] to ensure the safeguard of client files and electronic records:

> When it comes to paper files, the DLR applies to physical locks. For files you keep in your office, they should be kept in a locked cabinet behind a locked door. When placing files in your car, the files should be places in a locked file box, then locked into the trunk of your car. If you keep your notes, client files, data, and more on your laptop or tablet device, the DLR still applies. All devices (e.g., laptops, iPads) should all be password protected. If you password protect the files as well it increases the security of that information further. The devices should be kept physically secured in a trunk or in a locked office, for example.

Figure 7.9 Simple Steps for HIPAA Compliance

- Take client privacy and confidentiality very seriously. The penalties for violation are steep and there are felony charges that could potentially cause the loss of your license.
- Designate someone in your office (or hire an outside party) to create a process to handle PHI.
- Train your office staff on how to handle PHI, including under what circumstances PHI may be disclosed.
- Use consent/authorization documents that the client signs.
- Do not discuss **any** medical information with any third parties unless **written** consent or authorization has been obtained.
- Be careful when discussing a client's PHI with office staff; disseminate it on a need-to-know basis.
- Assign User IDs and passwords to anyone with access to electronic information (e.g., computer billing software, voice dictation programs).
- Contact your practice management software company and make sure the version you're using is compliant.
- Use passwords and security programs to protect and maintain computer files.
- For e-mail, obtain written consent from the client and use encryption software. Use electronic signatures to authenticate who sent the e-mail.
- Use auditing software to monitor who sent what and when.
- Create a policy for the destruction and retention of medical records that also includes e-mail communications.
- Design a client information sheet that explains the following: how you use their information; the storage method for client files; the circumstances under which you may disclose client information; and the procedure for clients to see or obtain copies of their files.
- Store all client files in a locked room or in a locked cabinet. Only allow authorized employees access to these files.
- Do not leave files in an area that is accessible by clients or unauthorized staff.
- Keep appointment books from view of anyone, except those directly dealing with client care.
- Get authorization from clients about marketing (including greeting cards, flyers, and newsletters).
- Present each client with a "Notice of Privacy Policies" form. New clients must sign a separate form indicating that they have received the Notice of Privacy Policies.
- Each client must sign a form giving consent for treatment, payment, and healthcare operations.
- When applicable, have clients sign an authorization for any and all release of PHI.
- Put confidentiality notices on all faxes and emails.

Informed Consent

If you have ever felt the powerlessness of undergoing a medical procedure without fully understanding what to expect, you know the importance of *informed consent*. If you have ever felt the frustration of not having your hair cut the way you specifically requested, you know the importance of informed consent.

Informed consent, a concept that arose in the medical field in the early 1960s, served as the initial nudge of a major shift in consumer empowerment known today as "patients' (or clients') rights." Prior to the establishment of informed consent, the patient was relatively powerless in relationship to a doctor's authority over medical and health care matters. Doctors and other medical professionals held a certain power over their patients simply because they had knowledge to which patients weren't privy. Diagnoses, prognoses, and procedures were secretive and mysterious; patients were the uninformed bystanders in their own health care.

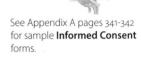
See Appendix A pages 341-342 for sample **Informed Consent** forms.

Because of informed consent, clients have the right to know about and fully participate in their own care. The client, or his guardian, must now give full consent for most care, except in emergencies where the client is incapacitated. The client also has the right to withhold or withdraw consent at any time. The consent given isn't considered valid unless the client is informed about all procedures he is expected to undergo, the reason for it, the possible risks and benefits, and reasonable alternatives to the procedure. Most importantly, the client must understand the information given.

It has become customary practice for the providers of many services outside the medical venue to practice the concept of informed consent. The consumer is now advised about what needs to be done or what is expected to happen before the service is rendered and the consumer must agree, either verbally or in writing, to the service. For example, when you take a vehicle to be serviced for an undiagnosed problem, the mechanic contacts you after the diagnosis is made and before the work is done to tell you what is needed and the estimated cost. You can opt to say, "Go ahead and do the work," or "Don't do the work." If more complications arise during the repair process, you're notified, and you must give your consent again. Like clients' rights, consumers' rights are protected now more than ever.

In theory, informed consent appears to adequately protect both the service provider and the consumer. Litigation is less likely to occur when the provider imparts information, offers an explanation of what is to occur, and the consumer gives full consent after being informed. Viewing informed consent **only** from a legally debatable standpoint is inadequate in the professional relationship that occurs between a somatic practitioner and a client. Informed consent between a practitioner and client provides the foundation and framework of an ethical and safe experience.

Informed consent also entails informing clients of what professional services you can legally and ethically provide as well as any limitations. Under the best of ethical conditions, informed consent is a twofold agreement in which the client and practitioner share an objective for the treatment or procedure and its outcome. The objective is explained, discussed, fully understood, and agreed upon by both the client and the practitioner before the treatment begins. Ethically speaking, the client needs to be *well-informed*, not *merely* informed. Most practitioners are very adept at offering information to their clients.

The Well-Informed Client

The following ideas are presented for your consideration, and as reminders, of the many ways in which we can keep our clients well-informed.

- Introduce yourself when a new client arrives for her appointment with a firm and friendly handshake and let her know that you're the practitioner with whom she will be working.
- Use a client agreement form to eliminate any misunderstandings about what your services are and are not.
- Be aware of why the client is seeking your services. Ask this question during the initial contact or add the question to your medical history form, but be sure to ask, "Why are you seeking these services at this time?" Follow this up in subsequent visits by asking the client at each pre-treatment assessment what her goal is for the session. When possible, meet her expectations; if it isn't feasible or possible, explain why.
- Explain procedures and invite input. A client reports on the medical history form that he is seeking massage to lower his stress and relieve his low back and hip pain. During the pre-treatment assessment you ask the client his goal for today's treatment, which is his very first massage experience, and he says, "To help my back pain." Before beginning the massage you inform the client: "After assessing you, (your complaints of pain, postural and range of motion assessments, and medical history), I would like to do a general relaxation massage treatment with some special focus to your low back and right hip area where you're experiencing pain. Since this is your first massage, I'll introduce your muscles to being massaged and use this first session to evaluate your response before I use deeper treatment methods. Does that sound like what you had in mind for today's treatment?"
- Do not assume that your client is familiar with your treatment process. Inform clients about what to expect by referring them to that section of your Policy Statement or offering them a "Welcome" form to read after they fill out their medical history.
- During the treatment, verbally inform the client when you're moving to more vulnerable areas, such as the anterior neck, medial thigh, and abdomen.
- Verbally inform the client when you're about to lean your own body against the table, or climb onto the table to assist your body mechanics or to facilitate stretches.
- Inform the client when your work deepens and check if it's tolerable.
- Get permission from the client before varying from the agreed upon treatment plan or using a new modality.
- Several minutes before the treatment ends, inform the client that the session is nearing completion and ask if she would like you to focus on an area that may need more attention.
- If a client is in a semi-sleep state, gently get her attention and tell her if you're about to do something that could be considered jarring (e.g., performing tapotement, applying stimulation to acupuncture needles).
- Keep in mind that there should be no surprises for the client. Remember that information, knowledge, and the right to refuse offer personal power to the client who is in a vulnerable or relaxed state.
- Inform the client about what to expect after the session. For example, when suitable, tell the client that he may experience soreness or tenderness the next day.
- Cover all bases so that neither you nor the client faces a situation without some preparation about what to expect beforehand. Let the only surprise be how much the client enjoyed the experience and how impressed she was by the way she was considered and nurtured during the treatment.

Informed Consent Form

Create a personalized Informed Consent Form, using the ideas presented in this section and the sample Informed Consent forms in Appendix A, page 341-342.

▌ Working with Minors

Working with minors requires special consideration. While legal definitions of who is a minor differ geographically, the purpose of all such definitions is protective. They establish a baseline for restrictions and safeguards that protect persons not yet recognized as adults.

Ethical standards also have a protective purpose, yet published guidelines often don't specifically address work with minors. Due to the intimate nature of somatic therapy, it's especially important to discuss how working with children and teenagers differs from working with adults, and to consider how ethical standards are maintained.

Special Considerations

While you should be even-handed about how you apply ethical standards to clients, you must certainly bring heightened awareness and sensitivity to ethical issues when working with children. One positive effect of laws regarding minors is to broaden the sense of responsibility toward youth so that all adults, not just their primary caretakers, share in this responsibility. In a session with a child, the practitioner may feel a similar broadening of responsibility for the child's welfare. It is helpful, then, for the practitioner to consider what special factors may clarify ethical decision-making to support the child's best interests. The three questions that begin this exploration are: What is the child's stage of development? Who is part of the therapeutic constellation? What are the therapeutic goals?

> "
> The ultimate lesson all of us have to learn is unconditional love, which includes not only others but ourselves as well.
>
> —Elisabeth Kubler-Ross

The Child's Stage of Development

Physical growth is, of course, a consideration in a session but it's only one of multiple arenas where the child develops. Emotional, cognitive, and social development also need to be taken into account. For example:
- Young people whose cognitive development is delayed may need the support of familiar people or places to receive the benefits of hands-on therapy.
- Girls who begin to menstruate at an early age may experience unresolved feelings about their bodies and generally don't develop a corresponding emotional maturity until years later.
- An infant who was separated from its parents immediately after birth for a prolonged period will likely have different needs and responses to touch therapy compared to an infant who achieved early bonding with parents.

By blending together, as much as possible, a complete picture of the child from these various aspects, a practitioner may design and implement a session that correctly meets the individual child's needs.

The Therapeutic Constellation

When a practitioner works with a minor, the therapeutic relationship expands beyond practitioner and client to include other caretakers. These may be one or both biological parents, adoptive parents, foster parents, social workers, or healthcare providers. Defining who is a part of the therapeutic constellation is an important early step when working with children.

The practitioner needs to know who is providing additional information about the child, who is helping to establish treatment goals, and to whom the practitioner must communicate about the progress of therapy.

Many practitioners value the autonomy and independence of their role in the therapeutic relationship. When working with minors, this individualism may need to be tempered for the child's best interest. The expanded therapeutic relationship can benefit the child by bringing together multiple concerns and multiple skills for the overall purpose of enhancing the child's wellbeing.

Any wide therapeutic constellation can raise complex issues of authority, responsibility, and decision-making. The practitioner determines how much to base the therapeutic encounter on what the child says and how much on what the adults say. In cases where the integrity of the caretakers comes into question, a practitioner may need to make the difficult decision to break therapeutic confidence. States require professionals who work with children to report cases of suspected child abuse and a practitioner must act ethically on behalf of the child, even if doing so may compromise the expanded therapeutic relationship.

Therapeutic Goals

A practitioner must consider the therapeutic goals in light of the other two issues, (i.e., the child's stage of development and the expectations of the care-taking adults). Elicit the child's input as much as possible in the process of choosing and evaluating goals. When children see their contributions as central to their healing process, therapy often proceeds more smoothly and achieves greater success. Specific goals with clear checkpoints and end-points, clearly communicated among and agreed upon by all parties, go a long way toward ensuring that ethical standards are maintained in the work.

Infants and Children

A strong educational component underlies most work with infants and young children. Part or all of the session may be devoted to how the family can utilize touch in a healthy way at home. When a practitioner works with adult clients, she has their implicit permission to touch by their request for an appointment. When she works with children, she must explicitly ask even the youngest clients for their permission before touching them, and model both listening for the child's cues and responding appropriately to negative cues. The practitioner also teaches caretakers to do the same at home, thus allowing children to develop a sense of autonomy about who touches them.

Any practitioner who works with children should both like children and relate well to them. A sense of humor is a great ally: young children tell you immediately and honestly what they think about your work. Young children also tend to respond quickly to hands-on techniques. Practitioners need to keep their expectations, plans, and timing flexible since a session may complete sooner than planned. Put a prorated fee schedule in place and clearly communicate your payment policies to the child's caretakers.

In general, a parent or other caretaker should always be present in the room when a practitioner works with an infant or young child. If the sessions become an established part of care, the caretaker may float in and out of the room while remaining nearby and accessible to the child. Occasionally, the practitioner may wish to interview the child alone and should ask both child and caretaker for permission.

Teenagers

Our culture doesn't offer many non-sexual ways for our young people to receive touch after the age of about 12. Manual therapies at this age can be a vital, positive part of a young person's changing body awareness and developing sense of self. They also provide our youth with a way to continue to receive the sustenance of nurturing touch—which feeds them physically, mentally, emotionally, and spiritually.

Preteens begin to develop more autonomy from parents or other caretakers and come to rely more on peer relationships for social and interpersonal support. At this point, young people may not wish for a caretaker to be present during their sessions and, yet, may not feel completely comfortable alone with the practitioner. An ethical way to approach such a situation is for the practitioner to ask the young client if she would like anyone else present in the room during the session. The presence of a friend or sibling can help the young client feel safer and more in control of the therapeutic encounter. If you're going to be alone with a minor, state very clearly to the minor and the parent together that you have no secrets in the treatment room concerning what you do, that the minor must feel free to tell the parent everything that happens because you do nothing in the parent's absence that you wouldn't do with the parent present. Also, urge the minor to tell you if anything is uncomfortable or doesn't seem acceptable.

During the teenage years, rapid physical changes are matched by the youth's constant adoption of different personality traits, philosophies, ideals, and values. A practitioner working with a teenager may feel that a different person is on the table at every session: this observation is close to the truth. Again, flexibility is the key. Continue to ask permission to touch and offer options when there are choices that don't affect therapeutic outcome: "Do you want to leave some or all of your clothing on?" "Shall the work be done in a standing, sitting, or lying position?"

In therapeutic situations, the practitioner is in charge, yet the client is in control. The practitioner must be in charge as the expert determining protocols and procedures. The client is in control because nothing may be done without the client's informed consent. The minor, still, certainly has the right to withhold consent, but it should be clear what is being chosen. Obtain input and alignment by asking questions such as: "What is the goal for today's session and how does that relate to the overall goal of our work together?"

Somatic practitioners can serve as important role models for teenagers in many ways. The practitioner who models self-care teaches the youth about body awareness and taking care of one's self. A young man who hears from his practitioner that "no pain, no gain" is a lie may later stand up to the football coach who tells him to play to the point of injury. Ethical professionals who treat young clients with respect and dignity reinforce their image as persons worthy of respect.

> In matters of style swim with the current; in matters of principle stand like a rock.
>
> —Thomas Jefferson

Parent vs. Minor

With a colleague or supervisor, describe and discuss situations where there might be a conflict between the desires of a parent and the desires of a minor.

▌ Declining Potential New Clients

Is it ever ethical for you to refuse your services to a potential new client? Of course, the answer is "Yes!" There are a number of situations where saying no to a new client may be the correct thing to do.

A Full Practice

Having enough clients to fill your appointment schedule well in advance is wonderful. Nevertheless, your refusal of new clients should be handled in such a way that the clients maintain a positive image of you and the profession. Remember your goal is to maintain a high quality of service for every client. Keep ready a list of the names and telephone numbers of other local practitioners whom you recommend. This list should be based on your direct knowledge of these practitioners, including the type and quality of work they do and that they're accepting new clients. Two examples of polite ways to tell someone that you aren't taking new clients are: "I appreciate your call and I am unable to accept any new clients at this time. I know several local practitioners whom you may call...." "Currently all my appointment slots are filled with established clients. May I recommend some nearby practitioners whose work is similar to mine...?"

Inability to Help

There are times when you don't believe you can help a specific client. Sometimes a telephone or pre-treatment interview makes it clear the client needs a specialized type of treatment or wants to work with a practitioner who specializes in specific populations such as pregnant women, athletes, or seniors. Also, the client may have a functional problem best addressed by a different type of somatic practitioner or the client may best be served by psychotherapy or life coaching. Unless you're trained in the specialty indicated or requested, you're ethically obligated to refuse treatment and refer the client elsewhere. Again, be prepared either with the name and number of an alternate practitioner known to you, or with suggestions of healthcare facilities, websites, or toll-free numbers where clients can find more information.

Many practitioners don't charge a new client for a first session if they discover their skills don't match the client's needs. If this occurs, you can say something like, "From the information you have given me, I believe you'll be better served by a specific modality I'm not trained in. You can find out more about this technique and obtain a list of local practitioners from...."

Countertransference

The most delicate reason of all to refuse treatment is when a practitioner experiences countertransference with the client. An ethical practitioner carefully examines such situations before making the decision to refuse. The countertransference may make itself known to you through the following ways: a feeling of great attraction or repulsion to the client; a sensation of intense dislike toward the client; a vague lack of affinity with the client. The fundamental question for practitioners to ask themselves is, "Can I give this client clear, caring, compassionate energy in the course of a treatment session?" If the honest answer is no, the client must be referred elsewhere.

Personal issues can hinder practitioners from working compassionately with clients. Especially in the earlier stages of one's career, a practitioner may bring unresolved issues into relationships with clients. As he gains experience and maturity in dealing with people, he usually resolves many of these initially disturbing issues. A supervisor or peer group can

See Chapter 1 pages 10-11 for details on **Countertransference**.

offer tremendous support, perspective, and wisdom. Usually the longer a practitioner stays in business, the broader the spectrum of people he feels comfortable treating.

Consider, for example, a client who is obese, has a disability such as an amputation, or has severe scarring from a burn. Ideally, these conditions would have no negative impact on a practitioner. If a practitioner knows he has difficulty maintaining a professional and caring attitude in this situation, he is ethically bound to refer the client elsewhere. This practitioner should also consider discussing his difficulty with a supervisor to see whether the personal issues can be resolved.

To refuse to treat somebody based solely on their disability is not only unethical, it's often considered illegal.

Regardless of experience, a practitioner may find herself attracted or repelled by a potential new client. When she determines that her best course of action is to refuse to work with that client, she needs an ethical, neutral, and non-hurtful way of expressing this refusal. The practitioner's statement should be less about her or the client and more about the appropriateness and quality of the service the client seeks. Following are examples where an inappropriate response is contrasted to a neutral, positive, ethical refusal.

INAPPROPRIATE: "I had a bad experience in my childhood with a relative who had a wartime amputation. I'm afraid I just wouldn't be comfortable working with you."

INSTEAD: "I don't believe my skills are developed enough to give you the standard of care you deserve. Let me offer you the names of practitioners with more experience in this area."

INAPPROPRIATE: "You really remind me of my former boyfriend. I'm working on my issues with him right now, so it's probably best if I refer you elsewhere."

INSTEAD: "I think my ability to help you is limited. I would like to refer you to a very skilled, experienced, and compassionate practitioner who can give you better care."

Refusal of Service

Identify reasons why you might refuse to work with a particular client. Discuss these with a colleague or supervisor for support.

Referring Out

One of the great mistakes practitioners make is to believe that they can do it all. Knowing when and how to refer clients to a more appropriate professional is as important as anything you do in a wellness practice. Awareness of your scope of practice, the limits of your training and knowledge, your personal and professional limitations, your areas of weakness, and your blind spots is an asset to your professional work.

In the beginning phases of practice (the first five to 10 years), some practitioners believe their work accomplishes almost anything if applied correctly. The saying "When all someone has is a hammer, everything looks like a nail" is an apt one for this professional practice phase. A seasoned practitioner in any field knows, or at least suspects, the limits of her work and regularly refers clients to other practitioners.

Consider the following examples: a seemingly simple neck and headache pain might turn out to be a brain tumor; a case of headaches could be meningeal irritation (meningitis) or even a bleeding from one of the vessels in the brain (a stroke); pain in the lower back at L_1 and L_2 may indicate cancer spreading to the spine; the sudden appearance of pain in the front of the thigh after a strenuous activity could indicate a blood clot in the femoral artery; and difficulty raising the arm above the head because of a protective pectoral spasm can indicate cancer in the lung.

Your motto should be, "When in doubt, refer out." Develop a network of professionals whose work you know to be of the highest quality. In the best of circumstances, you cultivate ongoing professional relationships with these individuals and communicate with them directly. Your clients and colleagues act as resources for the development of this network. Keep track of how your clients are treated and how they feel about the services they receive. Over time, you'll accumulate a list of reliable referral sources. If you're unfamiliar with someone's work, don't refer clients to them until you have received a treatment and can speak personally about the quality of their work.

Developing Your Professional Referral Network

- Create a list of healthcare practitioners in other disciplines with whom you have experience. Contact each one and ask if they're taking new clients, and ask their permission to be on your referral list.
- Make a list of techniques and modalities that you don't practice, or with which you're uncomfortable. Find practitioners within your discipline that specialize in these techniques and modalities.

▌ Dismissing a Client

A practitioner may appropriately decide to stop seeing an established client for any number of reasons. Although ethical considerations differ from one situation to another, the practitioner should consider in each case how best to communicate the decision to the client and whether referral elsewhere is appropriate. Sometimes, the best course of action is to review treatment goals and create a new treatment plan instead of "firing" a client.

If a practitioner is unable to treat a client for whatever reason, that practitioner should refer the client to another practitioner. It isn't appropriate to simply deny treatment to a client. If a client's condition is out of your scope of practice or requires modalities you don't prefer to utilize, refer the client to an appropriate practitioner who can help. If you don't like the client or have serious concerns about countertransference, refer him out, don't simply dismiss him.

If you're a primary care practitioner and a client doesn't pay his bill, you can't refuse to treat him on this basis; you must refer him elsewhere. In some professions refusal to treat a client is called "abandonment" and is illegal.

Discomfort

A practitioner should terminate work with a client who makes the practitioner feel unsafe or who makes continued sexual advances. Referring this client to another practitioner in the same field could pose ethical difficulties. More appropriate would be a referral to psychotherapy where issues of aggression or of infatuation with one's counselor frequently form a therapeutic fulcrum. In contrast, the hands-on session isn't a setting where such issues are dealt with and the practitioner can explain these facts to the client in a nonjudgmental way when communicating the end of the professional relationship. For instance, the practitioner might say the following:

> I find that your [sexual comments] interfere with the effectiveness of our work together. Since our sessions aren't an appropriate place to resolve these issues, I've decided the best course is to stop our work together. Let me offer you the names of some excellent psychotherapists with whom you might look at these issues more closely.

Transference and Countertransference

Situations can arise in therapeutic encounters where the intensity of transference or countertransference is beyond the ability of the practitioner to cope effectively. For example:

- The client becomes overly dependent or inappropriately demanding, and the practitioner is unable to set a workable boundary.
- The client suffers from some emotional disorder that threatens the practitioner.
- The client is a survivor of trauma, abuse, or incest, and the therapeutic session elicits hyperarousal in the client.
- The client asks the practitioner for help outside his scope of practice: "Can you help me not feel depressed?" "I'm angry and fight with people all the time. Will this work help that?" "I need to eradicate this cellulite. Will these sessions help?"

Discussions with a supervisor or peer group can help the practitioner determine when (and how) the practitioner could continue the therapeutic relationship by making appropriate changes, and when to let the client know their work together needs to end. Communicating this decision can be very difficult even when the decision to stop working with these clients is an ethical one. Affirm both the client and your work together while also expressing the limits of that work. In addition, the question of appropriate referral requires much thought. A same-field referral would be acceptable if you know the other practitioner has training and experience specific to the client's needs. For example, some practitioners hold concurrent licensure as psychotherapists or work closely with psychotherapists on certain issues. Otherwise, a psychotherapy referral as discussed in the last scenario may be most appropriate. The practitioner could say the following:

I've become aware that something you're asking for in your therapy with me (e.g., emotional support, memory processing) is outside my expertise. Although I feel our work together has gone well, I believe we've reached the limits of how much I can help you. I have enjoyed having you as a client and want the best for you as you continue your healing process; therefore, I'd like to offer the names of some excellent practitioners who offer a more suitable type of therapy.

Lack of Results

In a similar way, a practitioner may decide to end a therapeutic relationship because the client isn't benefitting from the treatment being provided. In contrast to the above scenarios, however, in these cases the problem presented by the client is appropriate to the type of work being offered. A client who suffers from chronic headache or low back pain, for example, can reasonably expect a somatic practitioner to offer techniques that may help the problem. Nevertheless, not all techniques are effective with all problems, nor do all practitioners possess the same training or skill level. So that both client and practitioner can measure the effectiveness of the therapy, set parameters by keeping records of predetermined checkpoints (number of headache-free days, level of intensity of pain, distance walked without pain) or by predetermining a certain number of sessions after which progress is measured. If these parameters indicate the therapy isn't working, it's appropriate for the therapist to terminate treatment and offer referral elsewhere.

We had the six sessions we agreed to when we started, and you've noticed very little change in your back pain. Clearly, the type of work I am doing isn't effective for you. I would like to suggest a few other practitioners whose work differs from mine and might better help you.

Completion

There is the happy circumstance where you finish what you can do for your client; your work was effective and the therapeutic goals were reached. In a process called benchmarking, where clear parameters are set around the work and progress is monitored carefully and charted accurately, it becomes easy for both practitioner and client to recognize the end of a phase of therapeutic work. It is the practitioner's responsibility to diligently track and document the outcomes of the therapeutic work, and to communicate the results with the client, including when the endpoint of the work will be, or has been, reached. Here, ending doesn't necessarily mean completely stopping the therapeutic relationship, although the client should certainly be given that choice. The practitioner can ethically present other options to the client—for example, ongoing maintenance sessions, or a change to another form of somatic work in which the practitioner is trained. Acknowledge the successful completion of specific therapeutic goals and give the client information about what can come next.

The problem you came to me with has been resolved. Congratulations on seeing this process through to its successful completion! I have enjoyed having you as a client and if you wish to continue sessions with other goals in mind, I would be happy to work with you.

Firing a Client?

Describe potentially uncomfortable situations in which you would need to terminate working with a client. Role-play these encounters and list actions you can take to overcome the discomfort.

Figure 7.10 Declining and Dismissing Clients

Reasons to Decline a New Client	Reasons to Dismiss a Client
• Practice is Full • Inability to Help • Countertransference	• Discomfort • Lack of Results • Transference/Countertransference • Completion

---

Client Policy Statements

This section reviews the topics discussed in this chapter, and guides you in creating policy statements for each. A policy statement is a useful vehicle for creating boundaries that encourage trust, safety, and comfort. Policies explicitly define the expectations for both clients and practitioners. They make managing a practice easier, circumvent potentially awkward situations, provide means for conflict resolution, and demonstrate professionalism. The policy statement also embodies the salient points from a practitioner's Code of Ethics, Scope of Practice, and Standards of Practice documents. Ultimately, a policy statement increases the chances for a successful outcome of the services provided.

Policy statements can be designed in various formats: resembling a letter, a page with bulleted items, or a combination of the two. Eight major areas to cover are: type of service; training and experience; appointment policies; finances; client/practitioner expectations;

"Standing in the middle of the road is very dangerous; you get knocked down by traffic from both sides.

—Margaret Thatcher

personal relationships; confidentiality; and recourse policy. Some of these sections may only be a line or two on the finished policy statement. Written policy statements set a professional tone, even if you don't have specific policies stated for every situation.

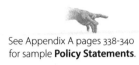

See Appendix A pages 338-340 for sample **Policy Statements**.

Periodically review your policies, delete ones that are no longer appropriate and add ones to further clarify your requirements. The main caveat with policies is: Do not have a policy you won't or can't enforce. If you alter a policy for a client, either on a onetime basis or if you change that specific policy permanently, make it very clear to the client what you're doing and that all other policies still hold.

Figure 7.11 Client Policy Statement Checklist

1. Type of Service (services, product sales, referrals)
2. Training and Experience (licensing, memberships, scope of practice)
3. Appointments (hours of operation, cancellation, lateness)
4. Finances (fees, tips, gift certificates, guarantees)
5. Expectations (procedures, draping, communication, attitudes, interaction, etiquette, illness)
6. Personal Relationships (dual relationships)
7. Confidentiality (HIPAA compliance)
8. Recourse

Type of Service

Provide a clear definition of services, including benefits as well as limitations. This section might include: areas of expertise; specialization; specific conditions your work addresses, such as headaches and back pain; target populations served, such as seniors or athletes; special equipment or products used; certain people with whom you don't work, such as pregnant women or people with certain medical conditions; and a description of the referral network of related professionals that you utilize.

Training and Experience

Describe your training and experience to increase the client's sense of safety and confidence. This section includes educational experience, organizational memberships, additional training, years of experience, specialty study, and licensure status. Although it may seem unnecessary for some professionals to provide this information, clients feel safer when they know the practitioner's experience with a particular problem or modality.

Appointments

Written, straightforward communication about your appointment time policies is a way of establishing clear boundaries. A policy statement should include the length of initial and follow-up appointments, as well as guidelines for scheduling changes, lateness, cancellations, and emergencies.

Finances

The exchange of money solidifies the professional contract between the practitioner and the client as it clearly indicates that the practitioner is providing a service to the client in exchange for a fee. Charging a fee helps clarify the distinction between personal time and work time. At the beginning of the professional relationship, clear communication about your fee policies is vital because many people have strong emotional responses to issues involving money. Financial policies should include the following: fee structure; sliding scale schedules; package plans; credit terms; insurance reimbursement; product guarantees and returns; bounced checks; gift certificates; and barter.

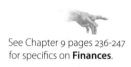

See Chapter 9 pages 236-247 for specifics on **Finances**.

Client/Practitioner Expectations

Clarification of practitioner expectations can ease anxiety for the client, as well as the practitioner. Create practice policies that include the procedural structure of a typical session, draping, communication guidelines, attitude, the level of interaction outside of the actual treatment, illness, and etiquette expectations.

Personal Relationships

Engaging in personal or social relationships with clients outside of the therapeutic relationship is difficult at best, and often leads to undue discomfort or even pain and suffering by the client. Dual relationships require enormous attention, maturity, and excellent communication.

The ethics of dual relationships varies to some degree among the professions. In psychotherapy, there is almost universal acceptance that dual relationships of any kind are unethical. While not deemed unethical in other professions, they're certainly discouraged. Any exceptions to keeping the relationship limited to one domain must be carefully justified and defined.

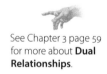

See Chapter 3 page 59 for more about **Dual Relationships**.

Some people have stringent policies about working with friends and family members. There is no right or wrong here, although it's easier if you don't need to accommodate dual relationships. You are the only one who can gauge your ability to keep clear boundaries. Even if you can work effectively in a dual relationship, the question still exists if the other person is capable of managing multiple roles. Another aspect of working with family and friends is that they're more likely to test your policies and limits—although not always intentionally. Clear policies make enforcement less awkward.

Sexual relations with clients is a blatant violation of most Codes of Ethics, and in many places is against the law. Policies that include a straightforward statement about the inappropriateness of sexual contact between the practitioner and the client contribute to an atmosphere of safety. The practitioner is responsible to ensure that sexual misconduct doesn't occur.

Confidentiality

Confidentiality guidelines for somatic practitioners generally state that information shared between client and practitioner during a session remains private. These guidelines are usually further interpreted to mean that client names, details of treatment, and information shared by clients during sessions aren't discussed by the practitioner with anyone else. These same rights apply to both verbal and written interactions you have with anyone other than the client. Your right to privacy statements should be clear and compliant with all applicable laws, and should include a statement on confidential recordkeeping (HIPAA compliance).

See pages 188-190 for more information on **Confidentiality and** HIPAA **Compliance**.

Recourse

What happens if the client is dissatisfied with the services provided or products purchased? Some practitioners refund some or all of a client's money if the client isn't satisfied. Others give another session without charge. Discuss the concerns with your client, regardless of your final action. Often, the dissatisfaction results from a lack of ongoing communication. Keep in mind that the power differential that exists in helping relationships may affect the client's ability to utilize a recourse policy. Because of this power differential, it's recommended that the policy statement include options involving a third party or mediator in the discussion. This kind of information serves to level the balance of power.

 Managing Your Client Policies

Write your Client Policies. Next, do the following activities:
- Identify the policies you might feel uncomfortable enforcing.
- Clarify how you handle the "bending" of policies (e.g., a client forgets her checkbook, a client who thought you were going to bill the insurance company).

Conclusion

Ethical practice management calls for high standards and personal integrity on the part of every somatic practitioner. The foundation is to be clear about your scope of practice and know the applicable laws. Your policies create the structure for a sound practice and identify clear expectations for yourself and your clients. In addition to you enjoying a sense of pride from maintaining an ethical practice, your clients will receive the best possible treatment and the whole field is enhanced.

8
The Team Approach

"Alone we can do so little; together we can do so much."
—Helen Keller

Office Ethics
- Codes of Conduct
- Policy and Procedure Manuals
- Client Custody

Working for Others
- Ethical Considerations for Employers
- Ethical Considerations for Employees

Care Coordination and Case Management
- The Five-Step Process
- Key Components for Effective Case Management
- Ethical Care Coordination in Specific Environments
- Handling Referrals from Outside Providers

Group Practices
- Common Ethical Issues
- Multi-Disciplinary Group Practices
- Specialty Centers

Spas
- The Franchise Phenomenon
- The Work Environment

Hospitals and Hospices
- The Hospital Setting
- The Hospice Setting
- Ethical Considerations in Hospitals and Hospices

Medical Clinics
- Integrated Complementary Care in Medical Clinics
- Adjunct Complementary Care in Medical Clinics
- Ethical Considerations in Medical Clinics

Key Terms

Business Association
Care Coordination
Case Management
Case Manager

Code of Conduct
Compliance
Conflict of Interest
Franchise Systems

Insider Trading
Intellectual Property
Legal Entity
Partnership

Working for yourself can be rewarding, yet working by yourself can also be lonely. Joining an environment with other professionals can be a great way to add collaboration and camaraderie to your practice.

Many wellness practitioners are joining forces with other healthcare providers to create associations, group practices, and partnerships, potentially sharing some overhead expenses. It is also becoming more commonplace to hire practitioners as employees and co-workers in clinics, hospitals, and franchise organizations. The other professionals in these environments may be practitioners of your same discipline, or they may practice various other complementary therapies. You may share facilities, equipment, or staffing. You may promote yourself independently, market as a group, or share clients as assigned by an employer.

These alliances can be quite beneficial for the practitioners as well as for their clients. Unfortunately, too many people develop these alliances or take jobs in companies without creating a proper structure to clarify expectations and guide interactions, thus creating an environment where ethical dilemmas arise.

The major areas for friction are: incompatible personalities; conflicting visions of the image of the business, the desired clientele, and the optimal business operations; marketing; client care; and finances. Working successfully with other professionals requires creating a clear and ethical plan that addresses these areas, including having a common vision for the establishment, as well as compatible healthcare philosophies and personalities. The practitioners need to agree with how the common business operates or how the separate practitioners' businesses can collaborate. Some situations lend more easily toward teamwork than others.

This chapter explores ethical dilemmas common to these types of team environments. We start by examining the team approach from the vantage of general concepts involved in working with other professionals, office ethics, and care coordination. Then we cover issues specific to working in different environments, such as group practices, spas, medical clinics, and hospitals or hospices.

Office Ethics

Corporations, business partnerships, and groups of professionals who plan to share a work environment benefit from conscientiously discussing, planning, and agreeing upon an office code of ethics that is suitable to each type of practice involved as well as to the shared setting. This code should be written, openly available, and regularly reviewed. The business should provide new members with a copy of the office code and encourage questions about how its guidelines are applied. Nevertheless, each practitioner and staff member in the group must assume individual responsibility for knowing if and where such guidelines exist, for reviewing them, and for applying them in the day-to-day work environment.

Office ethical codes exist along a wide spectrum. They may include laws and regulations that govern corporations, broad ethical strokes established by professional organizations, and statements of mission and purpose that guide a business. We examine the Code of Conduct and the Policy and Procedure Manual to illustrate the range of content that office ethical codes may comprise.

Codes of Conduct

Codes of conduct are designed to address applicable state and federal laws as well as established business and professional ethical standards. Codes of conduct refer practitioners to multiple regulatory and policy documents that the members of the business are expected to know and to follow. Complex codes of conduct are typically found in businesses in highly regulated fields (e.g., hospitals, clinics), in businesses that are publicly traded; and in businesses with a national or international presence. While you might not choose to develop a complex code for a smaller practice, you may adopt one from your professional association. If you work in a highly regulated environment, you'll probably need to sign a document that you agree to their formal code of conduct. Common policy areas covered by codes of conduct are conflict of interest, compliance, acceptable use of electronic resources, insider trading, intellectual property, professional misconduct, and relationships with vendors.

Conflict of Interest

Conflict of interest refers to circumstances wherein personal interests may conflict with the interests of the business. For instance, the possibility of personal financial gain may affect an individual's objectivity and performance on the job; or a person may be hired because of a personal relationship with an employer; or an individual may use his connection with the business for personal gain in other arenas. Many corporations and institutions require their staff to file regular reports of financial and other relationships that could be sources of conflicts of interest. Consider the following examples of conflict of interest:

- Your client has achieved his major goals with you, yet you're reluctant to end the therapeutic relationship.
- You hire your cousin's wife as a practitioner and feel compelled to book her more than the other practitioners.
- One of your employer's clients works for a large company that wants you to do chair massage and you do it, but don't go through your employer.

> It takes two flints to make a fire.
>
> —Louisa May Alcott

Compliance

Compliance refers to adherence to applicable laws and standards. Examples are compliance with licensure programs, accreditation organizations, occupational safety regulations, and building and fire codes. Procedures for reporting noncompliance are established, as are protections for those who report possible compliance violations. Consider the following examples of compliance issues:

- The location where you work requires an establishment license in addition to a professional practice license. If you notice that there isn't one, and you don't notify management, then you're complicit in a legal violation.
- The Occupational Safety and Health Administration (OSHA) requires you to have non-slip flooring but you show up to work and discover some of the carpeting has peeled. If you don't immediately fix it then you're non-compliant.

Electronic Resources

Electronic resources made available by a business include the following: hardware such as desktop computers, laptops, printers, scanners, or smartphones; software such as word processing, security and auditing programs, image manipulation, and spreadsheets; and network capabilities including shared drives, Internet access, telephone, voicemail, and email. These are assets of the business, and claims to privacy aren't enforceable if an employee uses these assets for purposes other than business.

Insider Trading

Insider trading refers to financial gains that individuals may make based on information about company stock not available publicly. Laws exist to prevent persons with inside information from manipulating investment markets for personal gain. For example, a client shares confidential information that a large medical device company is coming out with a new revolutionary product, and it'll be announced next week. It would be insider trading for you to go out and purchase that stock. These laws are based on the ethical argument that massive gains for a few create losses for the many in a field where fairness depends upon all players having equal access to information.

Intellectual Property

Intellectual property rules determine who owns ideas, discoveries, and improvements generated by individuals during their work. Corporations and institutions may have the legal right to copyright, patent, or trademark such work and may also have guidelines for distributing income generated from the work. Consider this example of an intellectual property conflict: you develop a way to track client progress that's used throughout an organization where you work, and then attempt to sell this product to other organizations without getting permission. Even though you created the tracking system, it was done while you were an employee and that employer owns your work product (unless you made a prior agreement otherwise).

Professional Misconduct

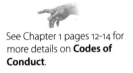

See Chapter 1 pages 12-14 for more details on **Codes of Conduct**.

Professional misconduct refers to violations of professional codes of ethics. Examples include fraud, theft, negligence, and practicing outside one's Scope. It is often a difficult choice to report knowledge or suspicion of professional misconduct, especially on the part of peers or close colleagues, but it's considered a cornerstone of ethical practice.

Vendor Relationships

Vendor relationships are potential sources of value not only to the vendors but to those in an organization who deal directly with the vendors. Policies may be formulated to ensure impartiality and objectivity in these relationships, and to manage the possibility that vendors may offer gifts, travel, or entertainment to acknowledge or encourage use of the vendor. An example of this conflict is a vendor who offers you gifts and a travel package in exchange for you recommending the use of their products to the company.

Policy and Procedure Manuals

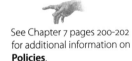

See Chapter 7 pages 200-202 for additional information on **Policies**.

Businesses and group practices that don't need a code defining regulatory requirements may instead prepare a manual of policies and procedures for the smooth running of the business. Some details may appear trivial, such as rules about parking lots and bathrooms, but they reflect the daily realities of shared space and time. A successful practice identifies potential problems before they arise and creates values-based and orderly methods for their resolution. Rules and regulations ought not to be arbitrary, but based on the desire to create a working atmosphere where respect for one another, and for the business, can flourish. When a group creates working policies on such a basis, they're, in fact, creating ethical guidelines for conducting the business. Of course, even though a Policy and Procedure Manual may not mention applicable laws and regulations, these still govern the conduct of the business owners and staff.

Specific statements for office codes are beyond the scope of this chapter, but the following elements and questions should be considered, and guidelines created, as appropriate.

STANDARDS OF BEHAVIOR FOR PRACTITIONERS
- Is there a dress code?
- Is there a policy regarding use of fragrances?
- What are the expectations regarding timeliness?
- How are absences to be handled?
- What are the expectations regarding sobriety in the office?
- What are the expectations regarding language in the office (e.g., profanity, offensive language, innuendo)?
- In what offsite situations are practitioners considered representatives of the office? What kind of image should practitioners exhibit in these situations?

RELATIONSHIPS WITH CO-WORKERS

- What hierarchy exists among group members? In what circumstances is this hierarchy invoked?
- What referral patterns are acceptable among practitioners? What behaviors are considered poaching clients?
- What lines of communication exist for resolving internal conflicts between practitioners?
- What are appropriate reporting avenues when practitioners suspect, or know of, unethical behavior on the part of a co-worker?
- What policies exist regarding trading services with co-workers? How are discrepancies in value handled?
- What guidelines are provided regarding personal relationships between co-workers?

RELATIONSHIPS WITH CLIENTS

- How is privacy maintained? What procedures are in place to ensure HIPAA requirements are met?
- What are the policies regarding tips and gifts?
- What guidelines are provided regarding personal relationships between practitioners and clients?
- Are there limitations to practitioners advertising in a common waiting room to all clients, or to an individual client who is waiting for a different practitioner?
- What policies govern client/practitioner relationships when the practitioner leaves the practice?

RELATIONSHIP BETWEEN THE ORGANIZATION AND THE INDIVIDUAL PRACTITIONER

- How does the business ensure practitioners have proper licensure, credentialing, and continuing education?
- What guidelines exist regarding scope of practice?
- Does the work environment encourage practitioners to become multi-modal or to stay within a single modality?
- Are procedures in place for regular peer or employee review?
- What are expectations concerning noise in the office?
- What is the expected use of parking facilities by practitioners?
- What constitutes overlap of services or retail competition among practitioners?
- What pricing policies exist to prevent undercutting of other practitioners?
- How does the business meet applicable laws regarding correct billing practices, payments of taxes, and other financial regulations?
- What recordkeeping responsibilities do practitioners have?
- What situations constitute a conflict of interest?
- What responsibilities do team members share for the care of common areas such as lobbies, waiting rooms, bathrooms, kitchen, or break rooms?
- What procedures are established to create a healthy, safe, and secure working environment?
- How does the organization encourage community involvement?

Client Custody

Who retains custody of the client when a practitioner leaves a clinic setting or wants to see some clients at another location? This question is one that often elicits emotional upheaval and unethical behavior. Many practitioners work in other practitioners' offices, health clubs, salons, spas, and clinics in the hopes of building up their private clientele. Problems arise if the expectations and boundaries aren't clear. Consider the following:

A physical therapist works at a health club. Several of her patients decide they would prefer to receive their sessions at home. She decides to do this. The health club director finds out and suspends the physical therapist.

Points to Ponder

What are the conflicts of seeing patients outside of the health club? How could she have discussed these issues directly with the owner or manager? What agreements can be made ahead of time to avoid problems?

Your ability to ethically take on private clients depends upon your agreement with the club. The club owner might not care whatsoever, particularly if she mainly views your services as an added value for membership. But the owner might be upset if the health club regards you as a significant revenue-producing adjunct or spends a lot of money marketing your services.

Another common occurrence is changing locations. You may no longer want to work at the hiring party's location.

A somatic practitioner was hired as an employee at a wellness center. After five years she decided to have a child and wanted to reduce her hours and see clients in her home. Since she was an employee, the center didn't have her sign a contract. She had been seeing some of her clients for years and established a deep rapport. She wanted to continue working with her current clients in her home so she notified the clients of her plans to leave and gave them her home telephone number.

The center's owner was angry and felt cheated because he had spent a considerable amount of time and money building the practice (the practitioner did very little marketing) and providing continuing education opportunities for all the staff. Ultimately, they came to an agreement and the practitioner paid the center the following percentage split for each client that she saw in her home: 40 percent for the first five sessions; 20 percent for the subsequent five sessions.

Points to Ponder

Is this a fair arrangement? How can you be sure you present a fair arrangement as an employer? How can you be sure you get a fair arrangement as an employee?

> The law of self-fulfilling prophecy says that you get what you expect. So why not create great expectations and the highest vision possible of yourself and your world?
>
> —Mark Victor Hansen

Avoid hurt feelings, and possibly a lawsuit, by clearly defining how you'll deal with the future allocation of clients. Some options include: the leaving practitioner pays a fee for the client files, either a flat fee or a percentage of a specified number of sessions that each client books; the practitioner who leaves agrees to not see the clients for a specified time (e.g., three or six months). Regardless of the arrangement, you must get clients' written permission to take their files.

 Whose Clients Are They?

Write two drafts of a Client Custody Agreement: one from the perspective of an employer; one from the perspective of an employee. Do the two drafts differ? If so, how can each be altered as a fair compromise for appropriate client custody issues?

▌ Working for Others

Working for others and working for yourself aren't mutually exclusive concepts. When we deliver quality and ethical work as employees, the most obvious result is that we keep our jobs, which certainly is to our personal advantage. At the same time, our quality work contributes to the success of the company, and a successful company gives us more opportunity to perform quality work. This cycle of success is the root of employment and economic health.

To achieve this success, employers and employees share responsibility for the ethical conduct of the business. The responsibilities of each directly impact the other; therefore, in this section we explore the broad areas of ethical responsibilities held by both employers and employees.

Ethical Considerations for Employers

The reality of the power differential means that, ethically, a business should take a protective role towards its employees. Laws and regulations provide this ethical framework, which is ideally completed through policies and procedures that demonstrate the business' respect for its employees and defense of their individual rights. Important areas where these attitudes must and should be expressed are in practices of fairness and diversity, safety, security, and integrity.

Fairness and Diversity

Employment opportunities are to be made without regard to race, color, religion, national origin, citizenship, age, sex, gender, sexual orientation, sexual preference, veteran status, marital status, disability, or other characteristics protected under laws and regulations. Reasonable accommodations must be provided for qualified employees with disabilities. In compliance with applicable laws and regulations, a business aims for a diverse workforce. Opportunities for advancement within the company should be clearly advertised and fairly distributed. Unfortunately, many establishments inadvertently foster discrimination when they ask clients if they prefer a male or female practitioner. Other companies blatantly violate laws by limiting their employment opportunities to a specific gender.

> "
> Teamwork is the secret that make common people achieve uncommon result.
>
> —Ifeanyi Enoch Onuoha

Safety

The employer has the responsibility to provide a safe environment for the conduct of the business. The environment includes: a building that is structurally safe and meets fire codes; safety mechanisms such as protective latex-free gloves, hand sanitizer, hydraulic tables, and anti-fatigue floor mats that help prevent workplace injuries. In addition, safety measures include policies regarding workplace violence that may address issues such as harassment, threats, aggressive behaviors, substance abuse, and reporting suspected impairment.

Security

In addition to providing an environment that promotes physical safety, the employer must provide means for securing the privacy and confidentiality of employees. Personnel records, private health information, and personal identifying information shouldn't be shared outside the business except as required by law or as authorized by the employee. Within the business, private information regarding employees is shared only on a need-to-know basis. The business has an ethical responsibility to provide devices that help ensure the security of stored information, such as secure computer terminals, password-protected folders, and locked file cabinets or rooms.

Integrity

A business that functions with integrity complies not only with relevant laws and professional regulations, but with its own stated purpose, goals, and mission. Advertising, marketing, pricing, and promotions should be transparent, honest, and fair. Situations that require ethical decision-making should be reviewed by a committee whose membership includes appropriate representatives of owners, managers, and employees. Ideally, the business provides and encourages employees to use a confidential means for reporting known or potential violations of fairness, safety, and security. Always ensure that those who report such violations don't suffer negative consequences to their employment.

Ethical Considerations for Employees

The characteristics of an employee-employer relationship are like those of any long-term, serious relationship. By agreeing to accept employment, an individual enters a world where commitment, loyalty, cooperation, and obligation play important roles. Hopefully the business earns these from its employees through its own ethical behavior; nevertheless, these qualities on the part of the employee aren't optional. The employees' commitment, loyalty, cooperation, and obligation remains with their clients and the services they provide. Finally, certain legal and ethical actions specifically come into play when the employee knows or believes that a business is failing to act ethically.

Commitment

An employee demonstrates commitment through action. Quality work and performance start by being on the job as scheduled, in a timely manner, and by performing work skillfully for all clients and in all circumstances. Commitment proves itself over the long term; it shows up through diligence, determination, honesty, and objectivity. From a place of commitment, an employee chooses appropriate behavior at and away from work. The committed employee doesn't use business assets for personal reasons, and deals fairly with ownership and staff as well as with clients, vendors, or others in the business relationship.

Loyalty

A loyal employee avoids associations that interfere with the ability to represent the company. Conflicts of interest are resolved by the employee if they arise, and the employee recognizes that the organization has the right to own ideas and opportunities created by the employee as part of the employment. The loyal employee communicates candidly and honestly with the employer through appropriate channels, but recognizes that those channels aren't invitations to second-guess or criticize the employer's decisions.

Cooperation

The success of a business' ethical code depends upon employee cooperation. Employees must cooperate with laws and regulations for a business to remain compliant, and in some cases, employees as well as the business can be held legally responsible for infractions that occur. Employee cooperation ensures that the business deals ethically with clients and the public. When employees cooperate with the vision and growth targets established by the company, the work of the business becomes more efficient and effective. Employee cooperation feeds the cycle of success for both employee and business.

Obligation

Employees are obligated to keep accurate records and submit truthful billing accounts. Employees must responsibly manage client information as well as business proprietary information, and must maintain confidentiality of this information even after leaving employment. An employee who knows or believes that legal, regulatory, or other ethical infractions are occurring in a place of business is obligated to take action. If reporting infractions in good faith through internal pathways doesn't lead to resolution, the employee is obligated to take those concerns to an appropriate agency outside the organization.

Figure 8.1 Ethical Considerations

Employers	Employees
• Fairness and Diversity • Safety • Security • Integrity	• Commitment • Loyalty • Cooperation • Obligation

The Perfect Work Environment

Make a list of what you consider the advantages and disadvantages of working for someone else. Then, clearly outline your perfect work environment.

Care Coordination and Case Management

Care coordination can take a variety of forms. One of the main advantages of working in a group practice, clinic, or hospital environment is the opportunity to participate in multidisciplinary case management. Clients are often better served when they have access to a variety of healthcare providers under one roof who actively work together in their care. However, many clients may also be under the care of one or more healthcare providers outside of your direct practice environment. Some care settings, such as hospitals or multi-specialty medical clinics, have designated case managers whose exclusive role is to coordinate care and services among providers. Furthermore, health insurance companies occasionally assign specific case managers, often specially trained registered nurses or social workers, to coordinate the care of complicated or higher-risk patients. Regardless of its form, ethical case management conforms to professional standards of conduct in coordinating client care.

Case Management Society of America

http://www.cmsa.org/

The purpose of case management is to help clients more effectively reach positive health outcomes. The Case Management Society of America defines case management as a collaborative process that assesses, plans, implements, coordinates, monitors, and evaluates options and services needed to meet a person's health needs.[1] Formal case management is typically an interdisciplinary, client-centered process that recognizes and addresses the unique needs and conditions of clients or patients on an individual basis.

The Five-Step Process

In somatic practices the case management process consists of five steps: assessment, planning, implementation, coordination, and evaluation.

ASSESSMENT is the process of gathering client information to identify needs and potential barriers to meeting them. Pertinent information can include a general health history, physical examination findings, and phase of the condition (subacute, acute, or chronic). Information about psychosocial issues, such as age, functional capacity, living situation, and social support systems can be important components of the assessment.

PLANNING is the process of setting up specific goals, objectives, and actions to meet identified needs. Individual plans usually differ among clients with the same condition. Clients and collaborating practitioners must communicate effectively to ensure that they're all working toward the same treatment goals. Without good communication, perceptions may differ dramatically, which can lead to unnecessary treatments and poor care coordination.

IMPLEMENTATION begins once the treatment plan has been formulated. Effective implementation is facilitated by ongoing effective communication between the client and providers, as well as among providers, to assess progress and changing needs over time.

COORDINATION of care is required if two or more providers are involved in the treatment plan or otherwise providing ongoing health care needs of the client. Once again, good communication skills and effective communication channels are required for effective coordination of care.

EVALUATION measures the quality and outcomes of treatment plans. Effective evaluation is an ongoing process. If a patient's case progresses smoothly and as expected, coordinated evaluation among providers may happen infrequently. If progress is slow, or if goals change or aren't being met, evaluation is imperative to guide modifications in the treatment plan. Ideally, the client should be treated until her symptoms are completely resolved or until she reaches maximum improvement.

Case management continues along the entire continuum of care. Assessment, planning, implementation, coordination, and monitoring/evaluation often occur simultaneously, with effective communication as the cornerstone of success. Once treatment goals are met, case management facilitates the transition to self-care or to alternate treatment modalities.

Key Components for Effective Case Management

The key components needed for effective case management are critical thinking, communication, and collaboration.[2] Clear lines of communication, time, cooperation, and shared values are required for this to succeed.

CRITICAL THINKING implies a systematic process for gathering, synthesizing, prioritizing, analyzing, and evaluating information. Reliable, accurate information about the client's case must be gathered and shared with relevant providers, and each provider should ideally contribute to the process within their scope of practice.

COMMUNICATION is the ability to send and receive information. Effective verbal and written communication skills are essential to effective participation in case management. Lines of communication should be clearly defined and easily utilized. Relevant documentation about client progress should be professional, accurate and succinct, and if electronic, should be HIPAA compliant.

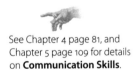

See Chapter 4 page 81, and Chapter 5 page 109 for details on **Communication Skills**.

COLLABORATION is the ultimate goal. The ideal environment for case management is one in which all practitioners working with a specific client communicate periodically about that client's treatment and progress. It should be clear who is primarily responsible for the case management process, be it the primary care physician, the senior provider in a clinic, a dedicated case manager, or another designee. Throughout the case management process, practitioners also empower clients by educating them about their care and involving them in key decisions.

Ethical Care Coordination in Specific Environments

Effective communication is the foundation of ethical case management. Regardless of the form that case management takes in your practice setting, preparation is the key to success. Update your treatment plans in a timely manner and be prepared to discuss them. Make sure that you're educated in the proper terminology to readily communicate with the other health professionals in their language regarding client care. Present your treatment plans concisely and with supporting information to gain cooperation. Be willing to compromise for the patient's best interest, setting aside self-interest. Keep the patient and collaborating practitioners informed, and educate them within your scope of practice. Above all, keep the process client-centered.

Single-Modality Clinics

If you work in an environment that only offers one type of major wellness care, such as a massage clinic, each practitioner should agree on the definition of case management or coordination, and what it entails, including the degree of interaction between the practitioners. Typically, these policies are written and accessible to all practitioners. Specific issues to consider include the following: intra-office referrals; cross-cover for established clients when the primary provider isn't available (e.g., vacation, last-minute appointments); standards for maintaining and storing patient records; lines of communication for care coordination (e.g., time and format of case management meetings, communication with healthcare providers outside of the clinic); and switching providers within the clinic (particularly when any conflicts arise, or upon a client's request). Consider securing an Independent Practitioner's Agreement, Employee Agreement, Partnership Agreement, or Associates Agreement that includes these issues, or verify that relevant policies and procedures are in place. Also, consider hiring an attorney to draw up or review the agreement, and, once signed, insist that all practitioners adhere to the spirit and specifics of that agreement.

Martha works in a clinic with three other independent massage therapists. The four practitioners share overhead expenses and a common charting system. The clinic uses a central answering service to schedule appointments. Martha decided to take a three-week vacation this summer and has two clients who need ongoing weekly sessions.

The first client was referred to Martha three months ago by his chiropractor for ongoing care of chronic pain after a motor vehicle accident. The client has made significant progress, particularly in the last few sessions, and has expressed a great deal of anxiety about switching therapists. Martha sends weekly updates to the referring chiropractor and plans to foster this relationship as an ongoing referral source.

The second client has been a regular client for two years. She is a busy executive with a rigid schedule. Martha has a firm standing appointment with her each week and the client wants to continue her treatments as scheduled during Martha's absence.

Martha arranges treatment sessions with two different therapists in the clinic during her absence. She asks Joseph to see the first client since he has experience with chronic pain patients and has worked with chiropractors in the past. She arranges three weekly appointments with Jessica for her second client, scheduling in advance and confirming the dates and times with both Jessica and the client.

Upon returning from her vacation, Martha reviews the charts of her two clients. She sees that the first client has continued to make progress, but unfortunately Joseph failed to send progress reports to the referring chiropractor. She finds only one documented treatment session for the second client. She checks the central schedule to find that the second appointment had been cancelled after Jessica tried to reschedule it, and the third had been cancelled by the client.

Points to Ponder

What types of agreements would facilitate effective care coordination in this situation? (Consider the process for assigning coverage, documenting effectively, and communicating relevant information in a timely manner.) How does having

clearly defined agreements about case management and care coordination affect the
ethical practice in a single-modality clinic?

Having written agreements regarding care coordination, particularly cross-cover for
established clients when the primary provider isn't available, helps to avoid mishandling
client care. Martha may have been more confident that her clients would have been cared for
appropriately if they had such written agreements in place.

Multi-Discipline Practices

Multi-discipline practice environments, such as integrative health clinics and physician offices,
serve a variety of clients and patients. If you work in an environment with primary and non-
primary care practitioners, many of the issues discussed above with regard to single-specialty
clinics still apply. However, it's even more important to be clear about the definition and
practice of case management in these settings, as practitioners of different levels of licensure
and scopes of practice will need to participate in care coordination. Lines of communication
between disciplines should be clearly established and it's imperative that the lead provider
or designated case manager be clearly identified. If a client requires a prescription for initial
or continued care, specific routes of communication must be established to communicate
ongoing assessment and progress. If a client wishes to continue working with you after a
specific prescription expires, the client must first be released from the clinic before he can see
you on a private basis.

A client is referred to a pain medicine clinic for the evaluation and treatment of
fibromyalgia. The clinic is staffed by a naturopathic physician, two chiropractors, a
nutritionist, an acupuncturist, and two massage therapists. It is the practice of this
clinic to hold monthly case management meetings to discuss the care plan for new
clients. The client sees the naturopath as her PCP. The client is assigned to the
acupuncturist for 12 weekly sessions.

After eight weeks, the client is showing signs of improvement. She seems to
be working well with the naturopath and the acupuncturist, and she is learning
new strategies to deal with her diagnosis. During the ninth session, she tells the
acupuncturist that she feels she has gained as much as she can from her work with
the naturopath, but she asks if she can continue her acupuncture sessions on an
ongoing basis. The acupuncturist explains to the patient that for her to continue
receiving acupuncture, he needs to discuss her request and treatment plan with his
colleagues during case management rounds. The acupuncturist asks her permission
to do so. She hesitates before confiding that she hasn't enjoyed her appointments
with the naturopathic physician; she gives permission, and asks the acupuncturist to
not relay this concern directly.

Points to Ponder

What would be your role in the next case management meeting and in the ongoing
care coordination of this particular patient? Who is primarily responsible for case
management in this situation? Who is responsible for ongoing primary care? How
would you handle the information about the naturopath?

It is important to always remain client-centered. The client care/case management team
must consider the needs of the client's condition, as well as the client's wishes. As an ethical
practitioner, you might encourage the client to discuss her dislikes with the naturopath, so that

the physician may have an opportunity to better meet her needs, or make necessary changes in the care of future clients.

A client self-refers to an integrative health clinic for non-specific low back pain. He undergoes a routine intake and screening process facilitated by the front office staff and is then referred to a massage therapist for treatments. After treating the client for a short time, the therapist realizes that the problem isn't progressing as it should, and refers the client to the in-house chiropractor. The chiropractor evaluates the patient and prescribes a course of treatment that includes twelve bi-weekly massage sessions for sciatica.

After three weeks of treatment, the client reports temporary pain relief from his chiropractic and massage treatments, but he isn't making the progress he had hoped. He confides to the massage therapist that he is very fatigued and has been losing weight. The massage therapist mentions this to the chiropractor during lunch the next week and suggests that the client's case be discussed at the clinic's weekly integrative case management meeting, facilitated by the osteopathic physician who owns the clinic. The chiropractor is initially resistant to the suggestion, but later agrees to bring up the case. At the meeting, the massage therapist relays the client's concerns to the group of practitioners from different modalities in attendance. The osteopath is concerned and schedules the patient for visit the next day. Radiographic imaging of his back reveals a tumor.

Points to Ponder

Who is responsible for case management in this situation? Who is the primary provider? In a multi-disciplinary clinic, how important is it to be knowledgeable about the scope of practice of the different practitioners in the clinic?

In this case, the chiropractor is the primary provider, but as such is responsible to discuss concerns with the client care team of this multi-disciplinary clinic. To better serve the needs of each client, it's important for practitioners to be knowledgeable about the scope of practice of each different discipline offered in the clinic.

Hospitals and Other Inpatient Treatment Centers

Many hospitals and other inpatient facilities, such as rehabilitation hospitals, skilled nursing facilities, assisted-living centers, and psychiatric units employ or refer to allied wellness providers. Patients in these facilities often have numerous conditions and are taken care of by multiple providers. In these settings, there is usually a dedicated case manager assigned to a panel of patients. The case manager coordinates care among providers, between providers and the patient, and performs ongoing needs assessment and planning—particularly during transitions of care (e.g., upon admission or discharge to the facility). Each individual provider is responsible for accurate and timely documentation of their assessment and treatment plans for the patients. In some facilities, the medical record is the central point for care coordination; in others, regular multi-disciplinary case management meetings are held. Some hospitals or similar institutions don't allow non-primary care providers to document in the patient chart, in which case the verbal reports are given through designated channels (e.g., the patient's nurse, physical therapist, or case manager). If you choose to work in a hospital or other inpatient facility, it's important to familiarize yourself with the care team and case management procedures, and be responsible for contributing within your scope of practice.

Matthew is a movement educator who works in the physical therapy department of a skilled nursing facility (SNF). Patients admitted to this facility are admitted from local hospitals and have special rehabilitation needs that require an inpatient setting prior to going home. He works with a multi-disciplinary team that includes an attending physician (MD or DO), a diabetes educator, a nutritionist, physical and occupational therapists, a registered nurse, and a case manager. Many of the patients are recovering from joint replacement surgeries and are seen only briefly each week by the attending physician.

Matthew and the nurse have daily contact with the patients. Matthew reports directly to the physical therapist, whose documentation in the patients' charts includes verbal progress reports from Matthew, but his activities overlap with occupational therapy goals as well. The team generally works well together and patients in particular seem to enjoy their sessions with Matthew.

Under pressure to better coordinate patient care, document clinical outcomes, and cut costs, the administration of the SNF is considering cutting Matthew out of the program because they don't really understand what he does and there's no clear documentation of results. The case manager asks Matthew to come up with a plan to document both his interventions and patient progress on patients recovering from hip and knee surgeries. Matthew proposes a progress note that includes 1) the treatment plan as prescribed by the attending physician, 2) specific goals as clarified by the physical therapist, 3) description and duration of his interventions, and 4) specific outcome measures, including patient satisfaction, pain scale, and range of motion.

Points to Ponder

In what other ways could Matthew participate in the case management of his patients while they're admitted to the facility? What is his scope of practice in relation to the other healthcare practitioners in the facility? How does this impact his ability to effectively communicate and collaborate with the other practitioners in the SNF?

Working in structured environments such as hospitals and inpatient treatment centers requires practitioners to follow direction completely, to accurately document and convey treatment information, to highlight patient progress, and to be vigilant about working within their scope of practice.

Handling Referrals from Outside Providers

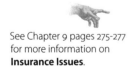

See Chapter 9 pages 275-277 for more information on **Insurance Issues**.

Many healthcare providers refer to allied wellness practitioners for specific conditions. In such cases, clients typically come with an established diagnosis. The referral may be a formal prescription for a number of sessions or treatments, or it may be informal, with no specific prescribed treatment. In this case, several issues relevant to case management must be considered. If a practitioner accepts referrals from outside providers, he also accepts responsibility for care coordination related to the care he provides. Timely documentation and communication of client progress to the referring provider in written form is a central component of ethical case management in this situation. Clients should give informed consent for this communication, and if the client declines, the referring provider should be informed, and the client should be directed elsewhere. In addition, clients should be asked if other healthcare providers should be included in case management. If expected progress isn't met, the referring provider should be informed as well. Policies and procedures, as well as HIPAA compliant modes of communication, must also be in place. If your services are covered by the patient's health insurance, special attention must also be given to documentation, and records must be provided if requested by the insurance company's care management department.

Janet is a massage therapist in a small town with an established reputation for providing high quality treatment to her clients. She is contacted by the case manager who works with Dr. Jones, a local family medicine physician. Dr. Jones has a patient that has difficulty standing upright. He would like to refer that patient for several sessions. This is the first time Janet has taken on a case-managed referral. During their first appointment, while conducting her regular intake interview, she learns that Joann recently had abdominal surgery and is experiencing severe back pain. Janet doesn't normally keep SOAP notes and proceeds with the treatment plan without thorough documentation. Several weeks go by and the case manager contacts Janet for a progress report because the physician hasn't noticed substantial change in Joann's condition.

Points to Ponder

What are the pitfalls of not keeping detailed treatment notes? How can you find out the types of documentation a referring provider wants? What are some questions you can ask a case manager to set up appropriate expectations? What policies and procedures must Janet have to ethically accept this referral and coordinate care with the patient's other healthcare providers? What are the potential obstacles to care coordination when working with a referral? How can you alleviate those obstacles?

Janet accepted the referral; so she also accepted responsibility for care coordination with Dr. Jones' office. Timely documentation and communication of Joann's progress would have demonstrated Janet's ethical case management, and would have alerted the physician to recommend altering the treatment plan.

Define an Ideal Practice Environment with Case Management

- Describe your ideal practice environment involving case management.
- Make a list of the potential care coordination issues in that setting.
- Identify the case management issues that might arise when coordinating care among different providers, both within and outside the practice.
- Brainstorm ways to overcome reluctance for associates in a group practice to incorporate case management.

■ Group Practices

Group practices differ from medical clinics and hospitals in the services they offer and the purposes of the practice. Group practices are often holistic healthcare centers and wellness centers where several modalities are offered, such as chiropractic, acupuncture, massage therapy, aromatherapy, yoga, movement therapy, and nutritional counseling. A sub-category of group practices are specialty centers that focus on one of these modalities. While medical clinics and hospitals have the goal of diagnosing and treating illness, group practices tend to focus on identifying imbalances in the body and musculoskeletal injuries that the various modalities can address, and on educating and guiding clients about preventive measures they can practice at home.

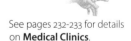

See pages 232-233 for details on **Medical Clinics**.

Common Ethical Issues

Three of the major ethical considerations that all group practices face involve legal issues, finances, and marketing. In this section, we focus on these issues and then explore the ethical aspects specific to multi-disciplinary and specialty centers.

Legal Considerations

Group practices can be formed legally in three ways: as an association, as a partnership, or as a single legal entity. The legal and operational ethical considerations are different for each, and practitioners should carefully review these to determine how much responsibility each individual member has by law.

In an association, individual practitioners under one roof each maintain their own separate businesses. Often the individual practitioners contribute toward common expenses, such as rent, utilities, marketing, and even the cost of hiring a receptionist. So long as the individual members only share common expenses and don't share revenues or profits, each separate business is separate for tax purposes as well.

If the association also shares revenues or profits, that association may be treated as a partnership, which requires different reporting for tax purposes. If revenues or profits are shared, the individuals should consider creating an entity, and reporting as an entity for tax purposes.

An association should also avoid holding itself out as a single entity or joint venture. If enough facts are cited by a complaining party, each member of the association could be liable for obligations of the other members. Filing partnership papers or creating a written partnership agreement isn't required to be legally considered as a partnership: the key to determining partnership status is the "appearance" that the business is indeed operating as a partnership, or representing itself as a partnership. Thus, you could be held responsible if someone were to file a lawsuit against an associate of yours.

Group practices can also be formed within one legal entity. In this case, all expenses, profits and liabilities are incurred by that entity, and allocated among the owners (although not necessarily on an equal basis). The entity may be a partnership, corporation, or limited liability company, depending on the goals of the individuals involved and various tax considerations. Each entity requires careful thought as to legal, tax, and practical considerations of the owners.

Pitfalls in a group practice can be circumvented by delineating in writing the rights and obligation of each individual. List all of the particulars that are important to each person in running the business. An agreement between members of an association should include the following: the purpose and major goals of the association; expectations and duties of each practitioner; how common expenses are allocated to the members; objective consequences for failure to fulfill obligations; procedures for handling problems (conflict resolution); and a dissolution (or buy-out) agreement. In the case of a group practice operating as an entity, the agreement should also include specific terms of allocating collection of revenue, as well as allocation of expenses. Note that the allocation of income should focus on actual collections, rather than what may be billed but not paid. Also, develop a general business plan, an agreed-upon Standards of Practice, and a Code of Ethics.[3]

Financial Considerations

Financial obligations can be a major source of entanglement in an association. In an association, often one individual is required to assume responsibility for common expenses (e.g., rent, utilities, telephone). If at all possible, include everyone's name on the lease and clarify the group's shared budget. Also include the following for an entity: prepare financial projections; have a written agreement of each person's financial obligations; determine how revenues and expenses are split; and designate who, in writing, is authorized to make minor decisions, major decisions, pay minor expenditures, and incur major expenditures on behalf of the entity.

Many group practices incorporate product sales. Although product sales are a great diversification method, three significant challenges arise: choosing the product lines; determining who is responsible for overseeing sales; and disbursing the profits, particularly when a client sees more than one practitioner in the group setting. Note: if your business is a partnership, the funds can be commingled. Be sure to create an action plan for product sales including goals and budget.

Marketing Considerations

Cooperative marketing is one of the strongest benefits to being in a group practice and is often an area where conflicts arise. Determine what percentage of marketing is done jointly. Develop a marketing plan with goals, target dates, and a budget. Before placing long term advertising (e.g., a shared directory advertisement), create a payment agreement to cover the possibility of an associate leaving.

In most group practices, each individual is responsible for booking his own clients. This gets fuzzy when new clients are garnered from shared marketing activities. Avoid misunderstandings, resentment, and unethical behavior by creating a new client booking policy that fairly distributes new clients among the practitioners.

Multi-Disciplinary Group Practices

A clear advantage of group practices is that practitioners of different modalities can integrate their therapies into individualized programs for clients to maintain health or address common health challenges. Practitioners have the opportunity to become knowledgeable about other modalities, establish professional connections, and experience a true team approach. Opportunities exist for mentoring and supervision, and wellness centers can model clear professional boundaries.

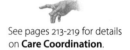

See pages 213-219 for details on **Care Coordination**.

A group practice may submit for insurance reimbursement, which is to the advantage of an individual practitioner who isn't recognized as a primary care provider. Practitioners must be skilled at charting client progress and at maintaining clear billing records for the group to meet regulatory and ethical requirements when requesting insurance reimbursement. Operation and marketing challenges are generally shared by the group.

Ethical Guidelines for Multi-Disciplinary Practices

- Carefully consider the other professionals in the practice. There should be clear alignment of your philosophy, values, and temperament with those of the group.
- Identify how active a role you wish to take in the running of the business, and communicate your preferences to the group.
- Consider the types of clients likely to be seen in the practice and honestly assess whether and how your modality would benefit clients by adding to the mix of therapies offered by the group.
- Assess the potential power and knowledge differentials between you and other group practitioners.
- Before joining the group, examine the various benefits of contractor or employee status, including how each status would benefit both you and the center.
- Clarify your own desired levels of interaction with other members of the group, and be prepared to invest time and energy in these relationships.
- Ask for a contract that outlines your financial obligations to the group and how profits are distributed.
- Insist that a code of conduct and/or a policy and procedure manual be written, available, and regularly updated.
- Clarify with the group the professional image that it desires to convey, and determine whether that image fits with your preferred modes of practice and client interaction.

- If a joint marketing plan is developed, ask that an agreement be reached regarding payment in case you or another associate leaves the group.
- Clarify parameters for working with clients outside the center.
- If your position requires you to sell products, ask for clarity regarding ordering and profit sharing, and regarding how much impact product sales has on your continued association with the group.
- Understand the existing dissolution agreement used in the practice or insist that such an agreement be created.

Specialty Centers

Specialty centers focus on one type of modality, such as acupuncture clinics, chiropractic groups, or massage centers. Specialty centers provide an excellent vehicle to make a modality more visible in the community and more widely available to persons who might not otherwise be clients. National franchises may bring the center together (see the following section), or local like-minded practitioners may combine their efforts. Whether local or national, specialty centers can have the advantage of offering sessions at lower prices than individual or group practices offer in the area.

Specialty centers can have high volumes of clients and, therefore, offer practitioners valuable customer experience and the opportunity to develop technical skills on the job. They may also provide continuing education opportunities that all the practitioners can benefit from. The center often provides supplies such as tables, oils, linens, laundry, and marketing. New practitioners, or those whose careers are in transition, may find a specialty center to be well suited to their practice needs, even though pay may be correspondingly lower when clients are charged lower fees. Peer support and supervision are advantages to working in a specialty center, but a disadvantage is that clients may develop loyalty to the center rather than individual practitioners.

Ethical Guidelines for Specialty Centers

Consider the following in addition to the issues listed above for group practices:

- Examine your reasons for associating with a specialty center. Your personal goals are important but must be balanced with the goals of the center.
- Remember that your commitment and loyalty to the center are keys to ethical practice. The success of the business is larger than the success of your portion of the practice.
- With all practitioners practicing the same modality, internal competition may arise. Develop and discuss policies and procedures to avoid or resolve competition.
- Decide how you can ethically make your services stand out from those of your peers. Some options include: specialize in a modality that isn't currently offered; enhance customer service with little extras, such as adding hot towels; promoting products that address the individualized needs of clients at home.

 Working Successfully in Groups

- Create an "ideal" partnership or associate agreement.
- Design a "New Client Booking Policy" that fairly distributes new clients among all of the practitioners.
- List potential reasons why you would be reluctant to refer clients to an associate.
- Identify reasons why an associate might be reluctant to refer clients to you. Designate options to counter this reluctance.

Spas

The spa industry has expanded in new and exciting directions over the last two decades. While the image of the local day spa remains most familiar, spas have also become common vacation destinations and are sought-after amenities at resorts, in luxury hotels, and on cruise ships. Dental and medical offices are including spa treatments to make their procedures more pleasant and attractive to their patients. Many spas have expanded their scope from simply furnishing beauty services to offering healthcare services. Estheticians, massage therapists, aromatherapists, acupuncturists, reflexologists, yoga teachers, nutritional consultants, and energy practitioners are commonly found in these spa settings.

Many practitioners work part time at a spa to augment their private practices. Working in these businesses requires conforming to a set image and structuring your treatments to align with the company's schedule, treatment protocol, policies, and philosophy.[4] Marketing is another area that is often a source of conflict. In a spa you don't have to do marketing or schedule clients, but there's often no guarantee that your work hours are filled. Many practitioners discover to their dismay that to increase the client flow they need to market their services.

To be successful in these environments, a practitioner needs to understand employer expectations, and understand the rationale behind the policies and procedures set by the employer. Certainly, these measures are set up to protect the client and the company, but, very often, they're set to protect the practitioner as well. One practitioner describes a helpful mindset when considering working in a spa environment, "I feel that when I work in a spa, the client is the spa's client and not my personal client. I usually am open to doing what is best for the spa. This keeps the spa going, and in the long run affects my ability to work."

The Franchise Phenomenon

As public demand has grown, even the image of the local day spa is growing and changing with corporations like the Red Door Spa and franchise systems like Massage Envy Spa getting involved in promoting day spas at the national level. CG Funk, Vice President of Industry Relations and Product Development for Massage Envy Spa says:

> With the increased public demand for massage therapy services, there is plenty of room for all types of businesses to open and be successful. National franchises are also contributing to our industry by creating more exposure of the work to a wider demographic population, which grows the industry for all of us. Franchising is being in business for yourself but not by yourself. Most franchises are owned by local small business operators, known as the franchisees. The owners live in the communities where their business is and contribute through creating jobs and bringing in revenue that helps fund local city efforts.[5]

Franchising is fast becoming a new and exciting business opportunity, not only as employment opportunities for practitioners, but also as an alternative for practitioners who want to own their own business. For those practitioners who want to be owners, private practice is no longer the only option.

In 2012, Massage Envy Spa provided 14.5 million services to 1.17 million members and 2.6 million guests. In 2013, they're providing 56,000 services per day. And that is only one of the many national franchise organizations today. Many people are now receiving massage that wouldn't have even considered it in the past, and probably weren't aware of the benefits even a year earlier. This industry has provided thousands of employment opportunities for massage therapists (and now estheticians), as well as tremendous visibility for all somatic practitioners at the national level.

According to Funk, working for a franchise spa may be a good option for practitioners who are new graduates, those that want to supplement their private practice income, those that don't want the responsibility of operating their own business, or those who simply want to work part time.

> *But to be successful in this environment, practitioners need to focus as much of their training and preparation efforts on communication and professional skills, as they do on their technique and style. These communication and professional skills need to include interactions with clients, front desk staff, other therapists, and especially with management.*[6]

A massage therapist had been working for a franchise spa for several months. Although he was trained in company procedures, including draping, he chose to continue with his own style of draping. During a recent treatment, a female client was uncomfortable about his draping and accused him of exposing her needlessly. The therapist insisted that the exposure was unintentional, and that his draping was appropriate and satisfactory. The company investigated and the therapist was terminated for not following procedures.

Points to Ponder

Why is it important for a therapist to follow procedures, even those as individual as draping style? What exceptions come to mind? What could the therapist or the company have done differently? Would it have mattered if the therapist was indeed following procedures?

In this scenario, the practitioner had no opportunity to defend himself. Had he been following the company's draping procedure, not only would he have made a defense against the client's accusations, but the company could have also defended him as a good employee who follows the rules. Many employees don't understand that operating within the structure set by the company is in their best interest. If both the employer and the employee are committed to creating an ethical work environment, it can be a healthy place for all those involved.

The Work Environment

Creating an ethical working environment is, of course, the mutual responsibility of spa management and employees. Ideally, spa management acts diligently to protect and serve the rights of both employees and clients. On their side, spa employees ideally commit themselves to quality work at all times and in all circumstances, and express loyalty to the organization by cooperating with policies and procedures, and avoiding conflicts of interest. Difficulties arise not just with actual lapses in these ideals, they also arise when suspicion and distrust surface within the organization. Both management and employees, therefore, need to practice transparency, honesty, and integrity in communications with one another.

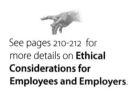

See pages 210-212 for more details on **Ethical Considerations for Employees and Employers**.

On one hand, the relationship between spa management and employees boils down to a question of autonomy. In most spas, practitioners don't have a choice about how many clients to see in a day, which clients they'll work with, or even which type of work is to be performed. Serving the customer is the spa's priority. Management expects employees to work to an assigned schedule, to expand their therapeutic repertoire by learning spa treatments outside their specialty, and to conform to the corporate image. On the other hand, spa management may offer the employee numerous benefits such as compensation based on seniority, commissions on product sales, health insurance, paid vacations, paid sick days, pension plans, profit sharing, and reimbursement for continuing education.

Perhaps the most serious ethical concerns in the spa environment surround issues of inappropriate touch and sexual misconduct. Management usually has a zero tolerance policy, meaning that if a client complains of sexual misconduct on the part of a practitioner, that practitioner is terminated without recourse. A similar policy might exist regarding practitioner complaints against clients who sexualize a session. Management needs to examine whether their policies disempower practitioners in these situations, while employees should know the limits of their legal rights.

Next we examine, more specifically, some of the ethical considerations that spa management and spa employees should be responsible for to create an atmosphere where cooperation and ethical behavior are encouraged and supported.

Ethical Guidelines for Spa Management

- Spa management is responsible for creating clear, written codes of conduct and policy and procedure manuals, and for ensuring that employees receive training that reviews these expectations.
- Management formulates employee contracts that clearly spell out all aspects of financial agreements, methods of compensation, and benefits.
- Management ensures that front desk and other support staff are educated regarding the types of treatments offered, that they understand the ethical principles behind scope of practice considerations, and that they're aware of basic contraindications to the treatments offered by the spa.
- Management does its best to design and decorate the spa environment in a way that doesn't elicit a confusing or sexual ambience.
- Management clarifies the types and means of communication that are appropriate among practitioners, as well as between practitioners and clients, and between practitioners and management.
- Management invests not just in modality training for its employees, but also in continued education in communication: interpersonal skills; HIPAA and confidentiality regulations; and avoidance of sexual misconduct and harassment charges.

Spa Legal Liability

http://www.theethicsoftouch. com/ ethics-in-the-spa- industry.pdf

Ethical Guidelines for Spa Employees

- Spa employees know the goals, mission, and standards of the spa; understand what actions on their part support those standards; and express their loyalty to the business through such supportive actions.
- Employees insist on the correct classification of their relationship with the spa, whether that is independent contractor or employee, so they legally meet IRS requirements.
- Employees clearly communicate with management concerning the treatments they're willing to do and the additional training they're willing to undertake.
- Employees are willing to conform to the corporate image to represent business success and unity to clients.
- Employees know the scope of practice parameters and contraindications to treatment, and maintain professional standards at all times.
- Employees maintain awareness of boundary issues and are diligent in avoiding dual relationships with management, peers, and clients.
- Employees are very familiar with HIPAA requirements and confidentiality measures taken by the spa management to ensure client confidentiality.
- Employees know and utilize the established means of communications to inform management of any ethical concerns that arise, and should be aware of their obligations, both legal and ethical, if management doesn't respond appropriately to their concerns.
- If sales are expected, employees base their sales pitches on honest evaluations of products or services that they feel support their modalities and client wellness.
- Employees are willing to research and create ethical marketing techniques to increase the visibility of their modality within the spa setting.

The Spa Environment

Make a list of ethical dilemmas that may be unique to the spa environment. Brainstorm ways for employees and employers to avoid or overcome those dilemmas.

Hospitals and Hospices

More and more wellness practitioners are finding themselves working in hospital or hospice settings, either as employees, as contractors, or as volunteers. The clinical and ethical considerations in these environments can vary greatly from the environments with which many such professionals are familiar. Adherence to HIPAA is more strictly enforced and more is at stake in the case of violations. Access to sensitive and detailed medical and health history information is greater. It is also typical to be working as part of team that is made up of a variety of other professionals like physicians, nurses, and occupational, physical, or respiratory therapists, working together within an established plan of care for each patient.

The Hospital Setting

Hospitals may be privately or publicly funded; may be for-profit or nonprofit; may provide care that is general or specialized in nature; may stand alone or be associated with a medical school or religious order; and may be small (10-20 beds) and community oriented, or large (over 1,000 beds) and international in reputation. Practitioners may treat patients with many conditions not seen in non-hospital settings, such as trauma patients, amputees, cancer survivors, burn victims, and patients preparing for or recovering from surgeries.

The demand in hospitals for wellness practitioners, and massage therapy in particular, is increasing at a rate that unfortunately challenges the speed at which most hospitals operate. This often results in haphazard hiring and poorly coordinated oversight of these practitioners. There may be a lack of understanding about the value and most effective manner of integration of hands-on therapies. Often considered something that is simply "nice" to have as opposed to clinically valuable, many hospitals are willing to engage somatic practitioners who have little or no hospital-specific training. Practitioners are asked to see patients without benefit of access to the medical record of those patients or to receive input from other members of that patient's medical team. They are brought in as a "luxury" to improve patient satisfaction measures, but their services aren't expected to measurably improve clinical outcomes. Luckily, many hospitals are indeed noticing improved outcomes. Practitioners and the professional associations need to continue to educate hospital administrators and doctors about the efficacy of wellness care. Additionally, hospitals are now forced to compete and are actually being mandated to demonstrate patient satisfaction. Wellness care is high on that list. Companies are being formed to manage these adjunct services.

In some hospitals, somatic practitioners are fully integrated as paid employees working within a funded program with full access to medical records. They are integrated with the other members of a patient's medical team, participating in delivery of an overall plan of care with an expectation that a patient's experience and trajectory have the potential to be measurably improved by the involvement of a properly trained practitioner. In other cases, practitioners are permitted only to work with ostensibly healthy staff members, often as part of a wellness program or a hospital's attempt to provide self-care options for clinicians.

The Hospice Setting

A patient may be referred to hospice care when a medical professional believes the patient's disease will lead to death within six months. Hospice care is provided to persons of all ages, from children through the elderly. A goal of a hospice referral is to provide comfort measures and daily care in the patient's home setting, but when necessary, the patient is admitted to an inpatient hospice unit or institution for more complicated or 24-hour care. Practitioners who are referred to work with hospice patients may see them in either or both of these settings and may follow patients on a weekly or bimonthly basis throughout the hospice admission.

Hospices have a better record than hospitals of accepting and integrating complementary therapies into their patient care routines. In hospice care, the concept of wellbeing extends beyond curing disease. Medical professionals in hospices regularly consider how to maximize patients' physical wellbeing within the limits of their illness, but also consider how to maximize their emotional, social, and spiritual wellbeing. Hospice professionals are willing and eager to welcome therapies that contribute to compassionate end-of-life care that helps mitigate patient pain and suffering, and enhances a sense of meaning and acceptance.

Generally, practitioners work in the hospice setting on a part-time basis. If not volunteering, practitioners usually work as independent contractors who receive a flat rate fee that doesn't include travel time to patients' homes. Last-minute schedule changes are common, so flexibility is essential. Being flexible in applying a modality is also essential, as patients are often bed-bound. An excellent working knowledge of contraindications for medical conditions is essential, and practitioners should request a clear working directive from the medical team, patient, and family regarding how to approach the work with each patient. Knowledge of medical terminology assists the practitioner to understand the medical team and to communicate concerns back to them.

Hospice work can be emotionally demanding, and practitioners should honestly evaluate their own readiness to undertake such work. Practitioners should maintain equilibrium in the presence of the patient and family. It is wise to have some outlet, such as supervisory or peer support, to help manage their own emotional responses to intense session work.

Ethical Considerations in Hospitals and Hospices

The way in which a practitioner is integrated into a hospital or hospice setting can have an important effect on the ethical considerations that might arise in his work. In these settings, the importance of information as a tool of ethical practice comes into sharp focus. If a practitioner is brought in as a volunteer with little or no access to health history or care plan details, that practitioner is being put in a position that is ripe for ethical dilemmas. For instance, what if the patient asks a massage therapist to massage a swollen limb? Is the swelling potentially caused by a blood clot? Could it be a complication of congestive heart failure? Maybe the patient simply bumped his leg this morning on the rail of his hospital bed? The patient may answer some of these questions, but perhaps not. Without access to more information, the therapist either has to deny care or make a potentially risky decision to work "conservatively" in hopes of avoiding harm. If the therapist is a contractor, she may have only spotty information. She may have access to other members of a patient's team, but not to the medical record.

It is important to remain cognizant of ethics by staying clearly within one's Scope. Patients in hospitals and hospices often receive care from many different people. It isn't always clear which clinician is responsible for which piece of care. As such, a patient may ask a somatic practitioner about his prognosis or perhaps about the reason for a certain test or medication. Even when that practitioner knows the answer to such out-of-scope questions it isn't appropriate for her to explain these to the patient. Medications are often given for off-label indications and prognosis is always a challenging topic that is best discussed directly with the patient's attending physician or nurse.

> It is one of the most beautiful compensations of life, that no man can sincerely try to help another without helping himself.
>
> —Ralph Waldo Emerson

Tim is a practitioner employed at a local hospital. His neighbor's co-worker passes out and is taken by ambulance to the hospital where Tim works. The neighbor knows that Tim works at the hospital and asks him to check on the co-worker's status and let him know about the co-worker's status.

Points to Ponder

What would you tell your neighbor? What if you find out the co-worker has significant medical issues, would you share that with your neighbor? What are all the ethical issues represented here?

It can be tempting, especially when it comes to personal relationships, to bend our ethical responsibilities. In this situation, we might think to ourselves, "What could it hurt? I'll just look the patient up. If it's really bad, I'll tell my neighbor I couldn't find anything." A person's privacy, medical or otherwise, must be respected. In fact, looking up a patient's medical information if you aren't providing direct care for that patient isn't only unethical, it's a direct violation of HIPAA.

A practitioner is working with a patient in the bone marrow transplant unit. The patient is under contact isolation precautions requiring all visitors, medical or otherwise, to wear gloves and a gown, particularly when coming into direct contact with the patient. As the practitioner works with the patient, a nurse comes into the room to check the patient's IV lines and she also adjusts the patient's blood pressure cuff. She isn't wearing gloves or a gown.

Points to Ponder

What would you say to the nurse? How could you approach this situation without offending the nurse, while protecting the patient's safety at the same time?

Wellness practitioners who work in a hospital setting often comport themselves with an overly-deferential manner that assumes that other members of the medical team "know better" or "must have a reason" for doing things a certain way. Obviously, the situation described above would need to be handled delicately to avoid offending the nurse who wasn't following the posted contact precautions, but your first responsibility is patient safety. You are responsible to the patient and to the hospital to ensure maximum safety. You would have to decide if you felt comfortable approaching the nurse directly to explain your concern or if reporting the situation to a unit director or patient care manager is more appropriate. It would also be important not to confront the nurse in front of the patient, if that's the approach you choose. However, having seen the nurse's oversight, you would be ethically bound to intervene.

A practitioner has been working with a hospice patient weekly for several months. The patient has recently become comatose, but the family has requested that the practitioner continue the sessions. The practitioner doesn't believe her modality is appropriate at this stage but is aware that it brings the family peace to see their loved one cared for.

Points to Ponder

How can you honor your knowledge of modality appropriateness, while honoring the family's wishes? Should you consider the family's wishes at all? Is it possible that the family's comfort also affects the patient's comfort?

The practitioner may wish to review her reservations about the appropriateness of the modality with the medical team, as well as with her supervisor or peer support group. If it's determined that the work is beyond her scope at this stage, she should decide whether the family would accept this news better from her or from the nurse or physician. On the other hand, even in the absence of direct benefit to the patient, it may be determined that the modality can "do no harm." The practitioner is ethically obligated to inform the family of this determination; nevertheless, continuing the sessions may indirectly benefit the patient by contributing to the family's wellbeing, and thus to a positive psychosocial environment for the patient.

The best framework for ethical clarity and practice is laid when you're integrated in a way that confers the privileges (and responsibilities) of being on staff, even if you're not. If the hospital or hospice wants you to interact with its patients using your professional skills, even as a volunteer, it must provide you with all of the tools it provides to other clinicians.

Ethical Guidelines in Hospital and Hospice Settings

- Know the appropriate use of, and safeguarding of, protected medical information.
- Know how, when, where, and with whom to discuss patient care specifics.
- You must be comfortable managing expectations and staying within Scope when a recommendation from a physician or nurse isn't congruent with what you know to be the safe, best practices for your discipline.
- You must be comfortable balancing patient expectations and requests with orders or recommendations from other members of the care team.
- Maintain clear boundaries with regard to fielding patient questions; know what you know and should know; know when to suggest that a patient or family member discuss an issue directly with another member of the care team.
- Honor the limitations of the "delineation of privileges" or whatever document makes your Scope within that facility clear. For instance, if you're trained in manual lymphatic drainage, but that modality isn't included in what you're authorized to do within the hospital, you may not employ that modality even when it's indicated by a patient's condition and would likely be beneficial.
- Use responsible, clear communication with patients and members of the care team regarding expectations around the results or effect of your work.
- Stay up to date on changes in policy or procedure that affect patient safety and execution of care plans.
- Understand what and how much to include in your notes in the medical record that detail the service(s) provided to a given patient.
- Always respect family privacy, especially when you're given access to the patient's home and intimate details of family life.
- Maintain clear boundaries to enhance professional and avoid personal involvement with patients and family members, even in the midst of difficult end-of-life scenarios.
- Avoid the imposition of one's own cultural, ethnic, and religious beliefs and practices onto a patient or family and instead maintain sensitivity to individual differences in these areas.
- Always be careful to recognize the power differential in emotionally charged situations and refuse to exploit this for personal benefit.

A hospital client has been released to go home and would like to continue sessions with you through your private practice. You can't accept insurance there and are concerned that the client will balk at paying the full fee. The client also doesn't wish for you to send records of these private sessions to the medical provider who supervised you and was in charge of his care at the hospital.

Points to Ponder

How could you set up appropriate boundaries with the client in this case? Would you consider altering your fees? Is it ethical to have separate fees for different clients? Are you ethically (or legally) bound to send records to the original supervisor in the hospital setting?

The practitioner needs to evaluate the relationship that has developed between herself and this client to clarify boundaries and the power differential. She also should consider her pricing structure and determine whether or not lowering her usual fee is a rational decision, and if so, by how much. Finally, the practitioner needs to re-examine HIPAA rules regarding patient autonomy in the sharing of medical records. If the practitioner believes it's important to report sessions to the medical professional, she must present a cogent argument to the client and decide on a course of action should the client still refuse to give permission.

A practitioner has been scheduled by the hospice medical team to perform a Reiki session with a new patient. The practitioner has just returned from a course in aromatherapy and, while interacting with the patient at the first session, becomes convinced that some of the patient's symptoms would be lessened by a specific aromatherapy treatment.

Points to Ponder

Is it ethical for you to offer a service for which you weren't scheduled? With whom should you discuss the new service, the patient or the staff who scheduled you?

It would be unethical for this practitioner to tell the patient or family about the aromatherapy treatment at this session, much less to administer it. After the session, the practitioner should approach the medical team with a description of the symptoms that he saw in the patient, an explanation about how the treatment might help, and a detailed description of the methods that would be used to deliver the treatment. If the medical team agrees that the treatment might be helpful, then the patient and family would be contacted for their permission.

Figure 8.2   Tips for Creating a Position within a Hospital or Hospice That Supports a Strong Ethical Framework

- No matter your level of integration, having access to the medical history, care planning, and impressions recorded by other members of a patient's care team is essential. A hospital wouldn't expect a physician to see a patient without access to this information. You and the patients with whom you work deserve the same consideration.
- Ask to be given privileges to chart in the electronic medical record. The other members of the medical team should see what you have done with a patient, and to benefit from your impressions and how they fit into the plan of care.
- Offer to provide brief "in-service" trainings to the clinicians in the facility or unit with whom you'll be working. Impressions of what various somatic therapies are and how they're valuable vary widely. Make it a priority to educate the rest of the medical team about what you understand the benefits of your work to be, how it might best fit into what they're already providing, and also invite them to offer suggestions and ask questions. A well-crafted, brief presentation delivered in a spirit of cooperation and openness can go a long way toward more complete integration on a day-to-day, operational basis.
- Ask to be included in hospital-wide notifications, trainings, and updates.
- Ask to be invited to Grand Rounds and other departmental and hospital-wide gatherings that relate to clinical decision-making and care planning, as well as those geared toward community-building and idea sharing.
- Ask to be affiliated with a department in the hospital that relates to what you do. Is the Physical Therapy Department a good fit? If you're working with oncology or surgical patients, maybe Palliative Care is where you should be. If the hospital has an Integrative Medicine Department, that is likely a good fit. Be wary of being assigned to Volunteer Services or Auxiliary. These departments don't typically provide what would be considered "clinical services" and are, therefore, not incorporated into the patient care picture in an essential way.
- Get connected with the Employee Health Department/Office to ensure that you have all immunizations and protections in place necessary to keep both you and the patients with whom you work as safe as possible.
- Establish a connection for professional supervision, either with hospital- or hospice-based colleagues. Many considerations in these settings are unlike those encountered in private practice or other outpatient settings.

- Call or visit your local hospitals and ask if they have practitioners on staff (or volunteering) within your specific discipline.
- Create a proposal for the appropriate hospital decision-maker that describes the benefits of adding your discipline to their patient care (include benefits to the hospital, as well as benefits to the patients).

Medical Clinics

Medical clinics are like hospitals in the sense that both are staffed by professionals who can assess, diagnose, and treat patients. The main differences between clinics and hospitals are in terms of scope. A clinic may be headed by a single practicing physician (a primary care provider, or PCP) while a hospital has a complex leadership hierarchy. Clinics have limited hours while hospitals are run 24 hours a day. Clinics work only on an outpatient basis while hospitals have inpatient wards. Clinics manage patients' wellness care and supervise home treatment regimens for chronic conditions. Hospitals provide some of these same services in addition to managing emergency and life-threatening conditions. When a clinic sees a patient who has suffered a severe trauma, or whose condition has worsened beyond the ability to be cared for by the patient herself or in the home, then the clinic refers the patient to a hospital.

The nature of a clinic arises from the combined skills of its staff and the purpose of its practice. A general outpatient clinic may have PCPs in several practice areas that provide primary health care for a community. Specialized clinics include rehabilitation centers, physical therapy clinics, sports medicine clinics, orthopedic physician's offices, and immunologist practices.

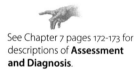

See Chapter 7 pages 172-173 for descriptions of **Assessment and Diagnosis**.

Many somatic practitioners work in these types of clinic environments in tandem with medical doctors or physical therapists. The concept of multi-discipline or multi-practitioner medical practices often provides exceptional client care. However, in reality there are two very different reasons for setting up multi-care practices, and manifest in two ways: as an integrated complementary care clinic, and as an adjunct complementary care practice.

Integrated Complementary Care in Medical Clinics

Integrated complementary care in medical clinics provides an environment where each patient has one chart for the office and may access all of the different specialty practitioners in the center. The designated case manager coordinates the patient's care plan between the different practitioners and oversees the progress. Each case is discussed at group meetings so that all minds involved can arrive at the best treatment(s) and ongoing care.

The medical clinic's business setup (be it an association, partnership, or single legal entity) may influence whether integrated somatic practitioners are hired as independent contractors or employees.

Adjunct Complementary Care in Medical Clinics

The main reason for adjunct complementary care in medical clinics is financial. Several practitioners of the same or different specialties join together to share overhead. They each maintain a separate practice with their own clients and really don't promote inter-office referrals. This lack of cross-referrals is often due to the fear of losing clients to another practitioner.

For example, a practitioner may have the option of renting a room in the PCP's office. The room may be shared with other practitioners, and the fee structure may be by the day, by the hour, or by the session. Advantages to the practitioner are the possibility of client referrals from the PCP and the potential for sharing marketing strategies. Generally, the practitioner, not the PCP, is responsible for needed materials or supplies. Practitioners in adjunct clinics are more likely to be independent contractors than employees.

Ethical Considerations in Medical Clinics

Major concerns about joining a medical clinic are: the possibility of needing to alter your style and scope of practice to suit the clinic's visions, policies, and procedures; and the issue of being hired as an independent contractor versus employee.

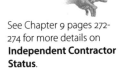

See Chapter 9 pages 272-274 for more details on **Independent Contractor Status**.

To avoid future ethical business complications, be sure the clinic attracts the kind of clients with whom you want to work, provides opportunities for you to use your favorite modalities, and allows you to work at the pace and in the style with which you're comfortable. Before working in this setting, determine if you can live with the clinic's policies for dress code, finances, logistics, practitioner/practitioner interactions, client/practitioner interactions, and marketing.

Most practitioners discover they need to alter their treatments in a clinic setting. The time you spend with clients and the actual work you do may be determined by the lead PCP. You could be told what to do, how to do it, when to do it, and the time allowed to work. You may even experience a sense of detachment from the client because someone else usually handles the greeting, scheduling, payment, paperwork, and, sometimes even, the follow-up. On the positive side, freedom from administrative tasks provides you with more hands-on time with your clients. In addition, your clients benefit from your association with the clinic because the setting provides access to managed care and possibly to state-of-the-art equipment that you otherwise might not afford.

Teaming Up

After reviewing this chapter, write down all of your personal and professional characteristics that would work well in a Team Environment. Then list all of your characteristics that wouldn't work well in a Team Environment. Are you currently working in the right environment for you? If not, what changes can you make to improve your conditions?

▌ Conclusion

Working in a team can be rewarding, and can also be fraught with complications and ethical dilemmas. Before embarking on this type of a path, review the ethical considerations for the different work environments. Determine which environments best suit your skills, personality, and preferences. Follow the suggested guidelines and create contracts that work well for everyone involved.

9
Business Ethics

"Hold yourself responsible for a higher standard than anybody else expects of you."
—Henry Ward Beecher

Attitudes About Money

Fee Structures
- Sliding Fee Scales
- Prepaid Package Plans
- Credit

Gratuities

Barter
- Direct Barter
- Barter Exchanges
- Financial Considerations

Gift Certificates
- Expiration Dates
- The Downside of Gift Certificates

Taxes

Product Sales
- Increase Profits, Revenue, and Bookings
- Make It Convenient
- Extend Your Treatment Benefits
- The Ethical Concerns of Retailing
- Nutritional Supplements

Referrals
- Acknowledging Referrals

Marketing Materials
- Exaggerated Claims
- Misleading Ploys
- Questionable Names and Titles
- Inappropriate Images
- Follow Business Regulations
- Misrepresenting Credentials

Social Media Ethics
- Social Media Policies
- Ethically Sharing Content
- What Happens In Vegas

Legal Issues
- Comply with Local, State, and Federal Laws
- Insurance Coverage
- Slander and Libel
- Copyrighted Materials
- Contracts
- Civil Lawsuits
- Employees and Independent Contractors

Insurance Reimbursement Issues
- Responsibility for Payment
- Preferred Provider Status
- Fee Schedules
- Timely Documentation
- Communication with Referring PCP

Key Terms

Boundary Violation
Business Page
Copyright Infringement
Defamation
Duty of Care
Ethical Dilemma
Fair Use
Fraud

Geotagging
Kickback
Libel
Malpractice
Negligence
Payer Discrimination
Personal Profile
Pin

Post
Power Differential
Self-Accountability
Sexual Misconduct
Share
Slander
Social Media Policy
Tweet

Running an ethical business challenges you to maintain healthy boundaries and to operate from deeply held values. Ethical conflicts can arise when you feel oppressed by laws and regulations, particularly those that are archaic or put unreasonable burdens on practitioners. Sometimes you may feel confusion about what is legal and what seems the right thing to do. Some practitioners may feel forced to find legal loopholes to justify their choices. These dilemmas require thoughtful choices. Truly ethical businesses require a commitment from the practitioner. The business reflects the person who runs it. *The Power of Ethical Management*[1] relates ethical behavior to self-esteem: people who feel good about themselves withstand outside pressure and do what is right rather than what is expedient, popular, or lucrative.

Business ethics covers the major ethical issues that relate to running a successful business: general finances; setting fees; tips; barter; gift certificates; taxes; product sales; referrals; marketing materials; social media; complying with local, state, and federal laws; regulating bodies; insurance coverage; slander and libel; contracts; civil lawsuits; employees status; and insurance reimbursement.

As with all ethical issues, running a business presents many choices, dilemmas, and challenges. In this chapter we review the concepts, beliefs, and information that affect your ability to build and maintain an ethical, professional, and solid business or business relationship.

▌ Attitudes About Money

Running a business that is both ethical and financially successful can be challenging since many people don't have a healthy relationship with money. We may wish it weren't the case, but money plays an important role in our lives. Some people innately handle money well while others find it difficult to balance their checkbooks. Few people are taught how to manage money. The only formal training people receive happens if they take economics, finance, or accounting courses. Ironically, most people taking those courses are the ones who are comfortable with the concept of money in the first place.

Consider the inaccurately cited biblical quote,[2] "Money is the root of all evil." The original quote is, "For the **love of money** is the root of all evil." Money is simply a medium of exchange for goods and services. Originally, people directly traded one thing for another. Money evolved as a method to simplify that exchange. Money is not a mystery. Unfortunately, we imbue it with emotional significance and other qualities because most of us don't understand how to relate to the concept of money or how to manage money in a rational way—and that's where trouble brews.

In her article on money operating systems, Lu Bauer wrote:

> *Yet, we all grow up dealing with money daily in a myriad of ways. We have had to develop our own guidelines and do our own learning, primarily by watching how money was handled in our families of origin. Unfortunately, this is often a case of "the blind leading the blind." Parents aren't even aware they're teaching those watching children. People also learn about money from comic books, stories, teachers, church, friends and their parents, family legends, radio and television shows, and advertising.*
>
> *If your family was struggling financially, you may have been led to believe that strong values and love were missing in those rich families on the other side of town. Also, you were probably told that it isn't okay to ask or talk about money. If your family was better off than others were, you learned not to show it. Most people grew up with an array of mixed messages such as: a purpose in life is to acquire as much money as possible, so you can attain a higher status and respect in society, yet you wouldn't want anyone to know what you had or to be seen as a "show-off." You may have been further confused by parents who demonstrated differing money styles; one might have been thrifty, even a hoarder, while the other might have been happily spending and acquiring. Such families have a lot of tension around money issues."*[3]

Many people in the helping professions proudly wear the "poor but pure" badge. Besides contributing to financial insecurity, this attitude often leads to questionable business practices. Many practitioners experience difficulty in charging appropriate fees for their services and many are uncomfortable charging anything at all. Income is often in direct proportion to one's self-esteem — especially for those of us in the healthcare field. It is imperative to recognize the difference between service and sacrifice.

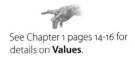

See Chapter 1 pages 14-16 for details on **Values**.

When a massage therapist first opened her practice, her fees were dictated by every hard luck story she heard. Her altruistic approach bankrupted her emotionally and drained her financial resources. What finally tipped the scales? She finally realized she was allowing her clients' money issues to be more important than her time. Several people had made comments such as, "I just can't afford to come here," and her heart strings were pulled and she scrambled to find a way to "help" them. Those same people would reveal during sessions that they recently went on a shopping trip, complain about how much it costs having their hair or nails done every week, grouse about how frantic having the new addition to their home has made them, mention an upcoming vacation, or leave and climb into a new car. It wasn't until she really began to listen and observe that she assumed the responsibility of her own life.

Points to Ponder

How does a situation like this rob clients of the opportunity to acknowledge the value of taking care of their health?

When it comes to money, everything is relative. An interesting shift occurred with the above scenario: when the massage therapist put a value on her services, so did her clients. Now she rarely receives complaints about her fees.

In his zeal to be "of service" a somatic practitioner felt it was his responsibility to provide his services to everyone who needed it. He worked 6-7 days a week, often charging at a sliding scale or *pro bono*. He had a substantial practice with very few clients paying his full fee. After years of dedicated work, he was still renting an apartment, driving the first car he bought, couldn't afford to take a vacation to care for himself, and had little savings for retirement. He felt good about helping so many people and realized he hadn't cared for himself. In so doing, he was now burnt out, worried about his future, and unable to focus as clearly on his clients' needs.

Points to Ponder

What example is this practitioner setting for his clients, family, and friends about prioritizing one's own health and wellbeing?

Balance is the key to service, as in life. Oftentimes, those in the wellness field care for others instead of caring for themselves. While it's noble to care for others, it's necessary to care for oneself in all aspects. This is a lesson that must be learned; otherwise, ultimately you won't help either yourself or others.

Suze Orman, author of *The 9 Steps to Financial Freedom* states:

> *Before we can get control of our finances, we must get control of our attitudes about money, feelings that were shaped by our earliest experiences with it. Opening ourselves to abundance— not only of the pocketbook but also of the heart is what's necessary for true balance and freedom.*[4]

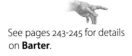

See pages 243-245 for details on **Barter**.

Create a journal about your attitudes toward money. What are your general feelings about the role of money? What was your family history with money and how does it influence your relationship to money today?

Fee Structures

The exchange of currency or barter is an integral aspect of the therapeutic relationship and helps establish boundaries. Many practitioners charge family members and friends a different rate than "regular" clients. While this practice is generally legal, it may pose ethical dilemmas. In addition, some practitioners charge different rates for cash paying clients versus those who pay with a credit card or bill their insurance company. Consistency of rates charged is the key. Unfortunately, even acts of kindness can lead to questions of financial impropriety.

A naturopath in a small city noticed that over the past year the other naturopaths had raised their rates. The dissenting practitioner decided that since he was making ends meet, he didn't want to burden his clients with an increase. Six months later he noticed that he wasn't increasing his client base even though he was charging a lesser amount than his competitors. He was also no longer making ends meet. He then decided to raise his rates in hopes that his current clients would understand. He received several comments from clients who felt his work was well worth the price. Interestingly, he also gained more calls from people inquiring about his services.

Points to Ponder

What if this practitioner had lost clients due to the increase? Do you think his getting more calls is a coincidence, or does having prices in line with other practitioners encourage customer confidence?

> Money motivates neither the best people, nor the best in people. It can rent the body and influence the mind, but it cannot touch the heart or move the spirit; that is reserved for belief, principle, and ethics.
>
> —Dee Hock

A delicate balance exists between charging too much for the services you offer or too little. Either way, your practice suffers. By charging too little, people will wonder whether there's something wrong with your skills or perhaps think that you're a novice trying to get started. Charge too much, and they might think that you're arrogant and they aren't getting their money's worth. It is essential to approach the following financial activities with thoughtful consideration: different rates for different clients; price reductions; sliding scales; package deals; and credit.

An acupuncture patient obtained insurance coverage for 10 sessions. At the end of the 10 sessions, the client had received relief but wanted to continue with maintenance treatments. The client asked for a reduced rate for the sessions. He told the practitioner that rate reductions are a common practice amongst healthcare professionals when a client pays in cash—after all, the acupuncturist wouldn't need to wait for payment and nobody else would know anyway. The practitioner stated that she bills all her sessions (cash, credit card, or insurance) at the same rate. It was unfair to expect a rate that was less than she charged her current cash-paying patients, particularly since she would be putting in the same amount of effort and skill that had brought the client to this point.

The patient left without booking a session stating that he'd think about it. The practitioner decided not to contact the patient about whether he would continue as she didn't want to compromise the value of her work or the relationship with other patients should they somehow find out.

Points to Ponder

Although this practitioner clearly takes an ethical stance, what if a client really needs the work and can't afford the regular rates? Is there a way for a practitioner to be both ethical and accommodating?

We discussed self-accountability in the Ethical Foundations and Practice Management chapters. The following scenario exemplifies the way in which the capacity for self-accountability determines financial ethics:

A physical therapist in private practice for eight years decided to raise her fees. While she enforced the increase with most of her patients, she decided not to inform several patients who had been with her for many years, allowing them to continue to pay the former fee. During the next two years she considered bringing those few patients up to the same rate as the rest of her patients but for various reasons decided not to raise their rates. Recently, one of the clients who wasn't affected by the increase had an appointment. At the end of the session, the patient handed the practitioner cash to pay for her session, and while the patient was in the restroom, the practitioner went to put the money away. As she did, she noticed that the patient had given her twenty dollars too much. It appeared that the bills were new and had probably stuck together. "Hmm," thought the practitioner, "Perhaps I'll keep it. I certainly deserve this extra 20 dollars since she saved a lot more than this amount in not being affected by my increased rates over the past two years. So, this isn't stealing. If I didn't count it and just put it away, I wouldn't even have known she gave me extra. She'll probably never realize that she gave me more than required...I deserve to keep it...it's her mistake."

The practitioner continued to ponder what to do. As she let herself explore the issue in her mind, she found her thoughts shifting to, "It is clear to me that if my business partner or another patient were there observing me when I discovered the extra money, there would be no indecision; I would inform the patient and give it back to her. Yet, here I am, with only myself to answer to with this ethical decision, and the answer isn't so clear as to what I should do. If I keep it, how will I feel about this tomorrow, or the next time I see her? Probably guilty and remorseful. How would I feel if she did this to me? Probably betrayed, and I would think she was dishonest and unethical. What would I do if a colleague brought this problem to me? I would tell her to return the patient's money. How could I face this patient again, knowing I didn't tell her about the money? What if she gets in her car and goes to get that $20 bill and she realizes she gave it to me? I'd have to lie and say I didn't notice. Now I'm stealing and lying."

When the patient returned from the restroom, the practitioner informed her about the extra money and returned her $20. When the patient left, the practitioner felt good about her decision, realizing full well how both ethics and accountability take on new meaning when the only one accountable is herself.

Points to Ponder

If this practitioner had the same rates for everyone, would she still have faced this dilemma? What other steps could the practitioner have taken to evaluate her own ethics and motives?

Offering different rates for different clients can lead to other ethical dilemmas. If you offer a rate to a client that makes you feel resentful in any manner, you may begin to justify lapses in your own standards. Thoughtful decisions about what you charge and why, along with self-accountability, lead to consistent ethical choices. You must be very clear about the nature of the price reduction (e.g., celebration, anniversary, referral thank-you, promotion) and follow the same policies for everyone.

A chiropractic patient recommended the chiropractor to a friend. The friend had several sessions with the chiropractor. The two friends were having lunch one day and during their chat, the one friend thanked the other for the recommendation as the chiropractor had greatly helped her. She mentioned that paying $35 a visit was really worth the relief she had gotten. Her friend was taken aback, as she was paying $45 per visit, but said nothing. Her chiropractic visit was the next day. She felt a little resentful and wondered why she paid more than her friend. She spent the evening debating with herself whether it would be appropriate to mention it to the chiropractor. When she arrived at the office, she was uncomfortable and couldn't relax during the session. The chiropractor sensed something was different but hesitated to say anything.

Points to Ponder

What situations could explain the differences in price? Which party was responsible for speaking up: the client who felt resentful or the chiropractor who sensed something was different?

In the previous scenario, the chiropractor might have been offering an introductory special or some other type of discount program. While this isn't unethical, the first patient now questions the chiropractor's motives and behaviors—which damages the therapeutic relationship.

Sliding Fee Scales

When a client can't afford your fee, sometimes you need to let the client go. Another option is to reduce the per-session cost by offering clients a prepaid package plan. Or, if the client truly has financial difficulties, you could consider working with a sliding fee scale.

Sliding fee scales provide an objective method for allowing certain people to pay a reduced fee for your services. Sliding fee scales can be awkward. It is tough to set one up in advance of the first session unless a client has said something to you while booking the appointment. In general, most practitioners don't advertise a sliding fee scale unless they work with a target market that needs it (e.g., people on meager fixed incomes).[5]

Usually what works best is to give parameters. A frequently used model that seems least offensive and fair is determining fees based on income level. For example, your sliding scale statement might look like this:

My standard rate is $75 per session. If this presents a hardship for you, then I will accept a sliding scale fee based on your combined family annual income level.

If the total amount earned is less than $15,000 annually the fee per session is $30, $15,000-20,000 = $45, $20,000-25,000 = $60, $25,000+ = $75.

Be cautious when offering any type of discounted fee or doing *pro bono* work. Keep clear boundaries. Make certain that you have lucid policies so that the therapeutic relationship doesn't get damaged, you don't feel used, and the client retains a sense of dignity.

Prepaid Package Plans

Prepaid package plans encourage people to book sessions more frequently, infuse extra income into your bank account and save clients money. Examples of prepaid incentives are: purchase three sessions and receive a $5 savings per session; purchase seven treatments and qualify for a 20 percent discount; and purchase five sessions and receive the sixth one free. The most important thing is to keep it simple. Do not overwhelm yourself and your clients with a plethora of options.[6] The main caution here is to limit the number of sessions in a package (a rule of thumb is three months or 10 sessions). You can always sell another package once the first one is completed. Consider the following scenario:

> A practitioner wanted to take a training course that cost $3,000. One of her regular clients knew about it and told her that she would be willing to cover the training cost for weekly treatments for one year. The practitioner was ecstatic! Everything proceeded fine until about the eighth month. The client missed one of her appointments. The practitioner called the client to find out if anything was wrong, reminded her of the 24-hour cancellation policy and told her that she would waive it this time, but any future cancellation without notice would be a forfeit of that week's treatment.
>
> The following month the client missed several appointments—again without notice. When she finally showed up for an appointment, the practitioner initiated a conversation about the behavior. The client made several excuses. Then she said that she felt the practitioner hadn't been giving her usual energy into the sessions and the client wasn't sure she wanted to continue.
>
> The practitioner considered the situation and offered the client to transfer the balance of the sessions to someone else. Unfortunately, the client felt the practitioner should have refunded the balance, was angry about the proposed solution and never gave those sessions to anyone.
>
> In retrospect, the practitioner said if she had to do it over again she would have refunded the balance of the sessions. More importantly, she would never agree to such a long-term contract again.
>
> ### Points to Ponder
>
> What other ethical consequences could arise from accepting such a large upfront payment?

Credit

Allowing a client to receive treatments on credit is rare in service professions. The three most common reasons for extending credit are: the fee has to be billed to a third party such as an insurance agency, attorney, or a client's employer; a client forgets his checkbook; or a client has cash flow difficulties.

When billing a third party, make the client sign a statement saying that if a bill isn't paid within a specified time (e.g., 60 days) the client is responsible for payment. Create a formal IOU with a payment schedule for clients experiencing cash flow difficulties.

- List your fees.
- What circumstances would prompt you to offer a sliding fee scale?
- What will you charge family members and friends for your services?
- If your family or friend rate is different than your standard rate, describe why.
- What types of package plans could you offer? What are the benefits and disadvantages?

Gratuities

The topic of accepting gratuities is complex. Some professions would never consider it because of the problems inherent with transference: since there is no guarantee that a client is feeling equal in power in the relationship, it's unwise and often unethical to take extra money. This includes extravagant gifts such as the use of a vacation home. The gray area concerns gifts that are more symbolic such as garden produce or homemade cookies. Graciousness is a delightful skill. It recognizes and affirms positive intentions. The acceptance of a flower can be a healing moment. However, if a client were to always bring something extra for you or offer you an expensive gift, it would be prudent to state that you're well compensated for your time and nothing else is needed.

Figure 9.1 Potential Ethical Issues with Tips

- Problems that are inherent with transference.
- Clients aren't certain when or how much to give.
- Clients can be concerned that the practitioner expects the same amount (or more) each time.
- Clients worry that they won't receive the same level of service if they don't give a tip.

Most people feel awkward about tipping. They aren't certain when it's appropriate or how much to give. Are you supposed to tip mail carriers, hair stylists, pet groomers, auto mechanics, estheticians, gardeners, and physicians? Do you tip them if they work for someone else, but not if they're the owners of the business?

Unfortunately, practitioners who work in settings such as spas often receive minimal remuneration and rely on their tips. To complicate matters, many spas now employ a wide variety of practitioners including acupuncturists, nutritionists, massage therapists, movement specialists, and physical therapists. This puts clients in a quandary about tipping protocol. Of course, if the practitioners were receiving appropriate fees for their work in these settings, tips wouldn't be an issue. Clients, however, aren't usually aware of the arrangements between the spa and the practitioner.

Many spas provide envelopes printed with the word "gratuity" for clients to leave tips. The manner in which this is handled makes all the difference. It is one thing to tastefully display the envelopes at the front counter; it's another to post a sign by the envelopes that says "I've helped make your day, now help make mine (hint, hint)."

Another downside to accepting tips is that it creates expectations: you don't want clients worrying about whether to give you a tip. Even worse is the anxiety clients might experience if they give you a tip one time and not the next. Will you think they didn't like the session as much? Will they receive the same level of service next time? This tension defeats the purpose of the work.

If you decide that in your setting, you elect a professional standard that doesn't accept tips, you can make a clear choice. If someone asks you about tipping, you can say something like, "I appreciate the acknowledgment and a tip isn't expected in a therapeutic relationship." You can also give the client options such as donating the tip to your favorite charity or starting a scholarship fund for people who normally couldn't afford your services. Another idea is to thank the client and ask her instead to tell her friends about your services. Remind the client that gift certificates are a wonderful way to introduce individuals to your services.

Gratuities can make you feel appreciated, yet money isn't the only way to express appreciation. Given that many people have money issues, it isn't necessarily the best form of gratitude. Encourage people to simply say, "Thank you!" and have that mean something.

To Tip or Not To Tip?

- When is it appropriate to take a tip?
- What are your parameters for accepting tips or gifts?

Barter

Barter is a cashless exchange of goods and services. This method isn't confined to primitive societies. For some, it's the preferred method of managing finances, while others use barter only occasionally to enhance their cash flow.[7] Bartering isn't a casual activity. According to the International Reciprocal Trade Association (the oldest and largest trade organization representing the reciprocal trade industry), approximately 300,000 companies in North America belong to an organized barter exchange. Those businesses transact approximately $4 billion in sales annually.

Technological advances in electronics have expanded barter from a face-to-face interaction to a global transaction. This enables a small business owner the opportunity to participate in an arena previously dominated by large corporations.

Barter affords a simple, legal method to conserve cash outlays. If you trade for something you need, then you can use your cash for other purposes. You may need your office rewired, your taxes prepared, flowers delivered, or your back adjusted. Bartering is also an excellent method for expanding your client base. Many people who've never received the services of a complementary wellness provider might be more open to scheduling an appointment if they didn't need to pay in cash. And even though you don't receive cash, the trade is useful and those barter clients may refer cash-paying clients.

> Weakness of attitude becomes weakness of character.
>
> —Albert Einstein

Direct Barter

Many healthcare providers already barter on a direct basis. They identify services and products they want and then approach appropriate business owners with a trade proposal. Quite often, a client initiates a barter transaction. These direct trades work best if the items or services are of equal value. You can use gift certificates for trades and get gift certificates or vouchers from the person with whom you're trading. For instance, if you're bartering chiropractic services with a printer, ask the printer to give you a voucher for the amount you normally charge for an office visit. When you're ready to do a printing job, you redeem your vouchers.

Here is another example: Let's say a restaurant owner wants to trade you meals for acupuncture treatments. You charge $65 per visit. One method is to have the restaurateur provide you with a $65 voucher for each treatment. Another idea is to transact a trade for a set amount, such as ten acupuncture certificates for $650 worth of restaurant vouchers (in varying denominations). The beauty of the latter idea is that the certificates and vouchers can be redeemed by anyone. If you don't want to eat $650 worth of food at that restaurant, give the vouchers as gifts or use them for trading with someone else. Your client does the same with the acupuncture certificates, ultimately bringing you additional cash-paying clients.

A successful barter arrangement requires that all parties feel good about the trade. This may be difficult to achieve if the client feels in a position of less power than the practitioner or if the client has difficulty speaking up for herself. In these cases, it's important for the practitioner to encourage the client to be totally honest about her sense of fairness in the arrangement. This is particularly important if the value of the services exchanged is subjective, such as the value of a painting for a struggling artist who has difficulty putting a price on her work. Sometimes a barter may be based on time rather than money. For instance, one practitioner may be trading with another who charges twice his fee but they're giving each other equal time. What the arrangement actually ends up being doesn't matter as much as having both parties feel good about the exchange they have agreed upon.

Two major problems with direct barter arise from inequitable trades and trading for goods or services you don't really need. For instance, you want to have someone to clean your office. You don't really have the cash to pay for that service so you consider approaching someone to barter. Although you may find an office cleaner, it probably won't work for long. The person is likely to become resentful when four hours of labor (at $15 per hour) equals one hour of your service.

The second problem, trading for items and services you don't really need relates to setting good boundaries. It might be tempting to accept a barter offer from a potential client, particularly if you feel that the only way the person will utilize your services is if you agree to trade. If this occurs, remind yourself that your time is valuable. If the trade isn't for something you want for yourself or for a gift, then you're essentially giving away your session. Both of these problems can be eliminated by membership in a barter network.

Figure 9.2 **Bartering Tips**

- Treat barter as cash.
- Issue gift certificates or scrip to keep track of trades.
- Carefully evaluate barter prices.
- Realistically assess your barter commitments.
- Set good boundaries.
- Join a barter exchange.

Barter Exchanges

Join a barter exchange if you plan to incorporate more than the occasional barter into your practice. Contact the National Association of Trade Exchanges (NATE) or the International Reciprocal Trade Association (IRTA) for listings of barter organizations in your city. Approximately 300 barter networks exist in the United States. The International Trade Exchange (ITEX) and International Monetary Systems (IMS) are two of the largest exchanges.

Essentially barter organizations work by members selling their goods and services to other members in exchange for trade dollars, which are valued at the equivalent of cash dollars. With each transaction, trade dollars are debited from the buyer's account and credited to the seller's account. The seller can then spend these trade dollars with other exchange members.

Barter exchanges function like a bank: they handle transactions; debit and credit accounts; charge fees; and send monthly statements. They may even offer a payment plan or extend a line of credit. You are given either a credit card or checkbook with which to make your transactions. A client getting a treatment from you either charges it and you log it with the exchange office (a similar procedure to processing bank credit cards) or the client writes you a barter check which you deposit (just like a bank check). The barter organization usually charges 10-15 percent commission (in cash) on the value of the actual trade. The commission is customarily applied against the buyer's account, but some exchanges split the charge between buyer and seller.

Before you join an exchange, check how many other people in your specific profession are members. You may want to consider groups that have a large enough member base as your potential client pool. For instance, it might not be the best marketing investment if the group is small and has multiple practitioners who provide your same service.

Barter Exchanges

http://www.natebarter.com/
http://www.itex.com/
http://www.irta.com/

Financial Considerations

Treat barter as cash; after all, it's taxable income. The trade dollars you spend on business expenses are deductible; the personal expenditures are usually considered draw or profit and aren't deductible. The barter exchange organizations report each member's income to the IRS via the 1099-B form.

Do not pay more for an item through barter than you would pay in cash. Before making a purchase, check prices with other vendors. Most barter members are ethical but some charge higher prices to trade customers than to cash customers. Also, don't accept bartering transactions that you can't fulfill. For example, a barter member wants you to provide ongoing wellness care to 50 employees. At first, this seems great until you realize that this would take between 16-20 hours per week of your time. This wouldn't allow you much time for cash clients. This transaction becomes more feasible if you know another practitioner who could work with you.

Creating Ethical Barter Transactions

- Describe instances when a barter exchange worked well for both parties.
- Describe instances when a barter exchange didn't work well for both parties.
- Identify what types of barter exchanges could work for you.
- How can you ensure that your barter transactions are handled ethically?

Gift Certificates

Gift certificates provide a surge of income into your practice and offer an easy way for clients to share your services with their family, friends, and colleagues. They can also be both a marketing tool to generate new clients and a goodwill promotion when given as presents or donated to charities.[8]

Gift certificates are a tool to increase your client base, so it's in your best interest that they get redeemed. Each person who uses a gift certificate can become a regular client. Thus the initial certificate (whether purchased or given as a promotion) can launch a wonderful business relationship and bring in thousands of dollars in revenue.

In today's time-pressed and hectic world, gift certificates for wellness services are growing in popularity. Many clients appreciate the convenience of this gift-giving option, and are enthusiastic about this unique and thoughtful way to support others' wellbeing. This section highlights the ethical concerns of selling gift certificates.

Figure 9.3 **Gift Certificate Benefits**

- Serve as a marketing tool to generate new clients.
- Provide a surge of income into your practice.
- Offer an easy way for clients to share your services.
- Serve as goodwill promotion when given as presents or donated to charities.

Expiration Dates

For more information on how to **market gift certificates**, please refer to the *Business Mastery* book.

http://BusinessMastery.us/

Many states have strict regulations concerning gift certificates: some don't allow expiration dates, some dictate how far they may be postdated, and several require that if the certificates aren't redeemed within a certain period of time, the money must be deposited with the state.[9] You can put an expiration date on gift certificates when they're used as promotions (no money has been exchanged), such as donating certificates to a charity auction.

Some people have advocated increasing one's revenue stream by aggressively selling gift certificates with very short expiration terms. Often the majority of certificates expire before being redeemed, and the practitioner receives the income without having to perform any services. While this scam might appear tempting, consider the long-term consequences of this and the ill will that this might generate.

When you sell a gift certificate, you're exchanging one form of currency for another, albeit not as universal as government scrip. A gift certificate sale is essentially a contract you have made with the purchaser to provide a service or product of a certain value. Confiscating that monetary value simply by creating a short-term expiration date demonstrates a lack of integrity. Indeed, making redemption difficult or unlikely is fraud.

For most people, a gift certificate is a significant investment. Your gift certificate sales will dramatically increase if you develop a system that allays concerns about purchasing something that might not be used. People feel more comfortable purchasing certificates that either have a flexible expiration date or no expiration date. Another approach is for the certificate to revert to the purchaser if not used by the expiration date.

A somatic practitioner gained four new clients because another practitioner refused to honor gift certificates after the expiration date—and this refusal was to someone who had spent $1,000 on Christmas gift certificates for two family members. The gift giver and the recipients felt extremely "ripped off" by the previous practitioner. Even though the new therapist uses an expiration date on her certificates, she calls the purchasers one month prior to the expiration date and suggests they contact the recipients. If someone waits until the last day to call for an appointment, she extends the expiration date for one month. If the recipient still doesn't redeem the certificate, it reverts back to the purchaser. She tells clients her procedure when they purchase gift certificates because she doesn't want their money to be wasted.

Points to Ponder

How ethical is it for a practitioner to refuse to honor gift certificates after they expire? What are the benefits to using gift certificates if the practitioner has to work so hard to get clients to redeem them in a timely manner?

The Downside of Gift Certificates

Some practitioners are concerned that gift certificates increase in value if not redeemed quickly (particularly if prices go up in the time between when the certificate was purchased and then redeemed), and thus they "lose" money. If you feel this way, consider putting the money into an interest-bearing account to make up for any fee increases. Another option is to put a dollar value on the certificate instead of a certain number of treatments. Many practitioners (reluctantly) admit that they don't always give their best service when a client pays for a session with a gift certificate (particularly when cash flow is tight). This is another example where self-accountability comes into play for the ethical practitioner.

An idea for circumventing the potential for a lack of enthusiasm on your part is to put at least half of all gift certificate revenue into a savings account and transfer the funds into your checking account when the certificate is redeemed. Otherwise, if you sell a lot of gift certificates, you could find yourself in the position of working for an extended period of time without receiving "new" income.

Ethical Gift Certificate Sales

- List ways to ethically sell gift certificates and manage those sales.
- Develop a policy to handle unredeemed gift certificates.

Taxes

Your financial belief system is the context for all your financial dealings. Taxation is a topic fraught with emotional charge. Many people resent the amount of money they pay in taxes (or how that money is spent) and use this anger to justify shady business practices. The two most common practices are concealing income (mainly cash payments and barter) and exaggerating expenses.

Charting makes it more difficult to hide income although we've all heard stories and seen movies where businesses keep duplicate sets of books. Beyond the simple fact that this is illegal, it makes recordkeeping a nightmare! Most practitioners wouldn't consider such an extreme action as keeping duplicate books or falsifying records. The more common occurrence is

> Laws control the lesser man. Right conduct controls the greater one.
>
> —Chinese Proverb

pocketing cash payments—particularly when it's unlikely that the client will return or if you don't chart and your clients don't ask for receipts.

Business deductions aren't always obvious and the thousands of pages of tax codes make this subject impenetrable for most people. The two areas most prone to entice people to be less than honest are purchases made by the business that are mainly used personally, and extravagant or unnecessary travel expenses. Keep accurate records and work with an accountant to find legitimate ways to reduce your tax liability.

A taxation area that many practitioners choose to ignore is sales tax. Unless you live in a state or province that doesn't levy sales tax, you're required to collect and remit sales tax on product sales—regardless of the volume. In the United States, contact your State Department of Revenue to apply for a Transaction Privilege Tax License. Most states charge a one-time fee of less than $20. The frequency of how often you must submit reports and the collected sales tax varies. Usually you're required to fill out a form on a monthly basis for the first year, then if the volume is low, it might get reduced it to quarterly or even annually.

Discuss tax collection requirements with the state (or province) as well as the company from which you buy products for resale (e.g., certain food-based products aren't taxed). Also, if you purchase products to resell you don't need to pay sales tax to the company that sells you the product. Unless you purchase products from out-of-state vendors, the companies often ask for your Resale Number, which is on the Transaction Privilege Tax License.

An ethical practitioner keeps precise records, declares all income received, refrains from inflating expenses, and accurately files governmental reports.

Figure 9.4 Unethical Tax Practices

- Concealing Income
- Exaggerating Expenses
- Not Collecting or Remitting Sales Tax
- Not Filing Appropriate Tax Forms

Product Sales

Somatic practitioners are in a unique position to provide adjunct client care through product sales. Retailing helps practitioners increase their income and provides clients with products to extend the treatment benefits to home. It offers convenience for clients, and that alone can reduce their stress.

Yet many practitioners are reluctant to sell products. They are concerned that retailing might be seen as unprofessional. They want to be respectful and not cross boundaries.

Product sales is a natural extension of the standard of care and healing already associated with somatic therapies, skin care, and personal training. A conflict doesn't need to exist as long as a few guidelines are followed. If you currently run a professional, ethical practice, then retailing can naturally follow suit. If you keep good boundaries, treat people with respect and fairness, and remain client-centered, you will manage product sales in the same manner that you manage the rest of your practice.

Most clients appreciate the opportunity to buy products from their practitioners—as long as the sales process isn't pushy and is relevant to their needs and wants. Clients will trust your recommendations, especially on those products used in the session itself. Educating your clients about products means there is no real reason to *sell* anything to your clients.

Figure 9.5 **Advantages of Retailing**

- Increase Profits
- Increase Revenue
- Increase Bookings
- Provide Convenience
- Extend Treatment Benefits to Home

Increase Profits, Revenue, and Bookings

Selling products in your practice is a great way to work smarter—not harder. You already have a relationship with your clients and retailing is simply another avenue of supporting your clients in their wellness. By selling clients the right products, you help them reduce their stress and improve their health. Retailing can actually increase the frequency of clients booking sessions. When clients use a product at home, it reminds them of their work with you, and that usually inspires them to book another session. Plus, if they share those products with friends, those friends are more likely to become clients.

Make It Convenient

Product sales also provide convenience for your clients. Make it easy for people. Most people are extremely busy and juggling so many things. They really appreciate you saving them from making a special trip to buy an item or having to go online and waiting for it to arrive.

Extend Your Treatment Benefits

Extend the treatment benefits at home by providing clients with products that they can use between sessions. This can be from a direct therapeutic point of view, such as a self-massage tool or a book on stretching, to recreating a relaxation response. Ideally, you use some of these items in your sessions so your clients associate those items with their experience of your work.

Sounds and scents are strong triggers for memories. This is particularly applicable to somatic practitioners and skin care specialists. For instance, let's say that in your session you played a certain CD, placed an eye pillow on your client's eyes, infused your massage lubricant with an essential oil, or used a special foot balm while massaging the client's feet. Those are all items clients can purchase for home use; every time they feel, smell, or hear those items, they most likely are transported back to the last time they experienced them—which would be while in a state of relaxation on your table. Although it isn't the same as receiving a treatment from you, it certainly helps extend the benefits of your work in-between sessions. Depending on the type of work that you do and your clients' goals, some of the products for clients to use at home can also be for a direct therapeutic result, such as keeping muscles loose, addressing trigger points, increasing flexibility, or reducing pain.

Product sales don't need to be limited to therapeutic items. Selling products that help clients feel pampered (and who doesn't need that from time to time) is also appropriate. Just imagine how lovely it would be for your clients to create a mini-oasis of tranquility in their homes.

The Ethical Concerns of Retailing

Product sales can be a lucrative adjunct to a practice, yet some disciplines discourage (or even prohibit) their members from selling products. This censure stems from a concern about the power differential that exists between practitioners and clients. Clients assume that you're an authority and may feel influenced to purchase products to please you or because they think you know everything. Even if you take great care not to exploit this power differential, you must nevertheless be careful not to manipulate or coerce your clients.[10] Ethical sales are based upon educating your clients on the benefits of certain products and allowing them the opportunity to purchase them from you.

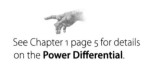

See Chapter 1 page 5 for details on the **Power Differential**.

A massage practitioner sells a line of essential oils at her office. She uses these oils in her own personal life and they have brought her improved health. Her passion and belief in these products is unerring. As a result, she wants to pass this along to her clients because she cares deeply for the health and welfare of each client she serves. Her office has a windowed front and she has hung a door-sized chart about the products in her window. Also, she has smaller sized charts, multiple brochures, and shelves placed all around her waiting area as well as in her therapy room. The charts and brochures all are advertisements for the products and have statements on them such as, "Try these. Get results. Never take antibiotics again."

Points to Ponder

Without ever saying a word to her clients about these products, what is the message that her office space is sending to her clients? Even though these print media forms are direct from the manufacturer and accompany her orders of product from the company, what is her ethical responsibility regarding the messages that these materials send to her clients?

Keep in mind your unique position as a somatic practitioner. You have a broad knowledge base about the body and what products can support clients in achieving their wellness goals. You have access to many superior products that the average client is unable to purchase at a local store or even online. Also, some companies only sell their products to practitioners and not the general public.

Most somatic practitioners spend at least one hour with each client. In that time you really get to know your clients' needs. Plus, the longer a client has been working with you, the better informed you become to help and recommend appropriate products.

Only sell products that you know are reliable, suitable for use by your clients, and are a natural extension of your business. For instance, if local statutes permit, it's totally appropriate for a somatic practitioner to sell healthcare products that are designed to assist in the relief of pain and promote wellbeing. Examples of these items are hot and cold packs, ice pillows, relaxation tools, support pillows and similar ergonomic devices, essences (such as aromatherapy), specialty lotions, self-health books and videos. In addition to these items, personal trainers and movement educators can also sell exercise tools.

Ethical product sales aren't about hype or "hard-sell" tactics. The point is providing your clients with easy access to high quality products that help enrich their wellbeing. As a healthcare provider, your clients depend on you to give them accurate information. You must know every one of your products well and convey that information to your clients. If your client really enjoyed the cervical hot pack you used during the session and wants to purchase one, you would educate the client on how to use the pack and under what circumstances not to use it. Your clients may lose faith in you (and no longer remain your clients, not to mention the loss of goodwill) if you fail to adequately inform them about the appropriate use, benefits, limitations, and possible side effects or contraindications of the products you sell.

Retail Mastery: Your Unique Position as a Therapist
(Webinar)

https://sohnen-moe.com/webinars/

If product sales aren't handled well, they can negatively impact your practice. The major issue here is: are you influenced in some way by the money that product sales generate, or are you selling products to clients simply because they need or want them? Exercise caution and check your motives to make certain that you aren't "pushing" a little harder because your income is down or because the multi-level marketing program you're involved with requires you to meet a targeted sales volume.

You can reduce the possible abuse of the power differential by restricting your conversation about products to before or after sessions. It is fine to mention the product during a session, such as, "Now I am going to use XYZ product on you. If you're interested in learning more information about it, we can discuss it after the session." The post-session interview is a good time to reference products. It is natural to recommend products that are appropriate to the client's goals when you're reviewing the treatment plan and any "homework" you might have for a client. This is also the time to ask for feedback on any of the products you used during the session.

Ultimately, selling products is no different than "selling" your services—simply share your enthusiasm about them. If you make your products visible, accessible, attractive, and affordable, your clients will buy them when it's appropriate.

Figure 9.6 Ethical Product Sales Do's and Don'ts

Do	Don't
• Make sure the products you carry are appropriate and wanted. • Find products that meet clients' goals and needs. • Know the products well. • Educate your clients on the proper use, benefits, and possible side-effects. • Restrict discussion of products to before or after the session. • Ask for client feedback. • Clearly label the cost of products.	• Don't overuse products. • Don't make product claims that the manufacturer doesn't make. • Don't manipulate or coerce your clients.

Nutritional Supplements

In the quest to diversify their practices, many practitioners sell nutritional supplements. The major concern is that practitioners may be working beyond their scope of practice unless they're a nutritionist, herbologist, or extremely well-versed in this subject.[11] The use of herbs and vitamins has expanded so much that a specialized industry term, "nutriceuticals," was coined and the government has its eye on regulation. In the 1970s, the Food and Drug Administration (FDA) attempted to reclassify chamomile as a narcotic—and almost succeeded. Comfrey became a target for a while and, more recently, herbal formulations are currently under scrutiny. The FDA on more than one occasion has said that certain supplements aren't safe. What qualifies a somatic practitioner to say that they are safe? Several times legislation was proposed in the United States to require a physician's prescription for these types of supplements. The bills didn't pass, but these actions serve as a warning. Clearly, most consumers don't want the government to take away their freedom to choose and purchase supplements from wherever or whomever they desire. Unfortunately, the more that people irresponsibly sell products without proper education, the more likely the government will intercede.

Some practitioners' waiting rooms look like small health food stores. It is highly unlikely that those practitioners know much about all the products they carry. Perhaps clerks in health food stores don't know that information either, so what is the problem? Essentially, the ethical and legal responsibilities significantly differ in a client/practitioner relationship versus a customer/retailer relationship.

If there is a product that you really believe in and want to make available to your clients, educate yourself on the product: the contents, suggested applications, possible adverse reactions, and contraindications. Keep in mind that just because something works for you, doesn't mean it's beneficial to the next person. Also, "works" is a tricky word. Beware of anecdotal evidence. Results aren't always proven or reliable. The possibility exists that the product could even be harmful to someone else. When discussing nutritional supplements with clients, you need to discuss the potential side effects in addition to explaining the benefits.

A practitioner spent a weekend at an educational meeting about a particular product line. She learned about the importance of balancing the vitamin and mineral supplements you take. She made the decision to sell some of these products because the information she gained seemed truly convincing. The information from the weekend meeting included data about balancing magnesium and calcium, and actually gave specific milligram dosages that women of a certain age should be taking. Most of her bodywork clients were women ages 40-65, many of whom had already begun experiencing issues with their bone health.

Once the practitioner began selling the products, she told clients about what she had learned about calcium/magnesium daily requirements and many of her clients purchased bottles of the products and began taking them based on what the practitioner had told them. A few months later, the practitioner heard from one of these clients who had purchased the magnesium/calcium. The client reported that she had begun to have major digestive disorders shortly after she began taking the product, went to her doctor, had lots of expensive medical tests, and the results were that the calcium/magnesium supplement was the problem. Her system was out-of-balance. Her magnesium was too high, and this resulted in the digestive issues.

Points to Ponder

What is the ethical responsibility of the practitioner? How could the practitioner have handled this before marketing or selling the supplements?

The more informed you are about the products you carry, the less risk is involved for yourself and your clients. If you're interested in herbs and vitamins, consider taking courses on the subject—or even pursue a degree in nutrition or herbology. Another option to ensure that you're providing your clients with information and products that are in their best interest is to team up with a nutritionist or herbologist. The marketplace is flooded with nutritional supplements and the general public is looking for direction. As healthcare providers, your clients naturally rely upon you to provide them with information, products, and services to enhance their wellbeing. Proceed cautiously when incorporating nutritional supplements into your practice.

- List the types of products that are appropriate to sell in your practice.
- List the types of products that are inappropriate to sell in your practice.
- Identify the types of products that you aren't certain are appropriate to sell; describe your concerns about each of these items.
- What experiences have you had in purchasing products from a healthcare provider?
- Describe how you can sell products without using "hard-sell" tactics or taking advantage of the power differential.

Referrals

As the healthcare industry continues to increase in specialties, referrals have become common among healthcare providers. This is good for the client as it's important to help them get the most specific and appropriate care. Somatic practitioners are getting referrals from other healthcare providers, and also from friends, family, and clients. A common ethical dilemma involving referrals is revealed in the following scenario:

> Wayne, a massage therapist, goes on vacation and sends several clients to his friend and colleague Carrie for treatments while he is away. One of the clients booked more than one massage with Carrie and after the second treatment, the client told Carrie she preferred her massage and wanted to continue to see her for treatments even after Wayne returns from vacation. The client asked Carrie not to tell Wayne about it.
>
> **Points to Ponder**
>
> Is it okay for Carrie to keep this client? What is more important in this situation: honoring a professional commitment to a colleague or honoring the client's wants or needs?

While Wayne did refer the client to Carrie, he did so with the expectation that the client would return to him. By referring the client, he is saying that he trusts Carrie's ability to take care of his client, and he trusts her professionalism. The unspoken commitment is to the professional relationship, and the ethical thing to do is to honor that commitment by referring the client back. It would be unethical for Carrie to keep quiet and continue to treat the client. For there to be a more ethical outcome, the client would need to tell Wayne that she prefers Carrie's massage and is choosing to end their therapeutic relationship. If Wayne is a true professional, he will support the client's decision.

Acknowledging Referrals

Thanking people for referrals seems straightforward, yet such a simple gesture can be easily misconstrued. The key is the nature of the business relationship. Consider situations where current clients refer new clients to you. Whether you give them a free session, a discount off a future session, a plant, a fruit basket, or even money, it still can be viewed as a kickback (although most of us hold it as a thank-you). Again, there is very little problem with these types of rewards because the client talking to a friend is usually on an equal power level.

It becomes an ethical issue when a person in a power differential relationship makes a recommendation to a client and the practitioner receives financial remuneration for the referral. Might the concept of a referral fee come to outweigh the client's need for the best possible objective referral? The bottom line is that a kickback is a kickback. Healthcare providers are responsible for serving the client to the best of their abilities. Accepting payment for referrals clouds that ability and puts their ethics in a compromising position. In all cases, this creates a conflict of interest. In many professions it's illegal; this practice of accepting payment for referrals, or referring to clinics or laboratories in which the provider has a financial interest, is known as rebating. Severe penalties can be levied on practitioners who violate laws of this nature. It is appropriate to refer within a health system network or preferred provider list. It isn't appropriate if the referral is based on the prospect of financial gain.

The gray area involves the little thank-yous. Be cautious so that there is no hint of impropriety. How much can you do as a thank-you without it appearing like a bribe? A holistic practitioner who is also a nurse states:

> As nursing employees, we were also prohibited from accepting personal gifts of any kind, even food, from the patients, from the medical staff, or from ancillary businesses such as pharmacies and home health agencies. These items had to be offered as "gifts at large" to the unit, or it was considered something like a tip, or even worse, a bribe. When asked for recommendations [referrals], the staff had to offer a list of all the agencies/professionals available in the area and decline to offer personal recommendations in their role as employees of a facility, since their referrals might be subjective, and reflect, for good or ill, on their employer.

Marketing Materials

Marketing materials are often essential to a successful practice. Done with good taste, accurate information, and honest intentions, these materials serve to enhance individual practice and the overall field. The major concerns about marketing materials are making exaggerated claims, utilizing misleading ploys, using questionable names and titles, displaying inappropriate images, not following regulations, and misrepresenting credentials.

Exaggerated Claims

Be certain that you can back your claims, including the verbal ones. It is impossible to know with absolute certainty that a given person will respond in a specific manner. Some clients present with symptoms that appear easy to manage but aren't. In addition, everyone has their own pace of letting go and healing. Avoid statements that promise results in a specific time frame such as, "You'll be better in just five sessions." Assuming that your techniques help with everything isn't wise, so don't say things like, "Oh, that isn't a problem. We can easily get rid of that." You might say, "In the past I've helped several people with this problem. This type of treatment may be very helpful for you, too, but it also may not work for you. It is difficult to predict a guaranteed positive outcome. I will do my best to help you and if it doesn't seem to be working in a [month, six weeks], I'll refer you to someone else."

Promising cures seems obvious to avoid, yet many practitioners approach or even cross that line. Check out brochures and advertisements by professionals in your field. The telephone Yellow Pages supplied these examples of statements that convey intent to help while avoiding blatant promises to cure:

We Can Help You with....	Offering Options, Quality & Sensitivity
Get the Relief You Deserve	Why Live with Pain?
Specializing in....	Feel Better Than You Thought You Could
Relaxation to Rehabilitation	We Can Help Give Back Your Quality of Life

Guarantees

Guaranteeing satisfaction is different from promising a cure. A clearly defined guarantee reflects confidence. Figure 9.7 is an example of how a massage therapist in Wisconsin found an effective way of guaranteeing satisfaction by posting this statement in her treatment rooms.

Figure 9.7 **Sample Client Satisfaction Statement**

Essential Massage Center Guarantee

- If you do not notice a reduction in pain or do not feel more relaxed after receiving a massage from one of our highly trained therapists, we happily refund the price of the session.
- Minor soreness, while not to be expected, does occasionally occur following a massage session. We fully expect that you will feel better within 36 hours.
- If after 36 hours you continue to feel that the massage has had no positive effect, your session fee is refunded.
- This policy applies equally to gift certificate clients.

Misleading Ploys

Sometimes words are misleading, so choose them carefully. We have all seen headlines that convey multiple, unintended meanings. Ask several people to read your promotional copy and tell you how they interpret your presentation. Clearly state the parameters when an offer has limits (e.g. "Good through March 15, 2020." or "Free to the first 10 new clients.") Avoid the "bait-and-switch" routine: don't offer a reduced price then claim that you have sold out or the offer expired; don't offer something for free then require the client pay something to receive the "free" service or product. Not only are these ploys unethical, they create ill will and alienate clients.

Questionable Names and Titles

Be sure to avoid gimmicky or inappropriate business names. Pain Eliminators might be catchy, but it sounds more like an *As Seen On TV!* product than a legitimate practitioner's business name. In addition, it would be hard to live up to the claim it appears to make.

It is also important to have a professional email address, rather than using your personal email. Ilovekittens@email.com is a very cute email address, but it may not be an appropriate address for a healthcare professional (unless maybe you're a cat doctor). In addition, suggestive email addresses like vixen@email.com or naughtygirl@email.com don't project a professional image, and seem to suggest a very different profession than health care.

Website names can be especially tricky. The business name could be perfectly appropriate, but when combined into a website address it may become very different. Read your web address in every possible way before settling on a title that ends up saying something you never intended. The best *worst* example is the Therapist Finder web address: www.therapistfinder.com.

Inappropriate Images

Marketing materials should be dignified and convey professionalism. Images should help potential clients feel confident and comfortable with you and your business. Think about what you want that to look like. Use professional pictures of yourself, your office, your products, and your services. Consider the following suggestions for any visual promotional product (e.g., business cards, fliers, brochures, display advertisements in directories and magazines, billboards, and television commercials):

- Hire a professional photographer to take pictures of you or your clients.
- Use high quality artwork. Be sure it's royalty-free or get reprint permission.
- Avoid sensationalism.
- Be sure your photos and artwork are not provocative: view pictures from all angles because sometimes images look fine from one direction, but suggestive from others.
- Refrain from using "glamour" shots.
- Make certain that photos do not portray results that you can't guarantee, such as showing someone in a wheelchair in one panel and running a marathon in the next.

Follow Business Regulations

Check your city, county, and state (or province) rules and regulations regarding marketing. For instance, some places have marketing regulations such as: your license number must be listed on all promotional materials; you can't use certain media such as billboards; or you're limited in the depiction of benefits.

Dr. Ross recently moved her medical practice from Arizona to Illinois. She acquired all the necessary licensing and certifications to practice legally in her new state. She decided to use the same marketing and advertising materials for her new practice, simply changing any reference from Arizona to Illinois. After a few months in her new practice, Dr. Ross received a letter from the Illinois medical board stating that she was in violation of the Medical Practice Act which prohibits the use of testimonials to entice the public. She had used testimonials on her website and in brochures because Arizona didn't have the same prohibitions.

Points to Ponder

How could Dr. Ross have avoided this issue? As a somatic practitioner, how could you know if such regulations also apply to you?

The above example illustrates restrictions to the medical community. However, somatic practitioners should always check state and municipality restrictions.

Misrepresenting Credentials

Honestly and accurately represent professional qualifications, competence, education, training, experience, and affiliations. If you list a specialty, be certain you back this up with appropriate credentials like the training and time invested in integrating the modality. Often practitioners cite numerous adjunct modalities in their promotional materials. A brochure that lists a variety of treatment modalities you practice is quite different than calling yourself a specialist or master in something—particularly after taking a weekend course.

Joyce recently took a weekend workshop, Beginning Shiatsu. She was interested in integrating Asian modalities into her already well-established deep tissue massage therapy practice. After the workshop, she decided to add ABT (Asian Bodywork Therapist) to the credentials after her name and began to practice some of the techniques she had learned. One of her regular clients decided to try a shiatsu treatment after learning about Traditional Chinese Medicine and the benefits of balancing the energies of the body (Qi). The client asked Joyce to tell her where her Qi was imbalanced and asked her to recommend dietary and lifestyle changes to complement the shiatsu treatment. Joyce didn't learn about Traditional Chinese Medicine in the weekend workshop she took, and so didn't feel comfortable discussing these aspects of her client's health. Joyce began to question her choice to call herself an ABT when there was clearly much more to be learned and practiced.

Points to Ponder

At what point or level of training could Joyce feel confident about using the ABT credentials? Why are credentials important, if at all? How can practitioners feel confident that they have had the proper training and invested the appropriate amount of time to integrate a new therapy or modality?

Identify Appropriate Marketing Materials

- Describe examples of marketing materials that you feel are in questionable taste.
- Describe examples of marketing materials that you feel are blatant examples of unethical marketing.
- Peruse a local directory for healthcare advertisements. Find examples that are ethical as well as ads that are questionable or that exaggerate claims.
- You took a weekend touch therapy course that is part one of a multiple series. It meets the CE requirements for renewing your license. Do you advertise this modality and list it on your business cards and brochures? What are your guidelines for listing a specialty in your repertoire of services?

▌ Social Media Ethics

Social Media has become such a big part of daily life; keeping the balance of business while participating in a "Social" arena can be challenging for some business owners who feel like they want to make it personal or have their personality reflect in the social media. The six social media websites currently considered to be the most popular are (in no particular order): Facebook, Twitter, YouTube, Google⁺, LinkedIn, and Pinterest.

When social media sites first became popular, they weren't designed to be used for business purposes. That soon changed and to date most social media sites offer a business page option. This can make it easier to separate your personal and business lives, and most do offer controls of who you allow to be friends and followers so that you can have a personal family friend connection separate from business. However, be aware of your privacy settings. When you make your comments public (even if you think you're making a personal post), you're actually making it accessible to the entire online community.

If your brand is also your name, you need to really be aware that people are watching you all the time. Your personal profile is subject to as much scrutiny as your business profile. This is because when people search on the social sites, they might end up on someone's personal profile rather than her business profile. Social media makes it difficult to separate your personal from business and therefore you should carefully consider what is being shared at all times.

Also, when you're a highly watched and followed member of an organization or facility such as a manager of a clinic, or a member of a board, you need to realize you're going to be subject to public notice at all times. As much as you would like to think people can separate the personal and business, they won't. Everyone—friends, friends of those friends, potential customers, customers, family, your peers, and supervisors—have access to what you post, tweet, pin, share, comment, like, and follow, and it's a direct reflection of your brand and image.

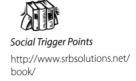

Social Trigger Points
http://www.srbsolutions.net/book/

Social Media Policies

It is always best to review the privacy policies, terms, and conditions of each social media website where you have a presence or are considering joining. Also, check to see if the social media platforms have account management features so that as your practice grows you maintain control of the sites and can delegate responsibilities to others.

Whether you're a single practitioner or work with others, you should create a statement of how you want your social media identity to be handled. Ideally, create a full social media policy for your practice. You may feel like the word "policy" is a dirty word, or is restrictive, or is a determent of social media engagement—basically the exact opposite of what you want for your practice. On the contrary, social media policies support, protect, and empower high-quality engagement.

Why a Social Media Policy is Important

Social media policies may not sound like the most exciting part of your practice, yet they are important to protect your clients, employees, and yourself. Most policies and procedures document the action steps to take for various situations: "if this—do that." However, for social media there's really no way to predict what situations might arise or how individuals handle them. Each social media network is an environment that changes daily. Therefore, establishing a social media policy can assist you to maintain an ethical guide for your practice and protect your practice.

Our judicial system is still in the process of interpreting the laws with regard to social media. This will more than likely take years until the interpretation process catches up with technology. Therefore, you as a business owner are operating without definitive guidance. Some of the more common issues for businesses using social media are client confidentiality, labor relation issues, brand hijacking, miscommunication, and spamming.

> A practitioner is contracted with a sports team to work with individual players. The team wins a big championship and the practitioner wants to leverage this win by posting the names of some of the individual players he helped. The team cancelled his contract and the practitioner was fined for mentioning the team and players without paying royalty fees or getting permission.
>
> **Points to Ponder**
>
> Should this be a breach of client confidentiality? Is it acceptable for the practitioner to leverage the fact that he works with the team as long as he doesn't specifically mention any one player?

Having corporate contracts is a great way to build your practice and can be best for leveraging your relationship with them to build your brand. Just be sure you iron out the details of what is acceptable. An even better situation is when you get recommendations from the owners, managers, or individuals from the corporation and are authorized to use their logos, testimonials, or letter of recommendations for your online marketing.

> A practitioner asks her friend to set up and manage social media accounts for her business. The friend creates business accounts using his own personal profiles on several social media sites. After several months, the two part ways. The practitioner doesn't have access to any of the social media accounts because they were linked to her friend's personal profiles and she has no control over what is being said about her business. All branding credit built through the business pages have to be re-created with new accounts.

It can be very tempting and seem like the simple path to hire or have a friend set up your social media accounts for you. Despite what you might be thinking, the accounts belong to whoever sets them up. They aren't transferable. Unfortunately, this is how brands are hijacked. That is why many of the social media sites have adapted their programs to include management or administrative levels for business accounts.

Consider this: if you wouldn't pay someone thousands of dollars to run ads in magazines, newspapers, and radio without your approval or direction why should your social media campaign be any different? Even though social media is a service that requires no direct fees from you, it still requires managing and guidance. You are responsible for your own practice. Ignorance isn't an excuse for poor business management.

Legal advice is important: ask a lawyer to review your social media policies. Legal review can be expensive however the alternative can be considerably more costly if you're sued. Review your social media policies every six to twelve months. Verify that the information is still relevant and if there are any legal updates that might apply.

Employees

The National Labor Relations Board (NLRB) has been involved in court cases regarding social media and labor relation issues. These court cases have been based on the National Labor Relations Act (NLRA) which was enacted to protect employee rights to organize. In the past, NLRA referred to face-to-face meetings or phone meetings. With the emergence of social media, it also applies to online. It is important to note that even if employees aren't unionized, they have the right to discuss conditions of employment with fellow employees.

Therefore, even a casual conversation on social media websites about working conditions may be protected under the NLRA. Each situation is viewed differently and until the courts have established guidance regarding these issues, be very careful about telling employees what they can and can't do on their own personal social media sites. Focus on setting an example by regulating your own actions first and foremost.

1. A clinic owner changes working hours and rates of pay. The owner discharges three of the ten practitioners after several posts were made on Facebook and Twitter between employees discussing their displeasure in the recent change. The owner felt it was a breach of confidentiality and it put the clinic in bad light to have them discussing it publicly. After reviewing the cases, the NLRB found the discharge to be unlawful because the practitioners engaged in protected concerted activity.

2. A practitioner attends a conference on behalf of the spa where he works. He takes photos and posts on Facebook an embarrassing incident that occurred at a social event involving another business. That same weekend he posts mocking comments and photos of co-workers during the event. The owner discharges the

practitioner for the postings. The NLRB finds the discharge for posting the photos and comments of fellow practitioners to be unlawful; however the discharge for posting the embarrassing photos about the other business was found lawful. Therefore the practitioner discharge was upheld.

Points to Ponder

When attending social events at a conference is it considered personal time or on the clock? Even if the postings were lawful, are they ethical? Are they professional?

3. A practitioner hires a receptionist to answer the phones and help with marketing. The receptionist posts some negative comments regarding the hours and pay of the job on her personal account on social media. The practitioner addresses the issues and the two decide it best to part ways.

Points to Ponder

Did the practitioner have the right to address the comments made on the personal profile? Should the practitioner have let the receptionist go in this case?

Because the social media realm is changing daily, it's wise to separate overall policies from site-specific guidelines. This saves you having to make constant changes. Keep your social media policies generalized. Establish roles and responsibilities, legal compliance and branding, and purpose and values.

Consider having two social media policies: one for using social media for your job, and one for using social media in your personal life. The social media policy for personal life should give guidelines about what can and can't be said about your company on a personal site. For example: trade secrets, client information, and even employee whereabouts might be strictly confidential.

You may want to encourage employees to act as brand ambassadors and provide helpful guidelines for talking about your practice online. Keep in mind that you're walking a fine line to require employees to use their own personal social media accounts to connect with your company online. They may choose to do so but it needs to be their choice. Also, before creating your policy, review the NLRA mentioned above.

National Labor Relations Board

http://mynlrb.nlrb.gov/

Develop a Social Media Policy

- Review the guidelines for social media websites.
- Create an overall Social Media Mission Statement for how you want your social media handled both for business and personal.
- Establish Social Media Policies for your personal and business accounts.
- Review the NLRA to familiarize yourself with acceptable language for social media policy.

Ethically Sharing Content

When you share content on social media sites, remember to follow some basic rules. No matter what the content (e.g. photo, article, quote), if you didn't create the content yourself, you're obligated to reference or credit the source of the content. When using the social sites, one of the best marketing strategies is to get people to share, re-tweet, or re-pin the content you post. You can also share from other social profiles. If you find something that you like and want to share, but you don't want to share from a particular profile, you can share directly from the source of the content. For example, The Massage Therapy Foundation shares a research study that is re-posted by your competitor. You find the reference on your competitor's profile, you can click on the link back to the Massage Therapy Foundation and share from that post.

Sharing Photos

When it comes to sharing photos, you aren't allowed to use just any photo you find on the Internet. Using photos without consent can result in legal matters or fines. There are royalty-free photo sites that allow you to use the photos for various purposes. Be sure to review the Terms of Use section of any of these sites. They offer specific guidelines on how to use the photos for free, including social media, website, and even print media. Typically, they just require you to include the website reference and the artist's name next to the photo.

Free Digital Photos

http://www.freedigitalphotos.net/

You can re-tweet, re-pin, or share a photo directly from a business or personal profile. However, don't download a photo to upload on your social media sites without giving credit to the page of the original post or without asking permission. Many photos that are posted like family photos with quotes, funny jokes, and such, already have the credit embedded on the photo. If they don't, be sure to include the credit in the description or comment area when you use it on your social media sites. This will save you many headaches.

By no means is it acceptable to download photos from a search engine or website without the owner's permission. Some people believe that if the photo exists on a search engine like Google it's okay to download and use for their purposes. This isn't the case. It could, in fact, lead to a very costly lesson.

If you want to promote products using your social media, most manufacturers will grant you permission and encourage you to promote their products on social media sites. However, you need to ask first and always remember to follow their guidelines for using their photos.

Most social media sites have instant sharing through cell phones. Most cell phones have automatic Geotagging loaded on phones. Geotagging is helpful for users to find a wide variety of businesses and services by location. However, if you upload a photo taken by a cell phone that is a client's or an employee's you might be giving away more information than necessary. Geotagging can be removed from photos and videos from the user's cell phone, or you can use software to strip the photos of Geotagging information before the photos are posted on your social media sites.

Sharing Article Links, Research Data, and Other Information

When it comes to sharing articles or information from websites on social media sites, you need to always include the URL (Uniform Resource Locator) with the post, pin, tweet, or share. For example, you find an article online about massage research reducing stress for infants and one of the benefits was it helped babies sleep better. You want to share this information with your followers. First post your summary, question, or opinion about this article then include the URL with the post. Here is an example of how this would be posted, shared, and tweeted:

Create shortened URLs

https://bitly.com/
http://goo.gl/
http://tinyurl.com/

> *Interesting new research finds that massage reduces stress levels in infants. One of the benefits is that it induces better quality of sleep for the babies. Read for yourself here:* www.titleofmagazine.com/titleofarticle.

Some social media sites, such as Twitter, have character limitations. Yet, many URL links are rather long. It is ethically acceptable to use website shorteners, such as bit.ly and goo.gl to shorten the URL. The shortened URL still takes readers to the article when they click on it; the shortened URL makes it user-friendly for you.

Posting on Social Media

- Create a post using a photo.
- Create a post using an Article link.
- Share a photo from another social media profile or page.
- Share an article link from another social media profile or page.

What Happens In Vegas...

Social media can be a very powerful tool for quickly building your brand and practice. The lines between our personal and business lives are fading. Most business owners haven't fully realized the challenges that can happen as a result of decreased privacy. Remember the Las Vegas promotion, "What happens in Vegas, stays in Vegas"? Well, today it might be more accurate to say "What happens in Vegas, ends up on Facebook, YouTube, Twitter, Google+, Pinterest, and LinkedIn..."

Most of the ethical problems around social media are due to ignorance rather than malice when it comes to business. Many business owners haven't fully thought through the repercussions of their online activities. By educating yourself and your staff about the uses of social media, you prevent many of the problems before they start.

Legal Issues

Legal issues vary by profession and locale. A professional practitioner who intends to do business for the long run wants to comply with all legal requirements. Attending to the legal aspects of a practice shows respect for the community, the field, the client's welfare, and the practitioner's own values. The principal aspects are: complying with local, state, and federal laws; maintaining appropriate insurance coverage; avoiding slander and libel; honoring copyright; negotiating and complying with contracts; minimizing civil lawsuits; and hiring employees and independent contractors.

Comply with Local, State, and Federal Laws

> Average people look for ways of getting away with it; successful people look for ways of getting on with it.
>
> —Jim Rohn

The two words "laws" and "regulations" make most people cringe at least a little bit. Few practitioners enjoy dealing with bureaucracy, even though the results are often beneficial. Complying with laws is usually straightforward—of course, this means being cognizant of the laws in the first place. Ignorance of the law isn't a good defense; in fact it's no defense. The difficulty arises when your values or morals conflict with one of those laws.

A reflexologist moved to a new city and was looking for a home/office. She found a house with a "mother-in-law" space that included a bathroom, small kitchen, and a separate entrance that provided privacy. This space was connected to the family quarters by a breezeway. The home was purchased prior to checking the city zoning codes. Surprisingly, she was restricted from using the space as the zoning board considered her profession a "medical" practice which required her to have office space in a professional building. Her home office granted privacy and separate restroom facilities. She believed she was providing what was necessary for her clients. In her opinion the regulation was unjustly classifying her as a "medical" practice. Her choices were to ignore the regulation and quietly build her practice, go before the zoning board and request a variance, or succumb to the regulations and allow her mother-in-law to move in.

Points to Ponder

Should practitioners just do what they want when a law or regulation doesn't match their values or morals? Which of the three choices above is the most ethical choice?

The two major options when encountering restrictive or archaic laws and regulations are to ignore them or change them. Changing the regulations is the best long-term option, although many people don't have the time (or possibly money) to invest in such a pursuit. The bottom line is that when you choose to disregard laws and regulations, you're acting unethically. At the very least, most professional Codes of Ethics state that you must abide by national, state, and local laws. Some people feel their actions are justified; nevertheless, the result is still a chink in their ethics. The other consideration is the extent to which you're in violation. The penalty for disregarding a regulation or breaking the law can be as slight as a modest fine or as severe as loss of licensure or even imprisonment. If you make a choice that technically violates a law, you must be prepared to pay the consequences. Investigate potential consequences before deciding what to do.

Insurance Coverage

Maintaining adequate business and malpractice insurance coverage is crucial; some localities require specific coverage. Accidents happen, and nature has been known to strike devastating blows; without proper coverage you could be out a considerable amount of money. The United States is a highly litigious society, and no one is shielded from the possibility of a lawsuit, even if his behavior is above reproach. A practitioner might win the case, but without insurance most practitioners would be hard-pressed to afford the astronomical costs of litigation. Be sure to carefully read your policy. For instance, some policies don't cover sexual misconduct while others cover the litigation costs but not the damages awarded if you're found liable. Also, some insurance companies will nullify a policy if the practitioner doesn't uphold all local, state, and federal legal requirements.

Figure 9.8 **Malpractice Insurance Issues**

- Make sure that it covers when an incident occurs, even if subsequently the practitioner no longer has coverage.
- Some insurance companies will nullify a policy if the practitioner doesn't uphold all local, state, and federal legal requirements.
- Most policies don't cover sexual misconduct.
- Some policies cover litigation costs but not damages awarded if the practitioner is found liable for sexual misconduct.

Slander and Libel

The two major forms of defamation are slander (verbal) and libel (written). Telling everyone about a bad experience you have had with another healthcare practitioner or denigrating a modality that you feel isn't beneficial is tempting. Most practitioners have overheard

Be careful of what you say so that you don't malign a colleague or aren't sued for defamation.

Make sure that you state your concerns about another professional or organization as your opinion. It is fine to be emphatic and say, "I won't do business with this person!" Always stick to the facts. The minute you start embellishing the truth you could find yourself in trouble. For instance, saying someone is a crook could be actionable, but stating that you never received payment or that you found the treatment to be ineffective is acceptable from a legal standpoint. Keep in mind that just because you don't work well with a particular practitioner, or certain modalities aren't effective for you or are contrary to your belief system, doesn't preclude others from receiving benefits. Determine your intent before saying anything that may be construed as "bad-mouthing" or gossip. These types of actions often reflect more poorly on you than the practitioner or modality in question.

Action can be brought against you if you try to interfere with someone's right to contract. The term for this is Tortious Interference with Contractual Relations. The measure is if you stated something that isn't true and contacted someone who is doing business with that person. For instance, you could be held liable if you know a clinic has hired a practitioner and you contact that clinic and bad-mouth the practitioner, causing the practitioner to be fired. Although a seeming paradox, this does align with the many professional Codes of Ethics that require members to report alleged violations by other members. Again, you can state facts, but be cautious about the wording. Gary Wolf, attorney at law in Tucson, Arizona, says, "Truth is the best defense for a defamation claim."[12]

Copyrighted Materials

Many practitioners copy materials to aid in marketing and client education without realizing that they're violating copyright law. If it looks copyrighted, assume it is. This applies to pictures and cartoons as well. The "fair use" doctrine allows limited reproduction of copyrighted works for educational and research purposes. The relevant portion of the copyright statute provides that the "fair use" of a copyrighted work, including limited reproduction "for purposes such as criticism, news reporting, teaching, scholarship, or research" isn't a copyright infringement.[13]

> Figure 9.9 **Copyright Guidelines**
>
> - Copying works for client education violates copyright law.
> - If it looks copyrighted, assume it is.
> - Copyright protects an author's right to obtain commercial benefit from valuable work.
> - Copyright preserves the author's right to control how a work is used.
> - Copyright law is mostly civil law.
> - Obtain permission to use the work from the copyright owner and always give proper credit.

Unfortunately, many practitioners and teachers take this to mean they can copy short sections of books or magazine articles to give to clients or use as handouts in workshops, classes, or free presentations. This is usually not the case.

The two main objectives of copyright are to protect an author's right to obtain commercial benefit from valuable work, and to preserve the author's right to control how a work is used. Copyright law is mostly civil law. Unlike criminal law, you aren't "innocent until proven guilty."

Also, be aware that new laws are being enacted to move some forms of copyright violation into the criminal realm.

Fair Use Factors

The law evaluates the following factors to determine if a particular use of a copyrighted work is a permitted "fair use," or a copyright infringement:

1. The purpose and character of the use. This includes whether such use is of a commercial nature or non-profit educational purposes.
2. The nature of the copyrighted work.
3. The amount and substantiality of the copied portion in relation to the copyrighted work as a whole.
4. The effect of the use upon the potential market for, or value of, the copyrighted work.

Although all of these factors are considered, the last factor is the most important in determining whether a particular use is "fair." Where a work is available for purchase or license from the copyright owner in the medium or format desired, copying all or a significant portion of the work instead of purchasing or licensing a sufficient number of "authorized" copies is unfair.

Almost all materials are copyrighted the moment they're written—a formal copyright notice isn't required. Copyright law makes it technically illegal to reproduce almost any new creative work (other than under fair use) without permission, and copyright is still violated whether you charge money or not. Facts and ideas can't be copyrighted, but their expression and format can. Ask yourself why you're reprinting (or recording) those materials and why you couldn't have paid for copies. Obtain permission to use the work from the copyright owner and always give proper credit.

Photocopy Request Information

Most authors/publishers gladly give permission to copy or excerpt material as long as it isn't part of a money-making venture. It is customary to send a request to copy a copyrighted work to the permission department of the publisher of the work. Companies such as the Copyright Clearance Center will obtain permission for you (for a fee of course). Permission requests should contain the following:

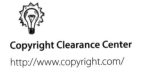

Copyright Clearance Center
http://www.copyright.com/

- Title, author and edition
- Exact material to be used, giving page numbers or chapters
- Number of copies to be made
- Use to be made of the copied materials
- Form of distribution (e.g., handouts, newsletter)
- Whether the material is to be sold

Contracts

Legal forms and agreements are an integral part of any business relationship, yet people often avoid written contracts. Whether you're interested in a one-time only interaction or a long-term affiliation, delineate in writing your roles and expectations. Clear written agreements serve several purposes: they help avoid problems; they provide a predetermined method for resolving conflicts; and they keep you focused on your goals.[4]

A binding contract doesn't need to be written on a piece of paper with the word "Contract" emblazoned across the top. In business arrangements all that is usually required is some written form (letter, memo, or a full-blown contract) that describes what is to be contracted, the terms of the exchange, parties' signatures, and dates. Keep in mind that once you agree to the terms of a contract, you're bound by it. Unfairness is rarely a legal ground for nullifying a contract unless it's outright fraud. Also, most states uphold verbal contracts as legal and binding.

Ideally, you would come to the negotiating process with a sample of your own contract and a checklist of key elements you want addressed, review the other party's contract, and create

> The dullest ink is stronger than the sharpest memory.
>
> —John Rickenbacker

a specific contract that is mutually agreeable to both of you. If the other party insists on only using her contract, make sure to obtain responses (preferably in writing) to all the items in your checklist. Verify that all parties initial each change whenever items to the contract are deleted or added. Rewrite the contract if it contains a significant number of changes.

You may be tempted to not write a "formal" contract for presumably simple transactions, particularly if it's just a "one-time" event, such as a cooperative marketing project or a short-term equipment rental. Yet it's usually those seemingly negligible occurrences that cause regrets. Invest the time in clarifying what is truly important to you in a business relationship. Even if you're currently involved in a business relationship and don't have a contract, you can always design one now. Each situation is unique and one contract won't suit all situations. Once you have the basics done, you'll find it much simpler to alter any contract.

Questionable behavior is rare when everything is working smoothly. The problems arise when one party isn't happy about something or when it's time to end the relationship. Some people let the "little things" accumulate until they explode. Contracts assist all parties in clarifying and maintaining ethical behavior.

Business relationships end for many reasons: one party wants to move in another direction; the association has run its course; the project is complete; the parties don't want to work together any longer. Most people don't know how to cleanly end relationships. You significantly reduce stress in ending a business relationship if your contract includes a dissolution clause that clearly describes how to terminate the association and what to do if there is an impasse.

Figure 9.10 Contract Checklist

- ❏ Names and addresses of all parties involved
- ❏ A short description and mission statements
- ❏ Summarization of contracted party's desired role
- ❏ A classification of the business relationship
- ❏ A description of what each party is to provide
- ❏ A timetable
- ❏ Location of where work is to be performed
- ❏ The duration of the contract
- ❏ Payment method and schedule
- ❏ Fringe benefits
- ❏ Opportunities for financial increases
- ❏ Insurance coverage provided
- ❏ Insurance coverage required
- ❏ Guarantees
- ❏ Financial obligations of the contracted party
- ❏ Conditions for termination of the agreement
- ❏ Guidelines for transfer of the contract
- ❏ Who retains custody of the client
- ❏ Arbitration
- ❏ Who is responsible for contract breach legal fees
- ❏ Contract communication contact information
- ❏ Signature lines and date the contract is signed

Dispute Resolution

The options for resolving a dispute with a business associate, a client, or a landlord include: ignore it; attempt to resolve it yourself; submit to arbitration; engage in mediation; take it to court. Stewart Levine details the following seven steps to conflict resolution in his book, *Getting to Resolution: Turning Conflict into Collaboration*[15]:

1. Adopt an attitude of resolution.
2. Listen carefully to each party's stories.
3. Allow a preliminary vision to arise with all parties.
4. Allow people to express their disappointment and then bring everyone into the current moment.
5. Agree (at least in principle) to create a new vision.
6. Design the new agreement.
7. Acknowledge resolution.

Many people are moving away from expensive, stressful, and time-consuming ways of resolving disputes. They are also reluctant to engage in the traditional "positional" dispute resolution where each person takes a position then uses a win-lose approach to getting what she wants. People are recognizing the many benefits in using interest-based bargaining, where parties engage in collaborative problem-solving that is based on the needs, desires, and concerns of each party. In that way each person fulfills his goals. Mediation is an extension of this idea and can be the best choice when those involved can't resolve a conflict by themselves; it provides the disputants with an opportunity to communicate and understand each other's points of view, create options, and control solutions.

Attorney Joan C. Calcagno states:

> When disputants participate in problem solving and decision-making, they're more likely to follow through with the agreement made to resolve the dispute. An enhanced working relationship is one of the many satisfactions that can result from a mediated solution to a dispute. Mediation is, at the least, less costly and time consuming over the long term and can be the way to finding innovative, mutually beneficial solutions, and preserving important relationships. Faced with a dispute, consider proposing mediation to the others involved.[16]

Civil Lawsuits

Many lawsuits levied against practitioners by their clients could be avoided by keeping clear boundaries, and using effective and compassionate communication skills. Luckily, the number of lawsuits filed against complementary healthcare providers is fairly low. This is reflected in the reasonable malpractice insurance rates. For instance, massage insurance policies can be purchased for approximately $150 per year; acupuncturists pay from $500-$2,000 per year; and chiropractic policies start at about $2,000 (depending on the state and inclusions).

When, after weighing the advantages and disadvantages, a client chooses to bring a civil lawsuit, time limitations may foreclose that action. These limitations, enacted at both the state and federal level, are referred to as "statutes of limitation" since they contain a specified time limit after which a suit may not be filed, regardless of the merits of the claim. Malpractice lawsuits statutes of limitation vary from state to state, but generally range from two to three years. Special limitation periods are often written into statutes that are tailored to specific legal avenues or causes of action.

Fairness underlies the rationale behind statutes of limitation. The enacting body or reviewing court attempts to balance the right of defendants to timely notice and settlement of claims with the right of plaintiffs to judicial resolution for civil damages. This balancing of interests can result in exceptions to the applicable statutes of limitations. The most commonly used exception in boundary violation cases is the discovery rule which suspends the running of the statute of limitations until the victim discovers or should have discovered the injury and its cause. The discovery rule benefits victims of boundary violations who may not connect the harm suffered to the offending practitioner until long after the damaging acts occurred.

If a client decides to pursue litigation, the process usually begins with filing a complaint in court. This document spells out the basic theories of legal duty and allegations of the

> " All human wisdom is summed up in two words: wait and hope.
>
> —Alexandre Dumas

practitioner's liability and damage to the client. In response to the complaint, the practitioner, usually through counsel, files an answer in which the practitioner responds to the allegations and asserts defenses. A prolonged period, known as discovery, follows the initial interchange between the parties to a lawsuit. During this period, both sides endeavor to gather (or discover) as much information as possible about the proof of the claim or the practitioner's denial/ defense of the claim. Although state and federal rules govern the extent of discovery, the scope is very broad. Friends and family of the victim usually become involved in the process and may be required to testify or provide other information to the practitioner's counsel.

The Discovery Process

The discovery period encompasses mechanisms discussed below. The stress of these intrusions into the victim's (and the accused perpetrator's) private life can be extreme and debilitating. Conduct this type of action ethically, focusing on your integrity and honesty.

INTERROGATORIES are written questions asked of either party and must be answered under oath. In most instances, the party answering the interrogatories provides a draft of the answers along with any corroborating documents to his attorney. The attorney then formalizes the answers which the responding party reads and signs, if correct. The attorney's duty is to present the information accurately and in the best possible light for the client. It is the client's responsibility to make sure that in doing so, the information is truthful.

DEPOSITIONS involve the oral examination of a witness during which an attorney asks questions that the witness answers under oath. Any person, including the parties to the lawsuit and others having information relevant to the lawsuit, may be summoned to a deposition. Typically, a deposition takes place in an attorney's office in the presence of the attorneys for both sides and a court stenographer.

REQUESTS FOR PRODUCTION OF DOCUMENTS are written requests by the attorney for either party addressed to the other party seeking the identification of documents that are relevant to the case. When a party responds to a request for production of documents, copies of the documents described are usually provided to the requesting party. In a malpractice case, a common document request would include the records of the healthcare provider and medical records of any prior or subsequent treating practitioner or physician of the client. The client's journals or other personal papers could be examined under a request for production. Keep in mind that you're legally obligated to provide the information even if the information may be damaging. The temptation may be great to alter or destroy documents; however, the risk, worry, and liability of being discovered isn't worth it.

REQUESTS FOR MEDICAL OR PSYCHIATRIC EXAMINATIONS are common. These involve examination of the client by a neutral physician or psychiatric practitioner if the client claims in the lawsuit that she suffered medical or psychiatric injuries. The examination provides an ostensibly unbiased opinion concerning the client's present condition, past history, and prognosis.

Malpractice Actions

The legal theory underlying most civil lawsuits filed by clients against exploitative healthcare practitioners is negligence. The most commonly invoked form of negligence action is the suit for malpractice. To prove a claim for malpractice, the client must establish four elements by a preponderance of evidence. This means that the client must prove that her version of events is more likely than not to be true. The quality, rather than quantity, of evidence determines whether the client has proven her case. The jury must determine whether one party's evidence is more believable, more trustworthy or more accurate than the other's, regardless of the number of witnesses testifying.[17] This represents a much easier burden for the client to satisfy than in a criminal case which requires proof beyond a reasonable doubt of all of the elements of a crime.

Remember that texts may be considered legal documents and can be subpoenaed.

The elements in a malpractice case that a client must prove by a preponderance of the evidence are:

1. a duty of care owed by the practitioner to the client;
2. a breach of that duty;
3. a causal relationship between the breach; and
4. damage to the client.

In malpractice actions, the breach of the practitioner's duty is determined by measuring the actions of the offending practitioner against what is expected from others practicing the same profession. Thus, the standard for judging healthcare practitioners is that they be "held to the standard of care and skill of the average member of the profession."[18] This measuring stick is called "the standard of care."

1. A client goes to a practitioner for a wellness treatment and when the treatment ends has difficulty getting off the table due to severe back pain that wasn't present before the session. This pain continues for several weeks and the client is unable to work. The client files a malpractice suit for pain, suffering, and lost wages. Through the discovery process, lawyers learn that 10 years ago the client suffered debilitating back pain for three months and couldn't work during that time.

   Regardless, the practitioner was still held liable. In this instance, had the practitioner done a thorough intake interview, it might have alerted him to this prior condition resulting in the exercise of greater caution.

Points to Ponder

How might the practitioner have avoided these consequences? How can you best conduct your intake interviews to account for thorough health history and allow for greater caution?

2. A person is involved in a car accident, goes to the emergency room and is diagnosed as suffering from a mild whiplash injury. Her major symptoms are general achiness and a mild headache. She makes an appointment with a practitioner in hopes of alleviating the discomfort. She experiences a moderate improvement after the first two sessions, but after the third one, she experiences an increase in neck pain. When she arises the morning following the treatment, she has severe neck and head pain and is unable to rotate her head more than a few degrees in either direction. She files a malpractice suit against the practitioner.

   The practitioner demonstrates that whiplash injuries can have a delayed onset of symptoms up to 2-3 weeks. The practitioner's notes clearly documented objective and subjective progress after the first two treatments. According to the treatment notes the same procedure was followed in each session. The case was resolved without any judgment against the practitioner mainly due to the evidence presented which included treatment notes and the testimony of an expert witness who confirmed the common occurrence of delayed pain onset in whiplash cases.

Points to Ponder

Could the practitioner in this case have avoided these charges? What kind of client education might you do to help whiplash (or other accident) cases better understand the pain and healing process of their injuries?

See Chapter 7 page 170 for information on the **At-Risk Practitioner**.

A practitioner breaches the duty owed to the client if the treatment rendered falls below the applicable standard of care. In the first scenario, the preponderance of evidence indicated that the standard of care was low, while in the second scenario it couldn't be shown that a causal relationship existed between the treatment and the damage to the client.

> **Figure 9.11** Avoid Malpractice Lawsuits
>
> - Gather and complete an accurate medical history from each new client.
> - Obtain as much information as possible from the other members of the client's healthcare team.
> - Have the client sign an Informed Consent sheet and other HIPAA paperwork.
> - Use common language when talking with clients.
> - Be courteous and professional.
> - Document every interaction (including phone calls) with a client.
> - If a problem occurs during a session, immediately discuss it with the client (and family, if appropriate), and don't have the client pay for further sessions.
> - Beware of high risk clients.

> **Figure 9.12** High Risk Client Characteristics
>
> - The sexually provocative client
> - The professional plaintiff client
> - The client with unrealistic expectations
> - The client who idolizes the practitioner

Employers' Liability

The employers of healthcare practitioners who commit boundary violations can also be held accountable for the actions of their employees under two distinct theories of liability: vicarious and direct. Vicarious liability, also known as the doctrine of *respondeat superior*, holds an employer liable for the acts of an employee. It is usually a prerequisite that when the wrongful acts were committed, the employee was acting within the scope of his employment. The theory holds the employer vicariously liable for someone else's behavior even though the employer didn't commit the act. Instead, the employer is deemed to have control over the employee when the employee is at work, even if the employee is working away from the place of employment or the employer isn't physically present at the time the wrongful act occurs.

By contrast, direct liability involves the employer's own negligence in hiring, retaining, or supervising employees. Consider this flagrant example of negligent hiring:

> A person with a long record of violent crime is hired as a security guard in an apartment complex and is provided with a gun. The person hired uses a master key to enter an apartment with the intention of robbery and shoots the startled inhabitant.

Points to Ponder

Should the employer be held accountable in this case? How can an employer take the necessary steps to avoid such extreme cases, as well as cases that are more subtle?

Clearly the employer has a duty to investigate the background of persons to whom weapons or access to property is given. Other potential areas of concern aren't necessarily obvious. A possibility that could easily occur is that of a healthcare practitioner who moves after losing his license for sexual misconduct and applies for a job at a clinic in another state. That new employer might be found directly liable for subsequent sexual misconduct by the practitioner if no inquiry were made into his background or if an inquiry was made yet no action taken. In many states, colleagues, supervisors, and referring professionals risk liability for victims' injuries when they knew or should have known of the misconduct and failed to take appropriate steps to stop it or warn the victim.

State Licensing Boards and Professional Organizations

Some victims of boundary violations by healthcare practitioners choose to file a complaint with the state licensing board (that regulates the profession) or with the professional organization of which the perpetrator is a member. These actions can be taken alone or in conjunction with the civil or criminal actions. One potential result of a licensing board complaint is the offending practitioner's loss of licensure to practice. This loss serves two purposes for the victim: to deprive the practitioner of a livelihood, and to prevent the victimization of others by the same practitioner. These results, however, aren't guaranteed. Often, state licensing boards don't possess the necessary resources to pursue all cases through adjudication. Secondly, a practitioner may forego her license but continue to practice. In many cases, the offending practitioner agrees to settle a civil case out of court for a sum of money as long as the victim agrees to refrain from reporting the practitioner to the licensing board.

A successful complaint to a professional organization might also result in revocation of the perpetrator's membership in the organization or some other sanction. As with license revocation, though, this event doesn't preclude the practitioner from continuing to practice. Although a potential benefit of an ethical or licensing board complaint may be confidentiality of the proceedings and findings, confidentiality requirements vary among states and professional boards. In those states that do maintain the victim's confidentiality, the victim may pursue these avenues without fear of public exposure. In addition, both of these options can be more "victim friendly" since the victim isn't cast in the adversarial role inherent in a civil lawsuit. A licensing board prosecutor typically presents a victim's case to a state board. The inquiry is more concerned with fact finding and determining whether the practitioner meets the criteria for licensing than with assessing the victim's emotional and monetary damages.

> Labor to keep alive in your breast that little spark of celestial fire called conscience.
>
> —George Washington

Who Pays?

One result of civil litigation is the award of monetary damages. In cases involving abuse by healthcare practitioners, the funds awarded help ensure that the victim of the abuse can afford treatment for the psychological or physical damages suffered. For a variety of reasons the most likely source of the funds used to compensate the victim is insurance, either of the offending practitioner or the practitioner's employer. Few practitioners can financially afford to pay a large monetary award. Furthermore, few people would risk the possibility of being held personally responsible for such payments. Most practitioners, therefore, obtain malpractice insurance if it's available to them. In most malpractice lawsuits, the insurer pays any judgment amount and provides the insured with defense counsel.

Even with insurance coverage, however, a practitioner may be responsible for some of the damages awarded the victim. If the practitioner refuses to settle out of court for a sum agreed upon by the insurer and the victim's jury award turns out to be higher than the settlement offer, the practitioner may be liable for the difference. The defense attorney assigned to the practitioner also represents the insurance company; therefore the insurer controls the case. If the practitioner wants personal representation, he can hire an attorney at a substantial cost.

Many malpractice insurance policies specifically exclude intentional acts from coverage. They also write exceptions into policies for sexual misconduct or set a dollar limit on any payments for sexual misconduct. Some require a separate rider for sexual misconduct coverage. Other policies pay for the costs of a lawsuit yet don't cover monetary damages if the practitioner is found liable for sexual misconduct. The insurer may also refuse to renew a policy once a sexual misconduct claim is filed.

These are important considerations both for the practitioner and the client. If the practitioner is denied insurance coverage, expenses incurred in defending against the claim (and the potential that a large verdict is returned) can lead to financial destruction and bankruptcy. For the victim, the lack of a reliable source of payment of damages can mean that he can't afford the treatment needed to recover from the injuries suffered at the hands of the exploiting practitioner. Thus, in an effort to avoid denial of insurance coverage, a victim's attorney focuses on boundary violations other than sexual contact to establish the practitioner's negligence. A knowledgeable attorney also seeks to avoid insurance exclusions or liability caps by raising other legal and public policy arguments.

Several other avenues for compensation may be available to victims. In some jurisdictions, the licensing board can order the practitioner to compensate the victim for treatment costs. In a criminal prosecution, the court may order restitution for the victim, or the victim may access funds from crime-victim assistance centers.

Legal or Ethical?

Determine if the following situations are legal issues or ethical issues. Then, discuss with a partner or colleague how you would react to each situation.

- The zoning ordinances in your area states that you can't treat clients in your home. You are in a tight financial situation. You want to turn one room in your two-bedroom domicile into a treatment room. What do you do?
- You read a flier that states: "Workshop to Help You Pass the Massage Licensing Examination." The charge is $35 for two hours of lecture and practice test questions. You know the presenters of this workshop. They were students with you at school and both did poorly in anatomy class, yet somehow managed to do well on their examinations. You suspected they had cheated in school. You heard that they were gathering test questions from the licensing exam by therapists who could remember the questions. What do you do?
- What would you do if you're changing the name of your business and discover that someone else in a neighboring city has an already established business with the same name? What if that person never registered the business name?
- What do you do if your client (or a colleague) tells you that she is considering working with a practitioner that you don't feel is ethical?

Employees and Independent Contractors

It is common for practitioners to be hired as independent contractors and not as employees. This is usually done because the clinic or spa owner wants to avoid the costs associated with being an employer. With employees, in addition to the responsibility of having enough money for their paychecks, the following needs to be done: match their FICA (Social Security and Medicare) deductions; pay FUTA (Federal Unemployment Taxes) which is calculated at a percentage of the employee's first $7,000 of wages annually; pay state unemployment taxes; provide workers' compensation; withhold state and federal taxes; deposit withheld taxes (the requirement varies from weekly to monthly to quarterly, depending on the amount); file regular returns; send W-2 forms to employees annually; and in most instances, offer benefits such as health insurance, paid vacations, sick leave, and retirement plans.[19]

The main advantage to those who hire independent contractors is that you aren't required to withhold income tax or social security tax from independent contractors. But, you must file a form 1099-MISC at the end of the year if you pay an independent contractor $600 or more during the year in the course of your business. Another advantage is that, in most instances, it's much easier and less risky to terminate a contracted practitioner than to fire an employee. Also, your liability is reduced in terms of malpractice if you have hired an independent contractor who is required to carry his own insurance.

The potential pitfalls of working with non-employees include paying a higher price for their services and not having control over their work in terms of timeliness and quality. Many clinic owners lament that the level of professionalism and camaraderie isn't the same among independent contractors as with employees. Plus, an independent contractor (by nature of the classification) is less likely to actively build your business—after all, she has her own business to pursue.

The Internal Revenue Service (IRS) guidelines for determining employment status are fairly clear when it comes to clerical staff: in most instances an office-person is an employee. A gray area exists in hiring healthcare practitioners. In researching numerous spas, clinics, and group practices, we discovered many of them walk a very thin legal line. A significant number of the so-called independent contractors that work for them would most likely be classified as employees under the IRS guidelines. Calling someone an independent contractor doesn't make it so.

Under common-law rules, anyone who performs services subject to the will and control of an employer, as to both what must be done and how it must be done, is an employee. It doesn't matter that the employer allows the employee discretion and freedom of action, so long as the employer has the legal right to control both the method and result of the services.

Two usual characteristics of an employer-employee relationship are that the employer has the right to discharge the employee and the employer supplies the employee with tools and a place to work. (Do not assume that you can get around this by having your "employee" provide his own specific supplies. "Tools" is a broad term that can include the equipment required in running a practice such as telephones and copiers).

If you have an employer-employee relationship, it makes no difference how it is described. It doesn't matter if the employee is called an employee, associate, partner, or independent contractor. It also doesn't matter how the payments are measured, made, or what they're called. Nor does it matter whether the individual is employed full time or part time.

The IRS has developed a list of 20 factors[20] that it uses to determine the status of employee or independent contractor. A practitioner can still qualify as an independent contractor even if some of these factors are present in the working relationship. The key elements to differentiating between employee status and independent contractor status in the healthcare industry involve the following: who regulates the type of work done and how it's performed; where and when the sessions occur; who determines the fee structure; who receives the money from the clients; who provides the equipment and supplies; who pays for client-related expenses; and who generates the clientele.

As an employer, you take a considerable risk by deeming a worker an independent contractor. If the IRS determines that your independent contractors are (or were) indeed employees, you may be required to pay fines (of up to 100 percent of the tax) in addition to the back income taxes and social security taxes. This can easily add up to a sizable amount. In the eyes of the IRS, it makes no difference if you signed an agreement that states you're contracting with an independent contractor—although a written agreement is advisable.

Minimize the risks of your independent contractors being reclassified as employees by taking the following steps: make certain independent contractors possess multiple sources of income; sign "independent contractor" contracts which clearly state the requirements of all parties while making it clear the contractors can pursue other clients; require contractors to provide their own tables, linens, products, music, and other supplies; allow contractors to set

> "
> Conducting your business in a socially responsible way is good business. It means that you can attract better employees and that customers will know what you stand for and like you for it.
>
> —M. Anthony Burns

their own schedules (make certain they work less than full time); have clients pay contractors directly; request copies of the contractors' tax returns; and require contractors to provide their own insurance and workers' compensation coverage. Complying with these suggestions still doesn't guarantee independent contractor status. If in doubt, you can request that the IRS determine whether a worker is an employee by filing Form SS-8.

If you decide to hire other practitioners as independent contractors, be sure to create a thorough contract. Hire a lawyer to review the contract. The several hundred dollars it may cost you in attorney fees is minimal compared to the potential fees and penalties the IRS are wont to impose.

Figure 9.13 IRS **20-Point Checklist**

An individual is likely to be considered an employee if he or she:

1. Is required to comply with company instructions about when, where, and how to work.
2. Has been trained by the company to perform services in a particular manner.
3. Has her services integrated into the company's operations because the services are critical to the success of the business.
4. Must render services personally.
5. Utilizes assistants provided by the company.
6. Has an ongoing, continuing relationship with the company.
7. Has set work hours established by the employer.
8. Is required to work the equivalent of full time.
9. Works on the company's designated premises.
10. Must perform services in the order or sequence determined by the employer.
11. Must submit regular progress reports.
12. Is paid in regular intervals, such as by the hour, week, or month.
13. Is reimbursed for all business and travel expenses.
14. Uses tools and materials furnished by the employer.
15. Has no significant investment in the facilities that are used.
16. Has no risk of loss.
17. Works for only one person or company.
18. Does not offer services to the general public.
19. Can be discharged by the company.
20. Can terminate the relationship without incurring liability.

Insurance Reimbursement Issues

Insurance coverage for complementary healthcare treatments is an evolving issue. Careful attention and recordkeeping can maximize the benefits for both clients and practitioners. This section presents several current ethical dilemmas for somatic practitioners in the areas of documentation, insurance billing, and communication with the healthcare team.

Responsibility for Payment

When is treatment finished? When does maintenance or wellness care begin? There is a fine line between the two, especially if the condition is chronic. By identifying guidelines for delineating treatment versus wellness care, you can ethically apply those standards to the insurance issue: who pays for care?

The insurance issue is often clouded by people's beliefs and bad experiences. For instance, many people feel that insurance policies or case managers limit access to manual therapy and prevent clients from receiving the number of treatments necessary to recover from their injuries. Therefore, in the seemingly few situations where authorized treatment exceeds the number of sessions necessary for healing, practitioners often feel justified in continuing to provide care. Certainly, the clients are willing to continue: manual therapy feels good and is effective. And it makes sense to continue; after all, an ounce of prevention is worth a pound of cure!

According to standard insurance definitions, treatment is warranted until the condition is corrected or maximum improvement is made. These definitions also state that treatment must provide the client with appropriate instruction for follow-up, self-care, and prevention of future occurrences. All maintenance and wellness care are the financial responsibility of the client unless otherwise specified by the insurance plan.

Sometimes it's obvious when the client has reached maximum healing: the client is pain free and fully functional. Other times, as with chronic pain, it isn't so clear. In such cases, wellness is determined by the client's ability to manage pain and successfully modify activities. The focus isn't on living pain free, but on quality of life: the client's ability to participate in everyday activities. Use these guidelines to determine when treatments are no longer necessary for resolving the client's condition:

- The client can function normally, or functional progress has plateaued.
- The client has no significant symptomatology, or clinical progress has plateaued.
- The client demonstrates self-awareness by identifying situations (e.g., activities, emotions) that exacerbate his condition.
- The client applies self-care techniques to limit exacerbations and to remedy exacerbations when they do occur.

Test your findings by discontinuing care for a predetermined length of time. For example, if after four weeks without treatment a client is sufficiently symptom-free and active, care can be reduced to a monthly or maintenance level of care. Ongoing treatment is warranted if that client experiences an exacerbation or acceleration of the condition in spite of performing his self-care routines.

Most clients who reach maximum improvement for their conditions would benefit from wellness care. Encourage the client to return monthly for wellness care (for a predetermined number of weeks or months) after terminating treatment. During that time, provide care as needed and fine-tune the client's self-care instructions. If the client's health deteriorates without regular care, you have a case to reinstate insurance coverage. If the client administers appropriate self-care and maintains his health status, celebrate his accomplishments and invite him to continue monthly or quarterly wellness sessions, or refer him to someone who specializes in wellness care.

Preferred Provider Status

Insurance carriers contract with healthcare providers in an attempt to limit who provides healthcare services and how much the carrier pays for those services. Insureds enjoy discounts such as reduced co-pays or deductibles that may be waived for receiving healthcare services from preferred providers. Often, insurance networks and insurance carriers can only support a limited number of providers. Set numbers of providers are credentialed for a given area based on the number of insureds that reside in that area. Once the quota is met, the network is closed to new providers.

Only credentialed practitioners are permitted to bill under the preferred provider contract. It is unethical and often illegal for non-credentialed practitioners to bill for services under the license of the credentialed provider.

Fee Schedules

Ethical billing practices include charging reasonable and consistent fees for services provided. It is tempting to charge higher fees to insurance companies because of the time and paperwork required for billing. However, it's unethical and in some cases illegal to charge insurance companies higher rates than clients who don't utilize insurance coverage for your services. This is commonly referred to as payer discrimination.

Unethical billing practices also arise when services are chosen because they cost more than other equally appropriate services, or when a practitioner bills for services that pay higher rates than the services actually performed. This course of action is tempting when insurance fee schedules delineate different fees for different manual techniques, as though one technique is better than another. For example, Healthy-We-Be publishes a fee schedule that charges $15 per 15-minute unit for therapeutic massage, $18 per 15-minute unit for manual therapy, and $21 per 15-minute unit for energetic therapeutic touch. It would be unethical for Healthy-We-Be to bill for four units of energetic therapeutic touch if other techniques were performed. It would also be unethical if they use only energetic techniques when other techniques could be equally or more effective.

The key to an ethical fee schedule is in its application. Be consistent and don't discriminate. Apply the same fee for the same service to everyone, regardless of the type of payer (this doesn't mean that you can't offer a sliding scale). Provide the service that is most appropriate to the client, despite the reimbursement rate for the service.

Timely Documentation

Unethical charting practices occur when weeks, months, or years later the chart is filled in because of a request for charts or because payment has been denied and rebilling requires copies of all treatment notes. Charting should be done in a timely fashion. It is difficult to remember a particular session after several other sessions have blurred the details.

The best time to chart is during or immediately after the session. Everyone has days, however, when the charts pile up and the practitioner doesn't get to them until the next morning. It is stressful but possible to recreate the session 24 hours later. However, few can record a session accurately weeks, months, or years later.

Communication with Referring PCP

As health care is currently structured, a physician or doctor, and possibly a nurse, naturopath, acupuncturist, or chiropractor (depending on the insurance policy and the state regulations), is considered a *Primary Care Provider* (PCP). The PCP is responsible to diagnose the client's problem, orchestrate treatment, and refer to adjunctive therapists.

Communication skills are essential particularly when you aren't the PCP yet are working under the referring PCP's direction, but not her supervision. Provide the referring PCP with clear, complete information so that she can give the client the best possible treatment.

Occasionally, you may find yourself disagreeing with the referring PCP about a client's condition or treatment. Do not express this disagreement to the client. Instead, state your views to the referring PCP calmly, professionally, tactfully, with the supporting evidence you have assembled. If your input isn't considered or if you find that you can't endorse the prescribed treatment, your best choice may be to withdraw from the case. However you choose to handle the situation, remember that the referring PCP is the final authority and that it is unethical to undermine the relationship between the referring PCP and the client. If the client approaches you with complaints about the referring PCP's approach to the treatment plan, support the client in addressing the issues directly with the referring PCP.

Permission to Consult with the Health Care Team

Protocol requires you to request permission from the client to exchange information with the other members of the client's healthcare team. In many states, practitioners don't need the client's consent to speak with referring providers. Nevertheless, it's a good idea to inform the client with whom information will be shared. When providing information to other practitioners, respect the client's confidentiality and limit those conversations to information pertinent to the client's condition. Omit your personal opinions about the client and any gossip or details that don't bear on the case. Refrain from discussing client cases in public where others who aren't bound by confidentiality might overhear sensitive information.

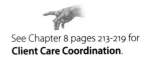

See Chapter 8 pages 213-219 for **Client Care Coordination**.

Conclusion

Running an ethical business requires that you maintain healthy boundaries, operate from deeply held values, engage in personal and professional development, set high standards, be client-centered, and review your business practices regularly. Ethical dilemmas are unavoidable in any business. You can be prepared for them and hopefully avoid many by following the suggestions in this chapter. It is definitely possible to achieve success while running an ethical practice.

10
Support Systems

*"No problem can be solved from the same consciousness that created it.
We must learn to see the world anew."*
—Albert Einstein

Helpers in a Helping Profession

Supervision
- How Supervision Helps Build Your Ethical Practice
- The Role of Clinical Supervision
- Essential Elements of Helpful Supervision
- Boundary-Setting Support
- How to Find a Supervisor

Peer Support Groups
- How to Start and Run a Peer Support Group

Mentoring
- Benefits for Mentors and Mentees
- Types of Mentoring
- Skills, Roles, and Responsibilities
- Setting Parameters
- Finding a Mentor

Mastermind Groups
- How They Work

Coaching

Internships, Externships, and Apprenticeships

Online Discussion Forums

Key Terms

Apprenticeship
Clinical Supervision
Coaching
Externship

Internship
Mastermind Groups
Mentoring
Online Discussion Forums

Peer Support Groups
Supervision

Overwhelming emotional and boundary dilemmas occur as a predictable aspect of the wellness practitioner's life. Practitioners must deal with challenging nuances of client care and interaction, thus self-care is central to maintaining an ethical practice. When a client's issues present themselves in such a way that the practitioner isn't prepared to handle, the practitioner can be overwhelmed, confused, and discouraged about her ability to do her job. Practitioners need a shame-free, trusting relationship with peers, a mentor, or a supervisor to sort out such dilemmas. This relationship protects clients as well as the practitioner. Ethical clinical practice for all somatic practitioners includes self-awareness, self-monitoring, and ongoing review of challenging or difficult cases.

Getting proper support to look at and deal with the everyday occurrences can help your career thrive and progress over many years. Multiple supports are available and often vary in both formality and cost. In this chapter, we highlight supervision, peer groups, mentoring, Mastermind groups, apprenticeships, coaching, and online discussion forums.

▌ Helpers in a Helping Profession

Helping is one of the main reasons why people come to careers in wellness care. The challenge is that for some people, helping others goes hand-in-hand with neglecting themselves. This leads to burnout, loss of clients, and even having to close a business. Understanding the needs that motivate you to help others can assist you in building a successful practice. There is nothing wrong with having needs; the problem is when your needs become the focus of your sessions and the client's needs take the back seat. Becoming aware of your needs and working to get them met outside of the client/practitioner session keeps the focus on the client and preserves the therapeutic relationship.[1]

It is easy to get caught helping others too much and giving of yourself willingly at the expense of your business, health, or your family. Perhaps you work longer than the allotted hour session thinking that the client needs more help and that doing so encourages the client to come in more often. You work after your scheduled hours thinking it's best for the client, when in fact it means that you're missing your children's soccer game or a family holiday.

Finances can be a source of challenges. Common examples of this include: charging lower rates and feeling like you need to be available to everyone no matter what their income; making money be the priority and have clients coming in more often than needed; and feeling resentful of the amount you charge or earn in a job.

Helping can imply that someone is broken and in need of fixing. Schooling often focuses on fixing clients. The idea that you can fix a condition or problem is very empowering and allows helpers to feel important and needed. We all have needs to feel important and needed, but when we get them met through the client/practitioner relationship, we risk creating issues in the therapeutic relationship that should rightly remain focused completely on the client.

How do you help? Why do you help? How can you help?

The following list of questions can be used to discover some of the issues behind helping:

- Do you often feel a need to have an answer for every question that your clients ask about their health and life?
- Do you have a difficult time seeing people in pain and feel that it's your responsibility to make it better or fix it?
- Do you often feel you're the only one who can help your clients and others?
- Do you often see the problems of others more clearly than your own?
- Do you find yourself giving advice when clients don't ask for it?
- Do you find yourself taking on the symptoms of clients and find yourself over-identifying with their pain?
- Do you feel like you always need to be available to your clients, friends, or family?
- Do you often put others needs before your own?
- Do you often find yourself telling clients your personal problems?
- Do you feel you get enough just from giving?
- Do you feel it's always better to give than to receive no matter what the cost?
- Do you feel guilty charging for your services?
- Do you charge lower rates thinking that people can't afford your services; or do you charge what you need to make a living?
- Do you often put off getting care for yourself?
- Do you often feel you don't have the necessary financial resources and enough time to take care of yourself?

More on the **Issues Behind Helping**.

http://www.
massageschoolnotes.com/
how-can-i-help/

Supervision

Supervision creates a setting for self-care, support, and nurturance. It is the right place for practitioners to receive appreciation for their good and useful work. It is a place to get your own needs met outside of the client/practitioner relationship and help you stay focused on your values, thereby creating a stronger framework for your business. Your business decisions are made easier when you understand and look at your own values and beliefs. Supervision assists you in maintaining a values-based ethical practice, reduces the risk of burnout, and helps you deal with burnout you may already be experiencing. The management of boundaries in professional relationships is complex. With increasing attention to boundaries, boundary violations, and professional misconduct in the practice of all healthcare professionals, and particularly in the touch professions, the fundamental importance of clinical supervision is clear.[2]

Supervision plays a critical role in maintaining the standards of the profession by helping to make practitioners more aware. The regulatory boards, licensing, and schools only start the process of being a practitioner. The concept of supervision is quite new for the somatic professions but more is being seen in each discipline. When the body is touched or when the body moves in ways that create more self-awareness, clients' feelings can become intensified, making it imperative that practitioners are skilled in dealing with their own feelings that arise as a result.

The clients who come for care and treatment have wide-ranging vulnerabilities, multiple needs, past relationship troubles, unrealistic hopes, and personal traumas. Practitioners also have these many needs and issues. An important and integral aspect of being a healthcare

> It's the we gotta syndrome: We gotta fix this up right away. We gotta call this person for advice. It's tricky because this impulse may arise from genuine empathy but the form of action is compulsive. Often what is happening is that we gotta get rid of someone's pain because it is hurting us too much.
>
> —Ram Dass,
> *How can I Help You?*

professional includes tolerating and managing feelings that arise in our professional relationships with clients.[3] Exploring your own vulnerabilities and needs helps you to see more clearly when your work is more about you than the client. Our own issues and blind spots can make this awareness difficult. The process of supervision can help us to be more aware of when sessions become more about us than the client.

Practitioners need to be involved enough to feel for and care for clients, yet distant enough to decide objectively on and implement the best course of treatment.[4] Inevitably, feelings toward certain clients affect practitioners by bringing them closer, pushing them away, confusing or irritating them as professionals. Particular clients may challenge their capacity to manage their feelings, expose professional blind spots, or touch on areas of personal vulnerability. This hampers practitioners' efforts to communicate directly and effectively, which impacts their ability to deliver the best care. Discussing these issues in a supervision setting helps to diffuse residual emotions and create balance.

Supervision isn't about having someone tell you what to do. In fact, it's quite the opposite. It is a person or a group of people who really listen to you and help you to feel heard so that you can feel more confident and secure in finding out what is true for you. These sessions focus on the needs of the practitioner. Supervision may also lead to consultation sessions for more specific help in ethical dilemmas, setting boundaries, and creating policies and procedures that support your business.

Supervision can provide a forum for taking a look at the underlying reasons why you want to help others at the cost of your health, time, or money. It can help you to learn how to be of more service to others.

How Supervision Helps Build Your Ethical Practice

Supervision and peer supervision groups can be a vital part of starting and running an ethical practice. Both options help practitioners deal with the many challenges that come up during the course of business. The process of supervision is really a way of getting your own personal and professional needs met so that you can work on developing and preserving the therapeutic relationship that occurs between client and practitioner. By learning more about your own values and needs, you can work to build a framework that supports your values (through boundaries) and learn to get your needs for appreciation and validation met in your own personal life or in the process of supervision.

Supervision also helps you build a vision of what your ideal client looks like and values. Your ideal client is one that makes you feel inspired, rejuvenated, and passionate about what you do. Clients who have the same values as you do can help you in the process of building your business. When clients already appreciate and value your work, they'll readily refer their friends and family members to you. They will come in regularly and won't have to be educated as much about what you do. They will be on time for the sessions and will respect your fees and time.

The less-than-ideal client often challenges your boundaries and may leave you feeling drained and exhausted. Clients who aren't willing to pay your fees, come late to sessions, or don't want to pay for missed appointments are much harder to work with and often receive less than your ideal work when you have to deal with these challenges. Supervision helps you see this picture clearly so that the boundaries you set through your policies and procedures can support you on the path to building your career. Your boundaries should be like the warm blanket that nurtures your business and helps it grow.

" If you take my advice, you will surely solve our problem. If you take my advice but fail to solve your problem, you didn't try hard enough. If you fail to take my advice, I did the best I could. So I am covered. No matter how things come out, I no longer need to worry about you or your vexing problem.

—Parker Palmer

The Role of Clinical Supervision

Clinical supervision has long been the primary professional training model for mental health clinicians[5], and more recently other somatic professionals have begun to recognize and use this forum to train students. Professionals who benefit from this type of supervision include massage and bodywork therapists, acupuncturists, chiropractors, physical therapists, physical therapy assistants, occupational therapists, athletic trainers, and other somatic practitioners. Clinical supervision is a valuable and necessary form of continuing education for all wellness professionals, and it's particularly important for practitioners who perform ongoing body therapy. Les Kertay, PH.D., states,

> If you're interested in doing work that has emotional and spiritual impact on your clients, then the most powerful way of dealing with the questions involved is to utilize ongoing professional supervision. Supervision isn't about being told how to do your job, rather it's a place to process your clients' work and your experiences of being with them.[6]

Clinical supervision can be done on a one-on-one basis or in a peer supervision group. It is often useful to have supervision in a small group of practitioners who are doing the same kind of work. Groups that include people of various disciplines that offer different views broaden the base of learning and create an additional support system for each member. If the practitioner is in a group situation where she can learn from others' experiences, it's possible to master the fundamentals of practice through witnessing others' learning, not relying exclusively upon her own professional trial and error. Hearing the fears and doubts of other practitioners who are feeling challenged by unusual client situations can help practitioners feel less isolated and alone. The people who are listening and providing support are doing as much work as those who are doing the sharing.

In a group setting, clinical supervision undertakes four functions: 1) addressing the relationship issues that arise between clients and practitioners; 2) functioning as a support group for the participants; 3) serving as a forum for didactic instruction on important psychological concepts (such as projection, transference, countertransference); and 4) training the participants in supervisory skills so that they feel confident continuing this helpful type of coaching by themselves at a later date without the supervisor.

> Sometimes our light goes out but is blown into flame by another human being. Each of us owes deepest thanks to those who have rekindled this light.
>
> —Albert Schweitzer

Figure 10.1 Group Clinical Supervision Functions

1. Address client/practitioner relationship issues.
2. Support the participants.
3. Provide psychological concepts instruction.
4. Increase practitioner confidence.

Identifying and understanding intense, sometimes objectionable, feelings in professional relationships is central to the management of professional boundaries. With inadequate preparation for managing intense, often startling, feelings, practitioners run the risk of over-identification, engaging in destructive behavior, or developing restricted practice styles that don't benefit themselves or their clients.[7, 8] Supervisors are well suited to assist practitioners with identification and management of their feelings around these boundary dilemmas. Consultations may assist practitioners in sorting out clinical and interpersonal dilemmas, thereby protecting competent care of the client. It isn't psychological counseling though. There is a fine line between sharing feelings and just being heard, and helping the person deal with the feelings which is the job of a psychologist or counselor.

The clinical supervisor helps the practitioner define his problems and questions. This can be a surprisingly difficult job for both supervisor and practitioner. When a practitioner feels disturbed by something, the task becomes naming that something precisely and figuring out what kind of help is wanted. There is an important distinction between how the practitioner sees the problem and how the supervisor sees it. Rather than offering advice and telling the practitioner what to do, a good supervisor helps the practitioner explore what is happening internally, define where the appropriate boundary is for the practitioner and the client, and determine what action might correct the situation. In general, these techniques, which draw on and validate the practitioner's problem-solving skills, lead to a more effective and empowering resolution.

Clinical supervision provides an opportunity to discuss with a more experienced, psychologically savvy practitioner how to best help a client while promoting increased self-observation and awareness. In a group setting, the supervisor often invites other members to help guide a colleague toward the core issue underlying the problem. Practitioners can increase their tolerance and understanding, and learn how to manage feelings in themselves and their clients through clinical supervision. Supervision is often a nourishing, protective, creative endeavor that greatly benefits the practitioner, the client, and the supervisor.

Essential Elements of Helpful Supervision

While the fundamental role of supervision in clinical practice is generally acknowledged, there is little consensus about the theory and structure of useful supervision.[9, 10] Formal training or curricula for supervisors is nearly nonexistent and there is no one prevailing theory or model of clinical supervision. The concept of supervision in somatic practices is fairly new and unexplored but there is a need developing as more people are becoming practitioners and having to deal with the many situations that arise during the course of a career. Most often, supervisors rely upon imitating the valued aspects of their personal supervisory experiences while trying to avoid the painful or negative aspects. The decision and responsibility of assessing the right fit between practitioner/supervisor, and the usefulness of the supervision, lies with the supervisee. Some clear ideas defining useful supervision have emerged from research,[11, 12] personal experiences, and anecdotal accounts.

1. Useful supervision includes an interpersonal climate of reasonable safety, including an atmosphere of warmth, respect, honesty, and support that allows a trust-based relationship to develop. A collaborative approach with a sense of mutual empowerment and openness to new learning for both parties is valued. Definition and clarity about the supervisory contract including time, fees, issues of confidentiality, evaluation, and learning goals are essential to establish a sense of safety and clear boundaries.

2. Supervision works best when the educational contract is as specific as possible and both parties communicate directly and clearly. The process of exposing and examining professional work and disclosing personal professional experiences commonly evokes feelings of anxiety or vulnerability. This is to be expected. Learning involves feeling like a beginner with a predictable sense of disruption as one transforms previous ways of understanding and integrates new material. These inevitable feelings of vulnerability, and perhaps ineptness, diminish with time and are coupled with a sense of increasing competence and self-confidence. Helpful supervisory experiences encourage the awareness that mistakes are an important part of the learning process. In a successful supervisory relationship, the sense of comfort and self-disclosure deepens across time.

3. Supervisory approaches that foster the personal and professional development of the individual practitioner are preferable. Supervisors who encourage practitioners to creatively answer their own questions facilitate the development of a competent professional. Supervisors who communicate that they believe they ultimately know the

best ways to understand and manage the clinical situation leave supervisees feeling incompetent, dependent, and unprepared for the complexities of client care.

Boundary-Setting Support

Consider the following examples illustrating boundary dilemmas practitioners have encountered and discussed in supervision. These scenarios depict the internal, interpersonal, and clinical process of formulating the dilemma and constructing useful boundaries through supervision.

Threatening or Dangerous Clients

In general, practitioners are advised to listen to their own anxiety as a reliable signal that a problem or client relationship deserves further attention and work. When possible, it's useful to identify the source of the anxiety. When a client presents threatening behaviors, the practitioner needs to assess whether the client presents a real, physical threat to the practitioner or the staff by evaluating the client's capacity for violence. Many somatic practitioners may not be competent or capable of assessing a client's dangerousness. A consultation with a supervisor or mental health professional may be necessary and indicated to assess a client under these circumstances, particularly if the client doesn't respond to verbal limits.

> There is only one corner of the universe you can be certain of improving, and that's your own self.
>
> —Aldous Huxley

An acupuncturist found herself feeling frightened and disgusted by a client, a 40-year-old divorced man who was a recovering alcoholic with a history of impulsive, aggressive behavior. Although he had always been in control in her presence at the clinic, the acupuncturist overheard the patient verbally abusing someone on the support staff. The acupuncturist wished to transfer the care of this patient to an associate in the clinic to avoid her anxiety and sense of intimidation. She understood that this patient had great difficulty with change and wondered if her wish to transfer his care was ethical and necessary. Did he present a danger to her and could she more effectively manage her anxiety and relationship with this patient?

With clinical supervision the acupuncturist became aware of her nearly phobic dread of this patient and explored what specifically frightened her about this man's behavior. Did this patient remind her of someone in her life? Did she have difficulty being appropriately assertive? While she understood it was her responsibility to set limits, she confirmed she was uncomfortable with confrontation and had little experience as a professional exercising her authority when it involved conflict. She realized her conflict-avoidance stance was a lifelong pattern in personal relationships and this patient might be triggering a personal set of experiences. The supervisor highlighted the practitioner's professional objective to become more comfortable with asserting herself in conflict situations, emphasizing the importance of these professional skills and responsibilities.

Through the process of supervision, the acupuncturist realized that several options were available to her. As a practitioner, it was her responsibility to educate and protect patients and staff, and seek mental health consultations if necessary around safety issues. To ensure competent and safe care of her patients and support staff, she needed to deal with her anxiety and difficulty with professional self-assertion through supervision. If she were unable to master her anxiety and assume professional authority with this man, despite specialized assistance and ongoing supervision, she might not treat this patient safely. If her sense of anxiety and terror with this man's anger continued to interfere with or compromise her clinical judgment, then she would have an ethical responsibility to refer his care to a colleague. This is the least desirable alternative, to be employed only after seeking assistance and trying to work with the patient and the professional issues that were raised for the practitioner.

Through direct questioning, modeling and explanation, the supervisor demonstrated how professionals might assert themselves by setting clear boundaries and establishing a safe environment for both practitioner and patient. With technical and emotional support, the acupuncturist decided she would try this approach and discussed with the client his inappropriate and scary behavior. While the client expressed his desire to air a grievance, he had little awareness of how frightening his behavior was to staff. He reassured her that despite his loud bark he wouldn't hurt anyone. Furthermore, he expressed that he had a low tolerance for the frustration that he felt while waiting for appointments that were even a little late in starting. The practitioner suggested that, in the future, he could keep his office waiting time to a minimum by calling the office ahead to see if she was on time or running behind. The patient liked that suggestion and also agreed to consider a referral to a mental health professional.

Points to Ponder

How might a practitioner gather more information to shed light on a client's behavior in a situation like this one? Would it be ethical for the practitioner to refer out to another practitioner if an amicable arrangement hadn't been made with the client?

A practitioner might also review a client's file and speak to the client to shed light on the client's behavior. Does the client have a history of violence and impulsive behavior? Against whom? Under what circumstances? How recently? Does the client currently use alcohol or drugs? Does the client have a serious mental illness? Is the client verbally threatening violence or behaving in an angry and threatening manner? All of these items, and more, can be used to determine the most appropriate and safest actions to take when dealing with a threatening or dangerous client.

Requests for Special Concessions

Deviations from usual practice (as demonstrated in the following example) may be a warning signal to practitioners.

A male bodywork therapist had a VIP client, a nationally known cardiac surgeon, who had injured his foot while on vacation and was facing many months of rehabilitation. The surgeon didn't want to travel to receive treatments and requested that the therapist make house calls. The therapist obliged, though he didn't usually make house calls, as he felt the client was a very important and busy man. However, the therapist found himself becoming annoyed as the surgeon regularly kept him waiting, causing him to fall behind in his scheduled office appointments. During the treatment sessions, the surgeon peppered the therapist with intrusive personal questions. The therapist struggled to respond in a professional and cordial manner while protecting his privacy. After the sixth session, the surgeon thanked him profusely for all his fine work and offered to the therapist and the therapist's family to stay in his elegant vacation home.

In supervision, the therapist identified the multiple ways in which his treatment of this client was exceptional and deviated from customary practice. He saw that treating this man at home under these circumstances was probably not in his best interest. With discussion, he became aware that deeply personal feelings and motives had shaped his clinical decision-making. His desire to be admired by an important man clouded his professional judgment. Envious of the surgeon's wealth and position, he wanted to share in the benefits of the wealth and status. This contributed to the therapist abandoning his professional standards and compromised the boundaries of his professional relationship with him. Additionally, he was angry with himself for his personal over-involvement, and angry with the client for the special treatment requests that he handled inappropriately.

The therapist became aware of how he had agreed to the surgeon's inappropriate behavior (keeping him waiting, taking calls during the treatment) to avoid disappointing him or provoking his disapproval. He didn't fear the surgeon's anger or any possibility of violence, but was afraid of his disapproval. The therapist's envy, unacknowledged longings, and wish to win the client's approval contributed to his faulty decision-making. The supervisor modeled more appropriate responses to intrusive questions, such as, "I'm not comfortable answering personal questions. Let's concentrate on getting your foot back into working order." The therapist's wish to have his client's approval, admiration, and material possessions was identified as an area for ongoing self-monitoring. The therapist focused his supervision sessions on self-monitoring and professional boundaries.

The therapist decided to decline the use of his client's vacation home. Thanking the client for the offer, he explained that he thought it was best to be clear about the professional nature of their relationship. He informed the surgeon that home visits and the late start of sessions didn't work in terms of his schedule and proposed that the surgeon receive treatments at the therapist's office. The client acknowledged the therapist's feedback, and together they came up with appropriate changes to their working agreement.

Point to Ponder

At what other possible points throughout the client/therapist relationship could the practitioner have asserted his boundaries? Is there a way the practitioner could have continued making house calls while maintaining boundaries at the same time?

If the therapist had noticed his personal involvement earlier, he might have declined the client's invitation to treat him at home, saying he didn't make house calls, instead recommending that he come to the office. In such instances, the client may resist and try to convince the therapist to make an exception to his normal practice. If that should occur, the therapist may share his thinking and rationale with the client, offering what he believes is the best care. Setting such a limit, of course, involves the possibility that the client will go elsewhere for treatment.

After identifying such deviations, it's always useful for practitioners to review the treatment rationale and decision-making process by posing the following questions. Is this the best course of action? What is gained and what is lost by this treatment approach or intervention? Is this a one-time occurrence or an ongoing process? What review process is in place to evaluate the usefulness of this unusual practice? What are the risks to the client, the practitioner, the treatment? Is this practice negotiated openly or does the practitioner feel coerced?[13]

Needy Clients

Clients routinely bring emotional personal dilemmas into the professional relationship, such as a low frustration tolerance, profound loneliness, and longings to be special to someone. Healthcare professionals must be equipped to manage the wide range of client behaviors and requests for treatment that may not be in the client's or the practitioner's best interest.[14] Clinical supervision is a valuable resource for assessing and monitoring the relationship aspects of care giving.

A 30-year-old male physical therapist had a 55-year-old unhappily married woman as a patient. She had been seeking frequent contact with him for numerous minor physical complaints. During office visits, the patient repeatedly requested to be physically examined beyond what might be necessary to evaluate her complaints. In addition, she came to the examination wearing bright red and black lace underwear.

Frightened and disgusted by his client's provocative sexual behavior, the therapist felt unsure how to address the issue.

With clinical supervision, the therapist identified his feelings of embarrassment and his anxiety about being vulnerable to an accusation of professional misconduct. The supervisor discussed the importance of clarifying the appropriate boundaries of the therapist/client relationship. Through discussion of the case, the physical therapist hypothesized his patient's seductive behavior to be an attempt to secure his emotional and physical attention or to repeat a history of sexual exploitation. He surmised that without seductive behavior and revealing attire, his patient might believe she wasn't worthy of his care. This understanding that his patient's behavior might be an attempt to express nonsexual needs in a sexualized manner, or that his patient confused care-taking with sexuality, helped the therapist to regain a compassionate, caring, protective stance with her.

The physical therapist decided to inform his patient that he would schedule monthly visits to discuss her status. Between these visits, if needed, he proposed to set her up with appointments with a physical therapy assistant. He explained that physical examinations would be deferred unless clearly necessary; instead, the visit would focus on her home therapy exercise program. The physical therapist chose not to comment directly upon his patient's clothing as this would likely shame and humiliate her. By identifying his patient's unsettling behavior and his own accompanying feelings through the supervisory process, the therapist formulated an approach that was both compassionate and protective of the patient, her care, and himself.

Points to Ponder

Did the practitioner handle this client appropriately and with care? How can you tell when a client is being provocative or needy? Is there a way to deal with these types of situations before the client's behavior becomes inappropriate?

Sometimes clients are undeterred in pursuit of personal relationships with healthcare practitioners or are stuck in repeating, maladaptive, interpersonal dramas with their care providers. Clients are responsible for their behavior and may require professional assistance to understand the limits of the professional relationship and what's acceptable behavior. Professionals may have to set limits assertively in a non-punitive manner, and document repetitive, inappropriate behavior, or sexual advances in the client's record. Open, direct communication with clients, consultation from colleagues, and documentation of the problem behavior and subsequent treatment approach protect the practitioner against litigation.

Personal or Sexual Advances

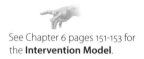

See Chapter 6 pages 151-153 for the **Intervention Model**.

Clients who have been sexually victimized as children may eroticize the professional relationship as they often confuse sexual contact with caretaking.[15] Practitioners may, on occasion, be confronted with requests for sexual favors, sexualized verbal conduct, and unwelcome overt sexual advances. While professionals may experience a range of intense feelings, including annoyance or anxiety about such overtures from clients, it's their responsibility to re-establish professional boundaries and set safe limits. Often, this involves the use of professional authority to educate the client about appropriate behavior and the limits of their relationship.[16]

After one month of weekly treatments with a female chiropractor, a male patient began asking the practitioner to go to lunch with him. The chiropractor wished to be sensitive to her patient's feelings and to educate him concerning her view of the professional relationship. She responded, "Thank you for the offer. I don't see patients outside the office. It is my policy not to mix professional and personal relationships." Despite her clear communication about the limits of the professional relationship, the patient persisted in asking her to lunch. The chiropractor felt a need to further educate her patient about his behavior and the professional relationship. She said, "I want you to stop asking me to go out to lunch. It concerns me that you don't seem to understand that our relationship is professionally based and won't expand outside the office. Your repeated requests for social contact distract from the professional care you deserve for your pain. If this continues, I may not feel comfortable treating you and will refer you to another practitioner."

Feeling upset and confused by his persistence; the chiropractor brought the situation to her supervision group. Through discussion, she realized just how unsettling these overtures had been to her and how it affected her care of this man. The supervision group helped her sort through her feelings and needs while exploring many options. With the group's consultation, she experienced herself as once again in charge and developed clarity concerning a plan of action. Most of all, it was enormously comforting not to manage this challenging situation on her own.

To the chiropractor's surprise, the patient didn't return for several weeks. She surmised that despite her best effort to be sensitive to his feelings while setting professional boundaries, that her patient might have felt injured, angry, or humiliated. Additionally, she suspected that her patient sensed her resolve and unequivocal stance about his overtures and that she would indeed refer him to another practitioner. When her patient returned for an appointment several weeks later, he commented, "I hope you're not angry with me. I like you. I know your work is effective and don't want to start over with a new chiropractor." The chiropractor responded, "I know you like me and I would be happy to continue to treat you. I'm hopeful the treatments will continue to diminish your pain. It is important that we have an understanding about how we're going to work together including the limits of our relationship."

After this conversation, the chiropractor felt some relief as her patient seemed to have realigned himself and she had a strong sense that he didn't want to jeopardize or lose their professional relationship. While she imagined her patient would consciously try to behave differently, she wondered if he might have romantic or sexual feelings toward her. As she reflected on this possibility, she experienced a heightened sense of responsibility to behave in a manner that wouldn't further stimulate romantic or sexual feelings and fantasies. She was certain that she would use her supervision group to continue monitoring the unfolding of the professional relationship and manage her feelings.

Points to Ponder

Should the chiropractor continue to treat the patient while still worrying that he might be having romantic thoughts or sexual feelings? Are the limits set by the chiropractor in this case sufficient to maintain the professional relationship? Are they too strict?

When a practitioner senses or has confirmation of romantic or sexual feelings from a client, scrupulous attention to professional boundaries is crucial. If a practitioner feels attracted to a client, careful self-monitoring of interactions and the safeguarding of boundaries is in order. Be alert, sensitive, and mindful of interactions with this client. By overly social or flirtatious conduct, a practitioner may signal that the professional boundaries aren't secure or that the practitioner is personally or sexually interested in the client.[7] Supervision is usually recommended when sexual issues are involved.

> Figure 10.2   Deciding When to Consult with a Supervisor
>
> - Does the care of this client deviate from the usual professional standards of care for this client's problem?
> - Are you aware of strong feelings about this client?
> - Are there behavioral indicators of favored or disfavored treatment status?
> - Are you confused or conflicted about the relationship aspects of this client's care?
> - Are you uncertain concerning the differentiation between professional and personal feelings, and where to construct the professional boundary?
> - Are you attracted to the client?
> - Is the client attracted to you?

How to Find a Supervisor

Supervision Sources

National Association of Social Workers (NASW)
http://www.naswdc.org/

American Psychiatric Association (APA)
http://www.psych.org/

American Psychological Association
http://www.apa.org/

American Nurses Association
http://www.nursingworld.org/

Finding a supervisor is often not an easy task, particularly in small, out of the way places where there are few therapists familiar with somatic practices. It is also not well recognized yet in many somatic professions, so there aren't many supervisors available. In some disciplines, you may find people who have been getting regular supervision sessions for over five years who may provide supervision sessions or lead peer groups. Psychotherapy disciplines have the longest tradition of providing clinical supervision and thus psychotherapists are excellent sources. Psychiatrists, nurses, social workers, psychologists, and counselors are likely to be experienced supervisors. Personal recommendations by a colleague or a valued teacher are also fine ways to secure names of potential supervisors. If a referral by a colleague or instructor is difficult to obtain, it's possible to contact state or national professional organizations to obtain names of professionals in good standing.

Interview Potential Supervisors

Many supervisors have websites where you can get a feel for their philosophy and what they're like. They may also have some articles and resources for you to review to get a first impression of who they are and what they do. Traditionally, supervision is done in person, but now you can hire supervisors located in other cities and states using tools like Skype and Google Hangouts to have face-to-face conversations with a potential supervisor.

You can start with an initial contact either by phone or email or video call to assess if the supervisor has time, is affordable, and sounds like a potential match. Then arrange a more formal interview or a first session. Some supervisors have questionnaires on their website that are sent to you when you're interviewing to help the supervisor also decide if you're a good match for what they do. During the face-to-face interview with the prospective supervisor you have an opportunity to experience how it feels to sit and speak with this person and gain an impression of how she thinks and works. Prepare questions in advance that you would like answered in this meeting such as the following:

- What has been your experience as a supervisor? How long? For what disciplines?
- Have you ever worked with, or supervised [name your discipline]?
- How do you describe your work as a supervisor?
- What is your fee for supervision? How long is the session?
- Are my discussions with you confidential? What are the limits, if any, of confidentiality?
- Can you give me the names of a few individuals you have supervised who would be willing to speak about their experiences?

- I would like to learn more about or want help with [list your professional or developmental concerns]. Is this something you can help me with?

These guidelines are designed to help you secure the best kind of supervisory assistance for your particular situation. If for any reason, even if it's difficult to articulate, you feel anxious, uncomfortable, or threatened in the initial meeting with the prospective supervisor, trust your intuition and look elsewhere. Seriously consider any visceral discomfort and reservations. Remember, there are other competent supervisors and you'll find one that is a better match.

Unhelpful Supervision

While one always hopes that supervisory experiences are helpful and productive, we know from research and anecdotal accounts that they can be positive or negative. Supervisors are professional role models and teachers. When they set positive examples and provide constructive guidance, and their supervisees take those lessons to heart, the effect on client care can be overwhelmingly positive. However, when supervisors evoke guilt or shame, pressure the supervisee to agree with their own personal opinions or preferences, or exploit the supervisee's vulnerability in any other way, both the supervisee and client care may suffer significant harm.

Elements of negative supervisory relationships include those that evoke intense negative feelings and are burdened with disrespect and lack of honest self-disclosure.[18, 19] Supervisors who abandon the role of teacher and treat the supervisees as clients aren't helpful. Supervisees who find themselves in a supervisory relationship characterized by these negative traits should seek other supervision. Remember, supervision should above all be helpful and enhance a sense of professional confidence, competence, and mastery. It should also be very satisfying.

Finding a Supervisor

- Recall an instance when talking to an individual or a small group was helpful in solving a problem.
- What qualities and values would you look for in a supervisor?
- Identify several situations or issues that you have experienced that you might want to take to a supervisor.

Peer Support Groups

A peer support group is a group of people in a similar career, who get together on a regular basis or a one-time situation to provide support in the form of sharing the struggles, challenges, and successes that arise on a regular basis. The leadership roles are rotated among the members or one leader can organize the group. The group often hires a consultant to work with them on a specific topic.

Peer support groups have easily identifiable advantages and some potential disadvantages. The strengths, limitations, and success of peer groups rest with the composition of the individual members and the clarity of the peer group contract. Members must agree upon the time, location, and frequency of meetings. The organizational structure and goals of the meeting and limits of confidentiality need to be defined and affirmed. Vague, ambiguous, overly ambitious, or ambivalent goals and structure often lead to difficulties. As with individual or clinical group supervision, an interpersonal atmosphere of reasonable safety including respect, warmth, honesty, and a collaborative openness is critical.

Competitiveness, criticism, inconsistency of members, absence of support and warmth all diminish the effectiveness of the group and the pleasure for the members. Potential

> There are high spots in all of our lives, and most of them come about through encouragement from someone else.
>
> —George Adams

disadvantages of peer group supervision include the varying commitment and inconsistency of attendance of members.

Peer support groups decrease professional isolation, increase professional support and networking, normalize the stress and strain of professional life, and offer multiple perspectives on any concern or problem. Intellectually stimulating and fun, peer support groups have the added benefit of being free (or mostly free) of charge.

How to Start and Run a Peer Support Group

Peer support groups can be formal or informal. The first step is for the group to decide on the format, frequency, and goals. This usually takes place in the first few meetings. Meetings can have a regular schedule or be held on an as-needed basis. An informal group usually gets together to talk and see what transpires. In this situation, there is no leader or goal to the group. A caution about informal meetings is that they may end up being venting sessions which may not be productive for the group. Just getting together regularly can be helpful to members of the group to reduce isolation and build connections with others in the same field. A more formal approach requires that some ground rules are set up for sharing and for getting support.

**Figure 10.3 Steps to a Productive Supervision Meeting
(Avoiding a two hour gripe session!)**

- Start with a Round Robin sharing: Each person is allotted a maximum of one minute to summarize a situation. No solutions get offered.
- Group picks a Case Presenter: There is usually one that stands out from the crowd. If not, someone can volunteer or select someone.
- Assign roles: Have a Moderator to monitor the time and tone of consultation, a Scribe to record solutions for the case presenter, and Consultants who initially provide feedback to the presenter and solutions, if asked for.
- Case Presentation: Present a case describing the details but omit or change pertinent information that may identify the client. Consultants and Moderator actively listen and provide feedback that they have heard and understand what has been presented. No solutions.
- Moderator (or Consultant) asks Case Presenter to formulate a key question for the group regarding the situation, specifically in terms of what type of help is needed.
- Case Presenter makes a request: The request can range from just being heard and supported, or asking for help with a solution. There are various methods for consulting, such as brainstorming, role playing, sounding board/gut reaction, best advice, or tip of the day.
- Consultation: Consultants share ideas or information based on the request of the Case Presenter. Scribe takes notes so the Case Presenter can concentrate on what is being offered.
- Conclusion: Case Presenter states which ideas were helpful, reports which of the suggestions were valuable, and expresses gratitude to the group.

by Dari Lewis http://www.anandamassagetraining.com/

A brief start-up consultation with a clinical supervisor or group specialist is helpful to define and establish the contract and framework for successful peer support group supervision. Many peer groups opt to have a clinical supervisor moderate their meetings on a regular schedule, such as quarterly or twice a year. This supervisor might also be appropriate to meet with individually when additional support is desired.

How to Get Participants

Getting people to commit to meeting regularly is often the challenge. A team leader can have the role of screening participants or it can be handled by the group. Meeting regularly with the same people helps increase the depth of sharing. When members don't show up, it can disrupt the group just as much as when someone arrives late for a meeting.

Many online tools exist for organizing a group, such as Facebook Groups, Meeetup, and LinkedIn. These online tools have event scheduling features that allow members to find meetings that fit their schedules and find local meetings. They offer RSVP features that also track members' attendance as well as providing a way to keep in touch in between meetings. These systems can also help get new members with the easy-to-use features they have for connecting people. Also, your professional associations and local schools might be good sources for participants.

Figure 10.4 Peer Support Group Success Tips

- Create a regular day, time, and location to keep things consistent.
- Create a privacy policy and confidentiality policy. What happens in a peer group stays in a peer group.
- Decide how formal or informal you want the group to be.
- Decide on whether or not the discussions are limited to one area or what the goal of the group is. Is it for talking about client issues or are issues such as business or marketing allowed?
- Start each group with short introductions and have each participant ask for how much time they would like to take in the meeting. If everyone wants time and there isn't enough time, a method for choosing who gets to speak has to be determined by the group. Often, when one person speaks, others have many of the same issues. Usually, the people who are just listening learn as much or even more than the person speaking.
- Set goals for each meeting. It can be to talk about ethical dilemmas or get help with techniques or get business and marketing support. It is about what the group needs at the time.

 ### Set Up a Support Group

- Set up guidelines for developing and running your ideal peer support group.
- Brainstorm topics for discussion in peer support group.
- Develop a series of questions you would ask a participant in a peer support group who is presenting an issue.
- Identify any areas or issues that you might be reluctant to discuss in a support group environment.
- List the advantages and disadvantages of peer support groups over clinical supervision.

Mentoring

A business or professional mentor is an individual, usually older, always more experienced, who helps and guides another individual's career development. Mentoring is a structured or informal one-on-one relationship that focuses on the needs of the mentee (person being mentored). The goal of mentoring is to foster caring and supportive relationships that encourage individuals to develop to their fullest potential. It can include learning, networking, and sharing of information and experiences. Mentors serve as role models for other practitioners. Mentoring usually doesn't involve a financial gain for the mentor. Mentors can be in the same field or in a field that is closely related. For instance, if you need to get more business experience find a business mentor. If you need help understanding bookkeeping or taxes, find a mentor with an accounting background. You need not limit yourself to one mentor.

Benefits for Mentors and Mentees

The benefits of finding the right mentor are many. A good mentor can be an invaluable career asset and greatly enhance your potential for success. One of the most valuable things a mentor can do is to help you take an honest look at yourself and identify areas where work is needed to achieve your goals.

People become mentors as a way of giving back to their community and to society at large. They may also do it to develop their skills as a teacher, manager, or consultant. An effective mentoring relationship also works in both directions. Mentors often build their own self-confidence by mentoring another person through the process of building a business. It is rewarding and gratifying to share experience and skills. Being a role model for others also helps your own personal and professional growth, particularly sharpening your leadership skills and communication skills. Listening is a major part of being a mentor. It is also an opportunity to be a part of the future of your profession.

For mentees, it can help to increase their chances of success, enhance self-confidence in their skills and knowledge, and build skills in business and managing ethical concerns.

> ### Figure 10.5   Mentoring Benefits
>
> - Sharpen communication skills
> - Increase self-confidence
> - Develop professional skills
> - Manage ethical concerns
> - Give and receive objective feedback
> - Improve overall success
> - Increase career satisfaction
> - Have an ally
> - Cultivate lasting friendships
> - Develop leadership skills
> - Be a role model
> - Give back to the community

Types of Mentoring

The two main types of mentoring are informal and formal. An informal mentoring relationship starts on its own. This occurs when you approach someone who you know is a leader or has the skills and training where you need help and you ask her to be your mentor. It can also happen in instances when you're receiving the type of work that you do and ask that practitioner to share hands-on techniques or business ideas with you.

Formal mentoring relationships are those that occur when they're assigned by a company, school, or association to help the mentee in a specific area in which the mentee needs help.

Skills, Roles, and Responsibilities

A mentor can have many roles and responsibilities such as being a teacher, a guide, a motivator, a coach, an advisor, or a door-opener for the mentee.

As a teacher, the mentor may need to help mentees with the basic skills they need in doing their job or in their area of expertise. It is important that potential mentors take time to analyze their skills and teaching abilities to see what exactly they can pass on to mentees. A good teacher works with mentees to discover where they are and where they need help instead of just putting out information and expecting it to be absorbed.

The basic root of the word education is from *educere:* to lead forth or draw out.

As a guide, the mentor helps to navigate the various career paths and options and works with mentees on things like politics at work, challenges in running a business, and working as a professional. At times, the mentor needs to motivate mentees and help them through difficult times or challenges. It could be helping them to complete a difficult project that has stalled or to pursue a higher goal in their career. A mentor can do that by providing encouragement.

As a coach, the mentor may be called upon to give constructive feedback to the mentees that may also be difficult topics to address. The mentor may need to give direct feedback regarding observations or experiences of the mentees' attitudes, behaviors, or treatment techniques.

As an adviser, the mentor helps mentees set specific goals for their career and for their immediate projects, and supports them to stay on track. Goals need to have a reasonable time frame for completion, so the mentees can experience success and build self-confidence.

A mentor's professional connections may also serve to open doors for the mentees and connect them to the right people that can help with their career, job searches, and in building a support system.

Mentees are people who are highly motivated to learn and achieve goals. They are passionate about what they're doing and will do anything to achieve their dreams, which is why they were probably seeking mentoring in the first place! They are open to constructive criticism and willing to look at themselves and make the necessary changes. They are usually risk takers or willing to learn to take risks with the help and guidance of a mentor.

Mentees provide the benchmarks to measure the success of the mentoring relationship. They determine the amount of help and guidance that is needed. Successful mentees apply what they learn and ask when they need more information or help.

Setting Parameters

The mentoring relationship also requires that parameters be set for the relationship to work best. Often, the most challenging element is the time commitment required to suit both parties: when to meet; where to meet; and how often to meet. Setting mentoring parameters provides an excellent opportunity to develop boundaries and learn about enforcing boundaries. It is important to respect each other's time and needs. Setting realistic goals keeps the relationship on track. It is vital to choose a mentor/mentee with compatible philosophies and needs. Mentors need to adjust their approaches to meet mentees' levels. For instance, a practitioner who is just starting out most likely needs more general assistance than a seasoned practitioner, while seasoned practitioners may need support with in-depth issues. The correct match and clear boundaries create a more effective mentoring relationship that allows the mentee to thrive without becoming too dependent on the mentor. Be aware of these issues as the relationship develops, particularly if it transitions into more of a friendship or if the mentee depends too heavily on the mentor.

Like coals in a fireplace, we keep our sense of character warm by contact with each other. Set any one of us alone on the moral hearth, and we'll pretty quickly turn to a cold dark cinder.

—Rushworth M. Kidder

Finding a Mentor

AMTA Mentoring Program Guidelines

http://www.amtamassage.org/
mentor/Mentoring-Program-
Overview.html

Sometimes a mentor can be found through a professional or trade organization. Also contact your *alma mater* to find out if it has a mentoring program in place. In most instances, the best place to look for a mentor is right in front of you, perhaps someone from work or in your professional circle whom you admire and respect. You might also know someone who doesn't do exactly the same type of work as you but is an expert in the same field. These are the types of individuals to approach first to ask if they would consider mentoring you.

Figure 10.6   Tips for a Successful Business Mentorship

- The mentor must possess a high level of expertise in the area(s) in which she offers advice or training.
- The mentee must be open to receiving feedback.
- Both parties must have the time to commit to this process.
- Determine the specific goals of the relationship and set a timeline for meeting them.
- Create an agreement about what is expected from each party during the mentoring process.
- Regularly check in with each other to see if the goals are being met and the relationship is still mutually beneficial.

Find Your Own Mentor

- Identify the types of support you would like from a mentor.
- Create a set of questions to ask when interviewing a potential mentor.
- List names of potential mentors.
- Describe several situations in which you might terminate using a particular mentor.

▌ Mastermind Groups

Joining a Mastermind group is a good way to strengthen your support system and widen your circle of professional acquaintances. Being involved in a Mastermind group is akin to having a volunteer Board of Directors that gives you guidance, support, and shares their proven success strategies. The concept of Mastermind groups was coined by Napoleon Hill in his book *Think & Grow Rich*. Hill defines Mastermind groups as the coordination of knowledge and effort in a spirit of harmony between two or more people for the attainment of a definite purpose.[20] Members of Mastermind groups serve as a confidential sounding board. They listen to business concerns and ideas are shared, analyzed, and honed. The strength of this type of group is that the members are committed to supporting each other. This synergy fosters amazing creativity and results.

How They Work

Mastermind groups usually consist of six to eight people, and no more than ten. The members are professionals with varied backgrounds, experience, and areas of expertise, or they can be from the same profession. They meet on a regular basis (weekly, monthly, or quarterly) to brainstorm with each other, give and receive feedback, bestow their secrets for success, set goals, celebrate their successes, and share their challenges. It is also a way to keep you on track and accountable with setting goals and completing them. As an added benefit, members often provide business leads and client referrals. You can really create a Mastermind group for any project or goal.

A Mastermind group can be set up so that responsibilities are shared by all members, or that one person leads all the time and even charges for the sessions. That is usually done by a person with more experience and who is willing to take on a leadership role. You can also have a Mastermind group where each person takes a turn at hosting a meeting. The host sets the agenda, coordinates schedules, handles the logistics (e.g., room set-up, refreshments), and facilitates the meeting.

If you're unable to find an opening in an existing group, you can create your own Mastermind group. You can use online video-conferencing tools (that are usually free) to meet with people when they're located in different areas or want to save the time of meeting in person.

▍ Coaching

The International Coach Federation (ICF), which claims to be the largest coaching credentialing and support organization in the world, defines coaching as "partnering with clients in a thought-provoking and creative process that inspires them to maximize their personal and professional potential."[21] The ICF goes on to describe a coach's responsibility as:

- Discover, clarify, and align with what the client wants to achieve.
- Encourage client self-discovery.
- Elicit client-generated solutions and strategies.
- Hold the client responsible and accountable.

Coaching is becoming more popular in many disciplines. A professional coach is similar to an athletic coach; someone who tells you what to do and how to do it, yet they're also much more than that. The main focus in coaching is to help people set goals and accomplish them. Appropriate coaching can increase productivity, time management skills, self-confidence, communication skills, team work, and improve the balance between work and personal life.

It is important to point out that coaching isn't counseling or therapy, which deals more with the emotional side of life and healing from painful experiences. Coaches help clients to set goals, follow through on commitments, and evaluate measurable outcomes related to personal or professional successes.

There are many different types of coaches to choose from. Life coaches can help you to achieve a successful balance between your personal and work lives. Career coaches can help you in deciding things about careers. Business coaches can help with starting and growing your practice from the basics (e.g., directing you how to get the right licensing), to the development and implementation of a business plan. Financial coaches can help you with your money issues and advise you how to set up your books and accounting systems. Leadership coaches can help you learn and practice the skills necessary to grow your business by adding employees, as well as become a leader in your profession and professional organizations.

International Coach Federation

http://www.coachfederation.org/

Internships, Externships, and Apprenticeships

Another option that is similar to mentoring and can ultimately lead into a true mentoring relationship is to intern or apprentice with a highly-regarded practitioner. These programs are systems of training practitioners in a structured competency-based set of skills. They usually accept applicants, and teach them how to work in a live setting. Internships are usually short-term, whereas apprenticeships can last up to five years or even longer. Interns often work for free and sometimes pay the trainer a modest fee. Apprentices are usually paid, with their salary increasing as they complete parts of the program. Most of these programs offer flexible arrangements to accommodate the individual's learning needs.

Many schools are integrating externship programs into their curricula. Externships are learning programs, similar to internships, offered by educational institutions to give students short practical experiences in their field of study. They are generally shorter than internships and last for approximately a few weeks to several months. Externs are closely supervised by practitioners who allow the externs to shadow them through their daily routines. This experience prepares students to transition from student to practitioner by allowing students to get a sense of the true workings of a practice. It also allows students to apply their knowledge in a real life setting, and gives them the opportunity to observe and ask questions.

Even when training programs include an externship piece, many beginning practitioners feel they need additional support after completing their training programs. Internship and apprenticeship programs are a great way to learn more of the "hands-on" portion of the training and to apply the theory and skills to actual real-life situations. More and more new practitioners are seeking out seasoned professionals to mentor and coach them from the beginning, but a structured internship or apprenticeship program can be more effective. Finding a clinic or skilled practitioner willing to administer one of these programs for continued training and support can make the difference to a beginning practitioner building the confidence it takes to become a skilled practitioner herself.

Online Discussion Forums

See Chapter 9 pages 257-262 for **Ethical Social Media Tips**.

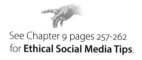

Online forums

http://www.facebook.com

http://www.linkedin.com

http://www. massageprofessionals.com

Online discussion forums are also a place where you can get more help. Facebook, LinkedIn, and other profession-specific forums offer more immediate help for specific situations. You can ask and answer questions on these sites.

One of the problems with these discussion groups is that statements can easily be taken out of context, and people can take seemingly impersonal statements personally. Caution is advised when posting online. With social media and public forums, you risk exposing yourself and your clients. People are losing jobs and insurance claims are being denied because of postings on various online forums and discussion groups. If you choose this route, make sure your privacy settings are optimal. Also, be sure to protect client privacy and confidentiality at all times.

Planning Your Perfect Support System

- Identify the key elements of helpful support systems.
- Create a detailed plan for developing your support system (supervisor, peer group, mentor, Mastermind group, coach, online discussion forum, or other support).

Conclusion

Supervision, peer groups, mentoring, Mastermind groups, coaching, internships, externships, apprenticeship programs, and online discussion forums are great options to get the support that you need in developing your career. What you get out of them is often about what you put into them. Technology has brought the world closer and the many formats, such as video conferencing, online forums, and social media tools, make it easier to get the support that you need. Yet, with all of these easily available tools for success, many professionals don't use them and therefore struggle. The more support you get in one or all of these venues, the better your chances of success—financially, mentally, emotionally, and spiritually.

11
Working
with Trauma Survivors

"What the mind forgets the body remembers in the form of fear, pain or physical illness."
—Louis Cozolino, Ph.D.

Understanding Trauma and Abuse
- The Potential for Harm from Uninformed Treatment
- The Core of Trauma and Abuse
- Types of Sexual Abuse
- Types of Physical Abuse
- Types of Emotional Abuse
- The Three Stages of Recovery
- Posttraumatic Stress Disorder
- Body Memories and Flashbacks

Benefits of Touch Therapy for Survivors
- Establishing a Place of Safety
- Rebuilding Boundaries
- Experiencing the Pleasure of Non-Sexual Touch
- Reintegrating Body Memories
- Enhancing Psychotherapy Collaboration

Prerequisites for Working with Survivors
- Practitioner Prerequisites
- Client Prerequisites
- Special Boundary Issues

Protocol for Working with Self-Disclosed Survivors
- Initial Contact: The Phone Interview
- The Physical Environment
- First Session Preliminaries
- Transition to Bodywork
- The Hands-On Treatment

Key Terms

Abuse
Body Memories
Boundary
Complex Posttraumatic Stress
    Disorder (CPTSD)
Consent
Dissociate

Flashback
Hyperarousal
Hypervigilance
Integrated Memory
Intrusion
Posttraumatic Stress Disorder (PTSD)
Protocol

Psychotherapy
Recovery
Secondary Traumatization
Survivor
Trigger
Unintegrated Memory
Vicarious Traumatization

On average, one of every five clients a practitioner sees has a history of some kind of trauma or abuse. Whether or not you're aware of it, in a large percentage of your sessions, the client in your treatment room may be a survivor of trauma. Even the client might not know it. To avoid ethical complications, every practitioner who uses touch needs basic knowledge about trauma and abuse survivors and a clear protocol for working with these particular clients.

This chapter offers practitioners ethical guidelines and techniques for working with clients who are survivors of physical, emotional, or sexual trauma. The technical and emotional skills needed to work effectively with this population are learned over time with ongoing training, supervision, and increased self-knowledge. Please note that the written information in this chapter isn't a replacement for in-class, hands-on training for working with this population. We strongly believe that any practitioner who chooses to treat survivors of abuse and trauma is ethically bound to seek continuing education and ongoing supervision.

If you choose to specialize in working with survivors of trauma and abuse, you'll find great rewards. But even if you don't choose this focus, we believe the following information is of fundamental importance to practicing ethically.

▌ Understanding Trauma and Abuse

Touch therapy can provide a valuable healing environment for the abuse survivor. Practitioners minimize the risks of retraumatization by being sensitive to the experience of the survivor and its effect on their work together. Psychologist Melissa Soalt eloquently describes the dilemma faced by the survivor as he enters therapy:

> Being present in one's body is a double-edged sword for survivors: on the one hand, working through the body can stimulate the trauma and evoke confusing or frightening feelings; on the other hand, it is this very ability to be present and in one's body that ultimately allows one to feel more grounded and thus safer and more in control.[1]

Many responsibilities fall upon the practitioner. When a practitioner begins work with an abuse survivor, she may be the first person to touch the client's body since the abuse. The practitioner minimizes potential errors and creates a safe environment for the treatment process when she has awareness and understanding of the factors surrounding abuse and recovery.

Sometimes, the client who is a survivor of abuse exhibits physical symptoms which indicate the presence of unresolved trauma. Examples of such symptoms include chronic fatigue, insomnia, chronic joint and muscle pain throughout the body, and a weak immune system.[2] Other reactions to the abuse experience are flashbacks and intense memories. It is useful for practitioners to understand the origins of these reactions, know how to recognize them, appreciate the contribution of the touch treatment to their resolution, and recommend other medical consultations when appropriate.

The Potential for Harm from Uninformed Treatment

Chris Smith, the founder of Trauma Touch Therapy™ and a survivor of abuse as a child, had some early experiences with types of bodywork that encouraged cathartic emotional releases. Although such releases may feel beneficial at first, Smith now believes that they ultimately increase rather than decrease the traumatization.[3] Smith is one of a large number of professionals who believe that bodywork undertaken in isolation from other therapies, or in a context that doesn't allow the client to integrate the experience, has more potential to harm than to heal. Following are several examples of the negative effects of touch therapy when done without appropriate knowledge and training.

A practitioner was approached by a client who wasn't in psychotherapy and wanted to address her abuse issues through bodywork. The practitioner had very limited training in working with survivors but wanted to assist the client in her healing process. In the course of their work together, the client began to have flashbacks during the treatments. The practitioner felt she should let the client fully experience these memory experiences and would process what happened afterward. After several weeks of treatment the client began to experience more uncontrollable, intense, and disabling flashbacks on buses, in the supermarket, and frequently upon entering the practitioner's office. The practitioner's lack of training in this area resulted in a damaging situation for the client and a lawsuit against the practitioner.

Points to Ponder

How do you know when to draw the line between being helpful and crossing into another's scope of practice? What actions should you take when a client's symptoms exacerbate? What steps could the practitioner have taken to protect the client and safeguard her practice?

This harmful situation occurred because the practitioner didn't understand that recovery from abuse proceeds in stages, and that her client was in a very early stage of this process. The practitioner also didn't understand the significance of the flashbacks and how to deal with them. Therefore, the practitioner didn't know what the client needed to proceed safely with her recovery. The client wasn't psychologically ready to delve into her past.[4] The boundaries and support systems necessary for effective treatment weren't adequately in place. She didn't realize the client needed psychotherapy and other support systems; she, herself, lacked outside supervision to guide her work when questions or difficulties arose.

In another instance, a practitioner performed deep and somewhat painful bodywork on a woman who was an abuse survivor. Only months later into the process did he discover that often, after sessions, she collapsed in bed for two or three days to recover from nightmares, light sensitivity, emotional pain, and turmoil.

Clients with a history of abuse often lack the ability to adequately protect themselves when a practitioner errs. Treatment mistakes occur when a practitioner works too deeply or inadvertently violates a boundary. Because survivors often have trouble recognizing their boundaries, they may ask for treatment that is inappropriate, or they may not let the practitioner know if they're feeling violated.

A woman came into a massage therapist's office and immediately began removing all of her clothing. The therapist quickly covered her with a blanket and gently asked her to dress again since they were going to start with an interview. During the interview and history the woman reported that she was an abuse survivor and only felt comfortable removing her socks and shoes.

Points to Ponder

How would you have handled this situation? What further trauma could have occurred if the practitioner didn't guide the client to put her clothes back on and conduct a thorough intake interview?

Practitioners must understand abuse issues and the process of recovery to structure the treatment session at a level appropriate for the survivor's needs. This determines how a practitioner approaches a session. The practitioner who works with survivors must possess a gentle and enduring patience, for the pace of the treatment may be very slow. For instance, a practitioner could literally work only on a survivor's hands or feet for two or three months.

Many clients report taking up to a year before they can have their backs and legs touched when they're unclothed. Patience can nurture healing, and well-informed care can minimize the potential for harm in the treatment process.

The Core of Trauma and Abuse

Before discussing how to work with clients who have been abused, it's important to understand what constitutes abuse and the complexity of its effects. Janet Yassen,[5] Coordinator of Crisis Services at the Victims of Violence Program at Cambridge Hospital and co-founder of the Boston Rape Crisis Center, defines sexual abuse as "unwanted or inappropriate sexual contact, either verbal or physical, between two or more people, that is intended as an act of control, power, rage, violence, and intimidation with sex as a weapon."

Physical abuse is defined as the use of force or violence to cause pain or bodily harm which is used as an instrument of intimidation, coercion or control. Emotional abuse is the infliction of emotional harm by verbal intimidation or neglectful behavior to intimidate, demean, or hurt another person. Mind control abuse can be defined as the act of undermining a person's free will through the control of behavior, information, thoughts, and emotions.

The trauma experience has a physiological effect, even if the trauma isn't physical in nature. The diaphragm and muscles of the chest contract, restricting breathing; muscles at the base of the occiput and pelvis often contract; energy frequently withdraws to the center of the body leaving the extremities cold; and there is an overall shrinking and contraction of the physical organization of the entire body.[6] Severe trauma may cause loss of muscle tone.[7] Symptoms of the breach in psychic integrity from abuse include depression and anxiety.[8] At its core, the intent of all abuse, whether sexual, emotional, mental, or physical, is the same: to dominate, humiliate, and gain control of another person. It is a traumatic event perpetrated by another person that violates the basic physical and psychic integrity of the victim.

Types of Sexual Abuse

Sexual abuse ranges from inappropriate seductive behavior and sexual touching to sexual intercourse. Sexual abuse includes rape, gang rape, date rape, partner or spouse rape, and incest.

Incest defines a specific kind of abuse which has particularly devastating effects. In the narrow, legal definition, incest is the sexual abuse of a person by a family member who is related by blood or marriage, such as a father, mother, uncle, aunt, sister, or brother. Within the psychological community, incest is more broadly defined to include sexual violations by trusted individuals with regular access to a child or care giving responsibilities, such as family friends, childcare providers, or clergy.

Sexual abuse rarely occurs as an isolated event. Violations are often accompanied by other types of mental, physical, and emotional torment. Emotional abuse such as putdowns, insults, demeaning comments, and sudden irrational acts intended to instill fear are common. In the case of incest, this may also include the withdrawal of love and affection or threats to hurt other family members as a weapon of control.

Sexual abuse can also involve more than one perpetrator or more than one victim. Examples of this include some religious cults and secret societies, or organized criminal activities such as pornography rings. These are systematic forms of violation in which the victims are subjected to sadistic torture and may be drugged to become compliant.

The Prevalence of Sexual Abuse

The statistics on sexual abuse are staggering and difficult for most people to fathom. The National Violence against Women Survey found that in the United States, one of six women and one of 33 men has experienced an attempted or completed rape as a child or an adult. Specifically, 18 percent of surveyed women and three percent of surveyed men said they

Keep a telephone list of the safe-house hotlines in your area.

experienced a completed or attempted rape at some time in their life.[9] The National Institute of Health, in its review of the reporting literature, estimates that one third of all females in the United States experience some form of sexual abuse during childhood. Studies of male victims are rarer, but the rate is likely to be as high despite less disclosure. Other statistics say that one-half of all women and one-third of all men in the United States have experienced childhood sexual abuse. These individuals are also at greater risk for depression and other health issues.[10]

To look at this another way, 18 to 20 percent of the United States population or approximately 50 million people had been sexually abused. In Canada, the 1984 Royal Commission on Sexual Offences Against Children and Youth reported that 22 percent of women and 10 percent of men experienced some type of sexual abuse before the age of 18.[11] Some professionals believe that these numbers are an exaggeration while others think they're low due to under-reporting. If these numbers are hard to believe, reduce the total by a factor of half, or even two-thirds, and the tally is still a frightening number. It is difficult to determine whether sexual abuse has always been this prevalent and is only now being more accurately reported, or whether it has increased due to the dissolution of the family and other social factors.

There have been several periods over the last hundred years during which sexual abuse has been exposed, discussed, and acknowledged, but it has only been since the mid-1970s that the social and political context has provided an ongoing, welcoming atmosphere for research and wide acceptance. According to Herman, the women's movement provided the political environment to support the ongoing research and recognition of the extensive existence of sexual abuse.[12]

Although more girls than boys are sexually abused, one research study finds that the number of boys who have been sexually abused is greater than previously thought.[13] Most of the abuse is perpetrated by men, although women do abuse both male and female children. Thus, a practitioner could generally expect that approximately one in five clients will likely be a survivor of sexual abuse, and many others were victims of other types of physical or psychological trauma.

> Our sorrows and wounds are healed only when we touch them with compassion.
>
> —Buddha

Types of Physical Abuse

Physical abuse of children is more common than imagined and shows itself in obvious forms such as violent beatings, corporal punishment, food deprivation, or aggressive tickling that doesn't stop. Other types of physical abuse include spousal battery, the threat of violence as a means of control, and the use of physical torture as discipline of spouses and children. More women are injured by battering than are injured in car accidents and it's estimated that each year millions of children directly witness acts of domestic abuse.[14] Physical assaults and muggings are commonplace as well.

All forms of physical abuse leave scars that close people off to themselves. Various forms of emotional and body oriented therapies can help these individuals reclaim themselves and their bodies.

Types of Emotional Abuse

Emotional trauma is experienced by everyone to one degree or another: a loved one dies; a love relationship ends badly; an accident occurs that severely curtails our activities. Most individuals experience these traumas and move on. However, when emotional abuse occurs, the extent of the trauma may go beyond the individual's ability to effectively cope. Whereas physical abuse inflicts harm directly to the body, emotional abuse inflicts harm to the psychological wellbeing of another.

We define emotional abuse as the infliction of emotional harm by verbal intimidation or neglectful behavior. Examples of emotional abuse include direct verbal threats, attacks, taunting, or belittling language used to intimidate, demean, or hurt another person. Emotional abuse occurs when a person, whether young or old, is regularly taunted, put down, shamed, berated, ostracized, or humiliated.

Emotional withholding and emotional neglect also constitute abuse. In children dependent on adults for their care, abuse may take the form of consistent lack of response to a child's emotional needs, the inability of the adult to express appropriate emotion to the child, or neglect. Other forms of emotional abuse include children being severely punished, dominated, or forced to perform acts which go against their humanity.

Usually victims experience strong feelings of fear, shame, rage, or despair. If the feelings are overwhelming, victims may enter a depressed or dissociative state in which they're cut off from some or all of their emotions. Emotional abuse is a means to overpower someone; it's always destructive and inevitably results in emotional scarring and long lasting self-esteem issues.

Cult Mind Control Abuse

The BITE Model of Cult Mind Control

http://TheEthicsOfTouch.com/pdf/BITE-model-cult-control.pdf

Cult mind control abuse occurs when people are subjected to an extreme form of abuse that involves creating an alternate identity which is programmed to depend on a person or totalistic system. This creates a dissociative disorder leading to a number of other trauma-related symptoms. Members are deceptively recruited into a destructive cult (religious, political, "therapeutic," or business). People who are born into such cults never get the opportunity to fully develop their own identity until they break away.

Mind control abuse includes the control of behavior, information, thoughts, and emotions to undermine a person's free will. Without specialized therapy, mind control victims can exhibit a host of psychosomatic complaints, as well as the following: identity confusion; black and white, simplistic thinking; difficulty with decision-making; fear and panic disorders; sexual problems; sleeping and eating difficulties. Cult members are often encouraged to cut off from family and friends, and abandon education and career choices. They tend to speak with cult jargon. They are either extremely aggressive in converting others, or are very secretive, deceptive, and evasive when asked direct questions.[15]

The Three Stages of Recovery

Clinicians have identified three distinct stages of recovery: establishing safety; remembrance and mourning; reconnection. Others believe that the healing process stages are less clearly defined and more fluid. Most likely, a continuum of the healing process exists. The three stages described by Judith Herman give practitioners a clear way to think about using touch while working with survivors in recovery. Throughout the therapy process, the survivor could move back and forth between stages two and three, or experience two stages simultaneously. Touch therapy may be appropriate in Stages 2 and 3 but is generally contraindicated in Stage 1.

1. Safety

The goal of the first stage of recovery is to establish physical and psychological safety.[16] The survivor learns to control his body and attend to his basic physical needs, (i.e., eating well, sleeping, getting regular exercise, having a safe place to live). As the client develops this immediate sense of safety, he can begin to exercise initiative and take charge of his recovery. It may take the client as little as a few sessions or as long as a few decades before he truly feels safe experiencing somatic treatments.

2. Remembrance and Mourning

The second stage of recovery involves remembrance and mourning. In the presence of safety, formerly unconscious, often fragmented, disguised, and deeply buried memories arise. Forgotten and painful memories heal by being reconstructed and transformed into an integral part of a life story. This stage of recovery can be profoundly painful and prolonged as the person relives the pains and horror of the trauma, and experiences the accompanying grief and loss. Herman observes the following:

> The telling of the trauma story inevitably plunges the survivor into profound grief. The second stage of recovery has a timeless quality that is frightening. The descent into mourning feels like a surrender to tears that are endless. But it is by the remembering, telling of their story, and grieving that the survivor can move toward integration of their trauma and eventually reconnect with ordinary life.[17]

3. Reconnection

In the third stage of recovery, the survivor begins to look to the future and imagine a whole, intact self. The survivor recognizes her trauma but isn't possessed by it. She feels more confidence in her ability to connect with the outside world and her capacity to appropriately give and withhold trust. A survivor in this stage often turns her experience into social action, having transforming effects on self and society.[18]

Safety in Recovery

- Why is working with a trauma survivor not advisable in the first stage of recovery?
- What are the elements of establishing safety in a somatic therapy practice?

Posttraumatic Stress Disorder

Traumas come with life. They create stresses which often encourage us to engage in self-exploration. Most people quickly overcome minor traumas, whereas other events take years to undo. Additionally, there is a category of traumatic events that goes far beyond the norm. Individuals who have gone through severe or repeated trauma may be in a kind of shock for the rest of their lives, while others work through the trauma by themselves or with help from others. The brutality of rape and war has been consistent throughout the ages. Now, the devastating aftermath these traumas create is beginning to be acknowledged.

National Center for PTSD
http://www.ptsd.va.gov/

Sexual, emotional, or physical abuse and trauma leaves profound and lasting effects on a person's psychological, cognitive, and emotional functioning. The impact and symptoms of trauma are known as posttraumatic stress disorder, or PTSD.[19] According to dedicated researchers, including psychiatrist Judith Herman who explored the effects of trauma in her groundbreaking book *Trauma and Recovery*,[20] similar effects of trauma are experienced by survivors of sexual abuse, political prisoners, kidnap victims, concentration camp survivors, victims of terrorism, and many soldiers who experienced combat in war. Other experts also include survivors of major accidents, childhood torture, and medical abuse.[21]

Symptoms

The National Center for PTSD summarizes the four major symptoms of PTSD as: hyperarousal, re-experiencing, negativity, and avoidance.

HYPERAROUSAL is a state of constant alertness to danger experienced by the survivor of trauma. The survivor's senses and body are poised to respond to the slightest movements, noises, or provocations. A survivor may react with extreme irritation or alarm to situations that impart little effect on others. Poor sleep is common. To the person in this state, all situations carry potential re-enactment of past traumas.

RE-EXPERIENCING is when past traumatic events recur as vivid memories interrupting the course of life in the present. "The traumatic moment becomes encoded in an abnormal form of memory, which breaks spontaneously into consciousness, both as flashbacks during waking states and as traumatic nightmares during sleep," writes Herman.[22]

NEGATIVITY refers to negative changes to beliefs and feelings that may come as a result of trauma. A survivor may avoid relationships as a result of distrust or negative feelings toward other people in general. A survivor who once felt close to others, or saw beauty in the world, may now see the whole world as a dangerous place.

AVOIDANCE is the state of actually avoiding situations, people, or thought processes that trigger memories of the trauma. The survivor may voluntarily avoid social activities, watching movies with disturbing content, or may even keep herself so busy that she doesn't have time to think about the traumatic event. The survivor may even avoid seeking help, to keep from having to talk about the event at all.

Involuntary avoidance occurs when the intensity and pain of an event is so severe that the survivor becomes numb and psychologically removed from the pain. The survivor registers the event in her awareness but in an altered state where she doesn't experience pain, attachment, or emotion. The person may describe it as going numb, going deaf, or leaving the body. Also known as *dissociation*, in this state, the trauma victim survives unbearable conditions from which there was no actual escape. One incest survivor described her experience of dissociation this way:

> After I knew what he was doing, I used to separate from him. I used to feel that if I could just get close enough to the wall, that he couldn't touch me (yet I knew he could), but I used to go inside the wall and it was like he was touching someone else. I would just turn off and get cold.[23]

This type of avoidance can also be experienced as hypervigilance, an overfocused narrowing of attention onto one idea, one part of the body, or a particular sensation or feeling. This constriction carries over to the experiences of the present, affecting the ability of the survivor to feel both positive and negative emotions, physical sensations, and attachments to others.

Complex Posttraumatic Stress Disorder

People experiencing posttraumatic stress disorder alternate between the opposing psychological states of hyper-awareness and numbness in an effort to gain balance. Until significant aspects of the traumatic memories are explored and integrated, the survivor is caught between complete forgetting and the constant fear of reliving the traumatic experience.

Herman coined the term, complex posttraumatic stress disorder (CPTSD),[24] for those subjected to prolonged, repeated trauma. Repeated traumatic abuse shatters a person's sense of self and relation to others. In an even more intense way, human contact, especially intimate contact, becomes associated with feelings of intimidation, pain, violence, rage, humiliation, disgust, shame, and betrayal.[25] Further, a person who has experienced prolonged abuse during childhood has no guideposts for judging who is worthy of trust or which situations are truly safe. As a result of the violation of physical, sexual, and emotional boundaries, a survivor of sexual abuse often has difficulty defining her personal boundaries with people in the present and is therefore at risk for further abuse.

Body Memories and Flashbacks

Trauma survivors often experience body memories and flashbacks. The following information is helpful even if you don't plan to specifically work with trauma survivors. You may not know that a specific client is a survivor, and a flashback could occur at any time. You help ensure a client's safety when you're prepared with the knowledge of how flashbacks occur and the steps to take when they occur.

A memory is a remembered past experience that may or may not be painful. Memories appear along a continuum of consciousness, ranging from an integrated memory to a brief, faint recollection that is gone in an instant (unintegrated memory), to a flashback which is out of the person's control. Memories can emerge as images, sounds, thoughts, emotions, sensations within the body, or any combination of these elements.

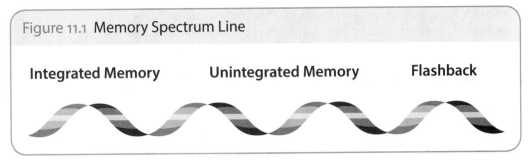

Figure 11.1 Memory Spectrum Line

Integrated Memory   **Unintegrated Memory**   **Flashback**

An **Integrated Memory** is a memory that may have been painful at one time but has been remembered, understood, and accepted. The person may not like the memory but doesn't fight remembering it and copes with the details of the memory without being overwhelmed by it. An integrated memory has a tolerable emotional charge that doesn't consume the person.

An **Unintegrated Memory** develops when a memory is so painful that parts of the memory are blocked and many of the details missing. If a memory is disturbing, it may appear and then be lost for periods of time. One person recalled having a clear memory that was painful, and then totally forgetting it within seconds—as if he were in a fog. Unintegrated memories stir up unresolved feelings and are usually quickly repressed.

Clients who feel indefinite, disturbing emotions when they're touched, are uncomfortable and don't know why. This can be the result of a painful memory that is triggered, but hasn't yet emerged into consciousness. Traumatic experiences may re-emerge, not as clear linear visual or auditory memories, but as vague emotions or felt body memories, such as the following: the pressure on an upper arm as the abuser guides the victim to a room; the heat and pain on a cheek from being slapped; the nausea and restricted breathing from being molested.

It can be difficult to distinguish which elements are part of the original memory when *Intrusion Errors* occur (i.e., when information that is related to the theme of a certain memory, but wasn't actually a part of the original episode, becomes associated with the event).

A **Flashback** is the experience of reliving or re-experiencing a traumatic event as if it's occurring or is imminent. When a flashback is triggered, concrete, distinct memories suddenly surface and intrude on the present. They can be triggered by touching any part of the body or by a particular emotion, sensation, or experience. Sometimes the smell of an essential oil or the cologne the practitioner wears is associated with a past event. A flashback can be experienced as a momentary flash of memory or a movie that the client is in. When this transpires, "the individual is awake but appears to be in a state of altered consciousness and often has subsequent amnesia for what takes place. The experiences last from a few minutes to several hours...."[26]

The client may have intense emotional reactions such as fear, sobbing, or feelings of rage with physical trembling. When the flashback is occurring, the person is dissociated from the present. The client can't tolerate the memory, splits off his consciousness, and is no longer psychologically present. When a flashback occurs, the task of the practitioner is to bring the client back to the present as quickly as possible.

Flashbacks differ from integrated memories. The body holds memories;[27] therefore, when an emotionally charged area is touched, long repressed memories may be evoked.[28] Certain areas such as the mouth, throat, neck, chest, abdomen, buttock, and inner thigh are more likely to hold memories of traumatic abuse than other areas. But this isn't always the case. One survivor described feeling very upset when her partner put an arm around her shoulder. She recalled her abuser putting his hand gently around her shoulder when the ritual of her abuse was about to begin in childhood.[29]

Many variations exist along the continuum from integrated memory to flashback. For instance, one has a faint recall of an event triggered by a part of the body being touched or by a smell or a sound, but nothing of substance is recalled. A person can also have a very clear memory and find it so unacceptable that she re-represses it and can't recall the memory later.

> The secret of health for both mind and body is not to mourn for the past, not to worry about the future, not to anticipate troubles, but to live the present moment wisely and earnestly.
>
> —Siddhartha Gautama

Here are some examples of how touch triggers different memory experiences:

- While her mouth and jaw were being massaged, one client described a memory of a very clear sexual encounter with her father. The client had no idea that she had been abused until that moment.
- Another client felt afraid whenever her left shoulder was touched. She only recalled the details of her abuse after years of psychotherapy.
- A third client had a momentary flashback triggered by a neck adjustment and went into a catatonic state for 20 minutes. This client was fully dissociated, not responding to verbal communication or touch.

When aware of the dynamics of body memory, the practitioner can help the client remember while remaining present and in her body. A skilled practitioner learns how to avoid inducing flashbacks and how to move the client back to the present if flashbacks occur.

While *The Ethics of Touch* covers many aspects of working with survivors of trauma and abuse, it cannot replace in-person training including boundary setting and flashback role-plays with a skilled teacher or coach.

Recognize Flashbacks

Recognizing when a client is experiencing a flashback isn't always easy. On one end of the spectrum, the out-of-control flashback can be frightening to experience and easy to recognize. Other flashbacks are quieter and are over fairly quickly. Recognizing these subtle flashbacks requires a practiced eye.

One of the keys to identifying a flashback is to look at the client's eyes. The pupils are often dilated and the client has a faraway look as if she is "out of it," extremely tired, or using drugs. She has left her body or is out of touch with feelings, thoughts, and sensations. She may only be in touch with feelings of the past experience. She may stare into space, curl up in a ball on the table, refuse to respond when asked a question, experience a loss of sensation (especially in the legs), begin to cry, flutter her eyelids, or talk incoherently. Phrases such as, "No, no, what are you doing?" "Who are you?" or "Don't touch me, I'm scared!" may be spoken. The body may suddenly tighten, stiffen, or shake uncontrollably.

Precautions

While any part of the body can hold body memories, physical touch to particular areas of the body is more likely to stimulate a flashback than others:

- In general, the "safest" areas to touch are the hands, arms, feet, legs below the knee, gently on the scalp and forehead, the middle and lower neck, shoulders, upper back area, and the mid-back. The lower back in certain individuals holds a high emotional charge because the muscles there move the pelvis and inhibit movement during unwanted sexual contact. Feet and hands can also be trigger areas if the client's abuse involved being held down or bound.
- Proceed with caution when working with the following areas: the deep, sub-occipital muscles at the back of the head; the buttocks; the front and back of the thighs. Some clients never want these areas touched.
- Consider avoiding the following areas except in consultation with the client's psychotherapist: inside the mouth; the front of the neck; the throat; the abdomen; the upper portion of the inner thigh.
- Avoid working on a woman's chest, the breast tissue, and the front of the pelvis (just above and to the side of the genitals). And of course, never work in or around the genitalia.
- Body position can also trigger memories and increase anxiety. Some clients may need to avoid receiving touch while lying on their backs, lying face down, seated, or lying on sides, depending on their body position during trauma.
- Entire regions of the body may be more hypersensitive, such as the left side, right side, front, or back. Even approaching a client on the more hypervigilant side may trigger a flashback.
- Certain techniques and qualities of touch may be triggers as well. Be sure to check with clients before using percussion or tapotement techniques (especially for physical abuse

victims), or gliding and friction massage strokes (especially for sexual abuse victims). Modify pressure with client's input as well.

Still, no matter how careful you are, flashbacks sometimes occur. Certain hand techniques or past associations with specific types of touch, such as a gentle touch on the shoulder, may trigger a flashback. In working with a client over a period of time, the practitioner may help minimize the likelihood of flashbacks. Remember, when the client is reliving a flashback, he may believe that abuse is about to occur or is occurring. The person may feel he is actually back in time re-experiencing the trauma. The practitioner, alert and conscious about his role in this situation, facilitates the client's awareness of the present and immediate surroundings. "Reliving" flashbacks doesn't offer the opportunity to learn from earlier experiences in a way that is useful.

Practical Application: Retrieve a Client from a Flashback

Follow these steps when you realize a flashback is occurring:

- **GENTLY BREAK CONTACT WITH YOUR HANDS.** Acknowledge that a flashback is happening before you do anything else. Say the client's name, e.g., "Rochelle, are you here with me?" and wait for a reply. If the client is in a flashback, there is usually no reply or a vague one that is uncharacteristic of the client's communication with you. Note: a flashback isn't the same as an emotional release, where you would likely maintain physical contact with a client.

- **MAKE VOICE CONTACT.** Using the client's name every time, say in a very calm voice, "Jane. This is Terry. We are here together." Or say, "Ralph, where are you right now? Are you here with me? This is Terry, I am here with you. We are having a bodywork session." Ask questions such as, "Do you know where you are? Do you know who I am?" If the eyes are closed, say, "Ann, can you open your eyes and look at me?" or direct the client to look at an object in the room. "Let me know that you hear me," is another phrase to bring a client back.

- **MAKE EYE CONTACT.** Eye contact is one of the best ways to stay in touch with a client especially because physical touch is often a triggering mechanism. Encourage the client to open both eyes and focus on you or an object. Eye contact is usually a very good way to bring a client back to the present.

- **COVER THE CLIENT WITH A BLANKET.** Create a safe, thick physical boundary around the body. Stand to the side of the table and make eye contact. The client's eyes are usually closed, or staring into space, not seeing you. The client may also cover her eyes with her hands.

- **FOLLOW CLIENT'S INSTRUCTIONS.** Follow instructions that the client has given you about how to respond if she goes into a flashback.

- **ENCOURAGE THE CLIENT TO SIT UP.** This often helps to re-establish an adult reality. Ask if the client would like to sit up. If the client isn't sure, encourage him to do so. If he says, "No," go with the client's preference. If you have the impulse to help the person sit up, first ask if it's okay. Do not touch a client in that state without permission. Instruct the client to sit on the table or move to a chair. Pull up a chair yourself and sit so you are neither above the client looking down, nor too close. Some clients are specific and ask the practitioner to sit off to the side, not directly in front.

- **TAKE TIME TO TALK ABOUT WHAT HAPPENED.** Do not probe for any details of the flashback. First, ask if the client feels able to talk about the process of what happened and what might be important from this experience to discuss with the psychotherapist. Then, talk together about what you're going to do next, whether you're going to continue the hands-on session, or stop. If the occurrence is a first for the two of you, it's usually a good idea to stop the hands-on portion of the treatment.

Points to Ponder

Do any of these steps make you feel uncomfortable? If so, what are some ways that you can gain confidence in these actions? What can you do to prepare yourself to appropriately manage interactions with a client who is experiencing a flashback?

> ### Figure 11.2 Retrieve a Client from a Flashback
>
> | | |
> |---|---|
> | • Gently break contact with your hands | • Cover client with blanket |
> | • Make voice contact | • Follow client instructions |
> | • Make eye contact | • Encourage client to sit up |
> | | • Talk about what happened |

Process Why the Flashback Occurred

Once the client has sufficiently recovered from the flashback, determine if you did anything to trigger the flashback. Was it something you said, a reaction to a specific part of the body you were touching, background music, or a scent wafting through the room? Gather as much information as you can in a gentle, noninvasive way. Ask if she felt or feels numbness in any part of her body, especially her legs. If numbing occurs, the effects of the flashback were very strong and are still occurring. This information influences your decision to continue or stop the hands-on part of your session.

If you choose to continue the session, check with the person frequently to see if she is present. Notice if the client becomes "spacey" and ask if she is beginning to feel numb physically, particularly in the legs.

If you choose to stop, leave the room and let the client dress before talking further. The routine of dressing and preparing to leave helps bring the person into the present. Call through the door once to make sure she is okay. Otherwise, you may return to the treatment room and discover that the client hasn't moved during your absence. When the client is finished dressing, sit down and have a more complete closure than usual. Ask what was and wasn't helpful when you were assisting the client back to the present. Ask what you could've done differently, if anything, to be more supportive.

Plan for Client Safety

Ask if the client has plans after leaving your office. The client should be with people with whom he feels safe. If the client feels too disoriented or dizzy to drive or to travel alone, ensure his physical safety by arranging for a taxi or for someone to pick up the client. Most people recover within a half hour, while others take longer. Help the client make emergency plans should another flashback occur. Talk about whom to call: a friend, partner, family member, psychotherapist, a hospital emergency room, or you.

Adjust Your Schedule

You may need to adjust your schedule and run overtime if a flashback occurs, particularly toward the end of the session. Extending a session shouldn't become a habit. If another client is waiting, take the first opportunity which feels appropriate to tell your current client that you're leaving for just a moment to tell the next client that you're running late. This lets the current client know that you're conscious of the extra time needed and also want to show respect to the person who is waiting. It sets a professional tone and helps both clients feel comfortable at the same time.

Follow Up

If you have an established collaboration with his psychotherapist, tell the client that you'll talk to his psychotherapist about what happened during the session. Suggest that the client call and talk with the psychotherapist the same day as well. If the flashback was more intense than those previously experienced and processed by the client, tell the client you'll call him later

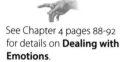

See Chapter 4 pages 88-92 for details on **Dealing with Emotions**.

> Grace strikes us when we are in great pain and restlessness... Sometimes at that moment a wave of light breaks into our darkness, and it is as though a voice were saying, "You are accepted."
>
> —Paul Tillich

that day (specify a time) to check on him. At the beginning of the next session, again ask the client what was helpful and what wasn't. You may hear different information.

Flashback Signs

- What are the signs that a flashback is occurring?
- What is the primary task of the practitioner when the client is experiencing a flashback, and why?
- Describe what "being present" actually means.
- Why is it important to maintain continuous communication when working with a trauma survivor? How might you maintain reasonably continuous communication without being intrusive?

Benefits of Touch Therapy for Survivors

As awareness of the prevalence of abuse has grown, an increasing number of survivors are seeking various touch therapies to help them reconnect with and reclaim their bodies. Psychiatrists, psychologists, social workers, and counselors are referring an increasing number of their clients for touch therapy. The practitioner who understands abuse and the healing process is prepared to respond in a helpful and knowledgeable way. Melissa Soalt, a psychotherapist and the founder of Impact (a self-defense training program), has worked with many survivors and observes the following:[30]

- Bodywork can be a very powerful adjunct to psychotherapy. The trauma from abuse typically results in dissociative numbing or repressive mechanisms that leave survivors feeling "empty" or vacant on the inside. With reconnection and integration (or a move toward wholeness) as primary therapeutic goals, working through the body can be a valuable tool toward this end. Because the body is such a direct medium, bodywork facilitates this process of re-entry and one's ability to feel more present.
- Bodywork can help survivors develop a friendly and compassionate relationship with their bodies. Sexual or physical abuse often leaves survivors feeling disgusted, shameful, or even violent toward their body, as though their body betrayed or turned against them.
- Bodywork helps survivors experience their bodies as a source of groundedness and eventually as a source of strength and even pleasure.

Working with a compassionate and skilled bodyworker helps rebuild survivors' sense of trust, and reconnects them with the possibility of other genuine caring relationships. When performed responsibly at the appropriate stage of the client's healing and with care and sensitivity, body therapy can be an important healing force in a client's life. Bodywork offers survivors a new and non-abusive way of being in touch with their bodies, a path to discover how their bodies feel, and a way to discern their general level of health.

> Great thanks are due to Nature for putting into the life of each being so much healing power.
>
> —J. W. von Goethe

Establishing a Place of Safety

When the survivor of abuse enters psychotherapy, establishing personal and psychological safety with the psychotherapist is a crucial first step in the healing process. A touch therapy relationship builds on this experience. A healthy bodywork environment creates another opportunity for the survivor to establish an environment where she feels safe with emotions and the physical self. Somatic work offers safe touch with dignity and respect in a nonjudgmental, non-sexual environment.

Rebuilding Boundaries

Somatic therapies can be helpful in rebuilding personal boundaries damaged by trauma and abuse. During this time the client reacquaints himself with his body through sensual awareness of how the body is organized and what sensations trigger trauma response. The process of learning about these boundaries and managing the bodywork session helps to integrate the sense of body control.[31] Eventually, the client stays grounded in his body while talking about the experience, bringing a new level of healing through reorganizing a negative body response into positive somatic memory.[32] The client has the opportunity to construct new boundaries as the treatment progresses. For example, the client sets important boundaries by simply telling the practitioner where to touch and where not to touch. By being in charge of the session, the survivor gains another piece of control of his life associated with the body. Each experience of inviting, choosing, and denying touch empowers the survivor.

A client described her experience of bodywork, expressing both the benefits and cautions needed to guide therapy in relation to boundaries:

> My "talk" therapist person suggested to me that I might want to start to draw some boundaries around places in my body where I just didn't feel that I wanted to be touched. That was the beginning of the physical healing part, to say, "No, I don't want you to massage below my waist and above my knees." I felt like such a baby having to draw those lines, but it was such an important part of my recovery. The more I was empowered, the more I could say "Stop" and "No." Rebuilding those boundaries was incredibly important to me. But there are still times when I roll over, if I feel like my genitals aren't covered up properly, it's like an alarm goes off somewhere in my head and I still have a lot of shame about saying what's going on for me in the moment.[33]

> ### Points to Ponder
>
> How would you approach developing a somatic treatment plan for a client with these restrictions? What other ways could you support a client in setting strong boundaries? What information would be helpful to receive from the "talk" therapist?

Rebuilding and maintaining boundaries are crucial for trauma survivors. Somatic practitioners can help facilitate the rebuilding process. Ideally, this work is done in conjunction with a psychotherapist.

Experiencing the Pleasure of Non-Sexual Touch

Touch that is neutral or pleasurable provides building blocks for a changed experience of the body. After safety has been established through repeated positive physical contact, the survivor usually begins to perceive the practitioner's touch as neutral and over time experiences touch without dissociation. Later on, pleasurable sensation which isn't sexual is usually experienced by the client. This capacity to experience pleasure in a relaxed parasympathetic state while receiving tactile stimulation brings an expanded sense of self and a trust in life experiences.[34] One client described her experience this way:

> Bodywork helped me learn how to be touched again—to relearn how to be touched. All the touch I had gotten was always abusive; sexually or physically abusive. I never knew that touch could be otherwise. Having a massage therapist helped me to trust again and eventually to relax. It was a wonderful way to learn how to go on to a normal life afterwards.[35]

See Chapter 2 pages 31-34 for more information on **Boundary Development**.

"
Healing may not be so much about getting better, as about letting go of everything that isn't you—all of the expectations, all of the beliefs—and becoming who you are.

—Rachel Naomi Remen

Reintegrating Body Memories

In conjunction with psychotherapy, touch therapy assists the survivor in reaching hidden memories and integrating them into his present experience. Abusive traumas from the past cause the survivor to dissociate from the body and this experience often recurs when the body is touched. Renegotiating somatic memory by replacing a negative physical response with a positive memory reintegrates the experience so that the client achieves a more balanced and positive state of body awareness. Therapeutic touch may trigger the recall of memories to be processed in psychotherapy.

As clients connect with their bodies in a more positive way, they experience improved body image and feel less shame. Practitioners may find that these clients take better care of their bodies as treatments continue.

Enhancing Psychotherapy Collaboration

Psychotherapists who recommend touch therapies for their clients see the bodywork practitioners as collaborators in the healing process. Many see touch as a valuable adjunct for some of their clients to reduce stress while others see it as a vital part of the task of reintegrating the body into the survivor's life.

In their collaborative book, *Embodying Healing*, Robert Timms, PH.D., and Patrick Connors, C.M.T., write, "Working with the body is a powerful means of sidestepping the conscious mind and gathering information directly from the unconscious fund of knowledge."[36] In their "psychophysical model," each professional brings separate skills and roles to the healing process. The psychotherapist helps the client integrate her emotional and cognitive insights, while the bodyworker helps the client increase her self-awareness and gain access to emotions and less conscious memories through direct touch.

Timms, a psychotherapist, describes the benefits of his frequent collaboration with Connors, a massage therapist, in the following way:

> Often I find clients are better able to make cognitive connections in psychotherapy sessions that follow bodywork sessions. In most cases, the client's characteristic resistances are lowered and she or he is more available for therapeutic insight.[37]

Melissa Soalt writes:

> In psychotherapy the therapist is often the one who holds the client's feelings until the client is more able or ready to have and own them. In this light, bodywork can both elicit feelings/memories and help survivors contain (i.e., stay with but not become overwhelmed by) these feelings, thus aiding in the psychotherapeutic process.[38]

Psychotherapists and bodyworkers collaborate in different ways. A sequential mode is when the client has a bodywork session in the first hour and a psychotherapy session in the next hour. A combined mode entails the psychotherapist and the practitioner working simultaneously with a client in one room, as described by Timms. (The combined mode, where psychotherapist and somatic practitioner work simultaneously, may present complex challenges, both rich in opportunity and possible difficulties.) Others work concurrently at separate locations, seeing a client weekly at their offices and communicating by phone as needed. Psychotherapists who regularly call upon touch practitioners to support their treatment plan usually interview the practitioners before they refer their clients to them.

Chris Smith's Trauma Touch Therapy™ method utilizes simultaneous but separate bodywork and counseling sessions. While the bodywork session may release memory and emotion, the counselor's role is to help the client integrate the experience in a meaningful way. In this manner, the practitioners in the two fields remain within their respective scopes of practice and avoid confusion of roles.

Find a Therapist

http://www.find-a-therapist.com/

Trauma Touch Therapy Certificate Program

http://www.csha.net/advanced/trauma.html

▍ Prerequisites for Working with Survivors

The undertaking of a course of any type of touch therapy is a journey of courage for both the survivor and the practitioner. It places many demands on both the client's and the practitioner's resources. Certain prerequisites are essential and others very helpful in preparing the practitioner and the client for their work together.

Practitioner Prerequisites

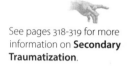

See pages 318-319 for more information on **Secondary Traumatization**.

The treatment of survivors requires a refined degree of self-awareness. Education to prepare for this type of work should include training in psychology, communication, sexuality, ethics, trauma, and counseling, as well as specialized hands-on techniques. The practitioner also benefits greatly from support networks that include peer counseling and supervision. Practitioners who lack information and formal training in working with survivors risk harming their clients and themselves. Untrained and unaware practitioners are likely to: impose their own assumptions, needs, and conflicts on their clients; retraumatize their clients during the bodywork session; and suffer what is known as secondary or vicarious trauma themselves.[39] Boundaries between practitioner and client can become blurred, and the boundary related to scope of practice can be unclear. In the book, *Victims of Cruelty: Somatic Psychotherapy in the Treatment of Posttraumatic Stress Disorder*, Maryanna Eckberg states that an experienced psychotherapist/bodyworker doesn't do bodywork on a client if the risks for transference, regression, or for eliciting sexual impulses are too great. She further adds that, "touch must contribute to the treatment process."[40] The untrained practitioner may casually give advice to a client whose real need is to receive a referral to another type of therapy.

Psychological Understanding

A basic knowledge of human psychology and specialized knowledge of issues related to abuse are essential to practitioners who wish to work with survivors. Fundamental psychological concepts relevant to the healing process include transference, countertransference, power differential, dual relationships, and boundary issues. Practitioners must learn how to deal with flashbacks, body memories, and psychological symptoms such as hyperarousal, intrusion errors, and dissociation. The experiences of abuse survivors intensifies all these psychological aspects of the therapeutic relationship, and often has unexpected effects.

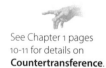

See Chapter 1 pages 10-11 for details on **Countertransference**.

Practitioners must understand the mechanism of countertransference. The untrained practitioner may project her own feelings about the client's history onto the client and assume that the client's responses are the same as the practitioner's. In doing so, the practitioner further disempowers the client and unwittingly adds to the client's sense of helplessness and hopelessness. Instead, the ethical practitioner learns to play a supportive role, helping the client find her own answers.[41] Practitioners who understand these concepts work safely and effectively, and identify ways to avoid re-enacting the very traumas for which the client has come to receive treatments.

Practitioners who work with self-disclosed abuse survivors respond to clients' needs in a helpful and appropriate manner. Clarification is always required beforehand about areas of the body to be touched, intensity of treatment, and whether the session can be done clothed.

Practitioners need to be sensitive to the messages a client sends (often without words) and create an empowering, non-hierarchical collaboration. The manner in which practitioners handle giving feedback and support to the client, and how the practitioners receive feedback from the client, is crucial in establishing and maintaining trust. The practitioners' reaction to a client's memories, inadvertent boundary crossings, and anger at treatment errors makes or breaks the relationship. Making mistakes isn't the problem because every practitioner makes mistakes. What is important is how the mistakes are handled. How the practitioner deals with his own feelings will be keenly perceived by the client's radar and will strongly affect the therapeutic relationship.

A massage therapist was giving a first treatment to a self-disclosed survivor of abuse. The client reported that her back was very tense. "Please work deeply," she said, "but don't go too far down, I don't want any work on my lower back." Everything went smoothly as the therapist massaged the client's shoulders and upper back, and he gradually moved downward. He planned to reverse direction right before he reached the lumbar area, but just as he neared the bottom of her rib cage, the client suddenly tensed up and said, "No!"

As the client burst into tears, the therapist, taken aback, lifted his hands. He felt a pull to try to figure out what he might have done differently to avoid upsetting the client, but quickly stopped himself, realizing that what mattered just then was connecting with the client and re-establishing a sense of safety. He took a deep breath and said in a clear, empathetic tone, "I'm so sorry. It seems like I accidentally crossed over into an area that wasn't okay for you. Would you like to take a break for a little while?"

"Just give me a moment," the client said. "I told you, I really don't want you to touch my lower back."

"That's right," said the therapist, "and I misunderstood what area was okay and what wasn't. I'm sorry about that." He then offered up a possible solution for moving forward. "Would it work for me to move the sheet further up, to make the boundary really clear? You can let me know exactly where you feel comfortable drawing that line."

The client agreed, and after a short break, she helped the therapist reposition the sheet. As the session went on, the therapist checked in periodically to make sure everything he was doing felt okay, and the client said yes each time.

At the end of the session, when the client was dressed, the therapist thanked her for letting him know when he had crossed a boundary. The client, in turn, thanked him for his respectful response, and made another appointment for the following week.

Points to Ponder

At one point, the therapist felt pulled to think about the past (what went wrong and what he could have done differently), but made a conscious choice to focus his attention on what the client needed in the present moment. Have you ever experienced this type of conflict? What helps you to stay present, and what gets in the way? How might the client have been affected if the therapist had gotten caught up in regret, self-doubt, or defensiveness? As a therapist, how can you be sure you correctly understand a client's boundaries? What are some other ways this therapist could have handled the unintentional boundary crossing?

The reality of practicing somatic therapies—particularly with individuals who have heightened sensitivities due to prior trauma—is that not all boundary crossings can be anticipated or prevented. Even when clients feel comfortable enough to assert a boundary, there may still be ambiguities or misunderstandings (for instance, in this scenario, different ideas about where the "lower back" begins). However, you can minimize any damage to the therapeutic relationship by communicating clearly, with skill, tact, and compassion. In fact, the relationship may end up significantly stronger than before; your constructive response to feedback goes a long way toward building and maintaining a safe, trusting environment.

Those who bring sunshine to the lives of others cannot keep it from themselves.

—James Matthew Barre

Issues and Motivations

Ethical practitioners strive to understand their own issues and motivations. Taking a closer look at why one chooses to become a touch practitioner is an important step. We all choose careers for different reasons. Awareness of conscious, as well as unconscious, motives helps the practitioner focus on what needs to be addressed to work effectively with a vulnerable clientele. Potential indicators that a practitioner's unresolved or neglected issues will interfere with the effectiveness of the work include making friends with many clients, or talking about oneself and one's life with clients, or having difficulty telling a client that the practitioner can't help. Consider the following:

1. A practitioner decided to work with the body because his family never touched him after he was 12 years old, except when he was punished. And, as an adult, he was only touched sexually. He wanted to learn about touching that wasn't punitive or sexual.

2. A practitioner spoke of how she was never verbally intimate or physically close with anyone in her family and that her work satisfied her need for non-sexual intimacy. She also realized that she was using her work as a way to avoid developing intimate friendships.

3. A practitioner realized she needed to re-enter therapy after learning she was overstepping her clients' boundaries by asking invasive questions. Her questions related to her own intense curiosity and weren't really relevant or useful to the therapy. In other words, her interventions with the client served her needs and not those of the client.

Points to Ponder

Is it ethical for a practitioner to use her touch practice to fulfill her own need for non-sexual touch or intimacy? How can you investigate your own issues and motivations, to prepare yourself to be an effective and appropriate practitioner?

Clarity about where and how the practitioner gets her personal needs met for touch, intimacy, and sexuality is an important aspect of preparing to work with survivors. Undergoing personal psychotherapy is an excellent way for the practitioner to explore her level of awareness about these issues as well as the ability to communicate effectively. Psychotherapy is a good place to investigate and understand one's own unmet needs before and during the work with survivors because of the many strong feelings that may arise during this process.

Ethical Dimensions

The ethical dimensions inherent in bodywork are intensified in working with survivors. Many touch practitioners who actively work with trauma survivors incorporate a code of ethics that is similar to that for psychotherapists. Having a clear ethical code that is thought through and adhered to is an important part of a practitioner's commitment to the survivor and the survivor's healing. Practitioners keep the treatment client-centered by paying careful attention to ethical boundaries including: relationships with clients outside the treatment context; respect for the client's confidentiality; precision with financial dealings; willingness to admit mistakes; and honesty if the situation goes beyond the practitioner's expertise.

Secondary Traumatization

Psychotherapists sometimes experience secondary traumatization when they work with survivors of abuse or psychological terror.[42] This is sometimes true of children of survivors as well.[43] They may even take on some of the symptoms of posttraumatic stress disorder (PTSD). A somatic practitioner may also experience the fear, outrage, and despair of the survivor client—particularly if her practice includes a large percentage of trauma victims. She may feel suddenly helpless in the face of the client's pain and emotions, emotionally vulnerable, and unable to protect herself well. Secondary traumatization is often referred to as vicarious traumatization, yet the latter is best described as a cumulative transformative effect of working with survivors of traumatic life events.

During a session, if a survivor chooses to tell the practitioner about abuse experiences, the sharing may stimulate uncomfortable feelings in the practitioner or memories from the past. If a practitioner feels overwhelmed by something a client says, a countertransference is probably occurring. The practitioner should process these feelings, memories, or countertransference in a supervision session, in psychotherapy, or with a colleague. Sharing these kinds of feelings and thoughts with the client is inappropriate. Practitioners need a process to work through the feelings stimulated by their clients' stories of abuse, or their unresolved feelings will impair their effectiveness.

Considering Traumatization

- How can you recognize secondary or vicarious traumatization in yourself?
- What can you do when you feel overwhelmed with a particular client?
- What steps can you take to deepen your understanding of trauma and its physiological impacts?
- Identify several resources to support you and your clients.

Supervision and Support

Setting up solid support systems for oneself before working with survivors is essential. Many issues and difficulties occur for the experienced practitioner, as well as for the novice: transference and countertransference; feelings of vicarious traumatization of the practitioner; and tricky situations in which the client unconsciously tries to reenact the abuse. Arrange for regular supervision with a psychotherapist who is an experienced supervisor and who has worked with abuse survivors. Ideally, this person has some familiarity with somatic therapies as well.

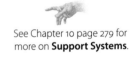

See Chapter 10 page 279 for more on **Support Systems**.

Define Practitioner Requirements

- Describe the three most crucial practitioner pre-requisites for serving trauma survivors.
- What are the fundamental requirements for serving survivors of abuse? Are these in place for your practice? If not, how can you provide them?
- Identify helpful and unhelpful motives for working with trauma survivors.

Client Prerequisites

Clients need to be in a place in their therapeutic process where they'll gain benefit from bodywork. They should be in therapy and at an appropriate stage in their recovery. Clients must be ready and strong enough to deal with the increased intensity of the psychotherapy process that touch therapy often elicits.

Engaged in Psychotherapy

Before beginning treatment with an abuse survivor, it's important to confirm that the person is working with a psychotherapist and that the psychotherapist has agreed that it's a good idea for the survivor to receive your type of treatment. Psychotherapy is the primary therapeutic relationship for working through survivor issues. (Survivor groups are also an essential part of the recovery and therapeutic process.)

Appropriate Stage of Recovery

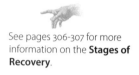

See pages 306-307 for more information on the **Stages of Recovery**.

Bodywork is generally most helpful as part of the third stage of recovery (reconnection), when the client is integrating her trauma experience and when she is building connections with the outside world.[44] Bodywork is sometimes helpful during the second stage of recovery (remembrance and mourning) as a means of making contact with the body, learning to like the body, and, in some cases, to help recover memories.[45] The psychotherapist and client decide together if the time is right for a collaboration.

When treatment is undertaken too soon, it may trigger memories that the client isn't prepared to handle. In these cases the client often experiences the hands-on work as recreating the trauma experience. There may be episodes of escalating intrusive symptoms, crying, sleep disturbance, and increased flashbacks.[46] Bodywork is generally inappropriate during the first stage of recovery (establishing safety), which requires very careful building of trust and safety between the client and psychotherapist. When repressed memories emerge from a client who is accustomed to receiving touch therapies as regular part of his health care, the practitioner may need to educate the client about the wisdom of suspending touch therapy during the initial stage of recovery.

Consent to Communicate

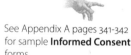

See Appendix A pages 341-342 for sample **Informed Consent** forms.

A client's psychotherapist and touch practitioner should consult regularly during the body therapy process. This may happen only at important junctures or once each month if the client is securely into the third stage of recovery. In other instances, weekly contact may be required. When a client experiences a flashback or a very strong memory during a treatment, it's useful for the practitioner, as well as the client, to communicate this to the psychotherapist. The psychotherapist may also make helpful suggestions as to where the bodywork might be concentrated at different points in the therapy. The client must be willing to give consent for this communication. This permission should be given in writing at the beginning of the first or second session and kept in the practitioner's files for his protection.

Before the work begins, the client must understand that sessions are confidential and only the psychotherapist, practitioner, and supervisor involved discuss the client's sessions. Some clients may feel most comfortable if the practitioner openly discusses which details he will be sharing with the client's psychotherapist.

Special Boundary Issues

Certain boundaries are built into the practitioner/client relationship that are quite different from those between friends, colleagues, or family members. How they're understood and applied has a profound effect on the quality of relationships with clients. This is particularly true for working with survivors of sexual abuse. Melissa Soalt describes her observations:

> Because abuse disrespects and destroys one's boundaries, survivors typically have poorly developed boundaries. To feel "safe," many survivors resort to a familiar isolation and erect dense protective barriers. Conversely, survivors often describe feelings of defenselessness and vulnerability that are equated with having "no skin" of one's own, and therefore, having no internal shock absorption. Everything feels "jarring" and triggering and personal. Creating flexible and appropriate boundaries can be extremely challenging for survivors.[47]

The boundaries of survivors have been crossed and broken repeatedly. Because of this past abuse, survivors often don't consciously recognize boundaries and protect themselves. Consider this example:

> I wasn't only molested by my father, but by my grandfather on my father's side. It was somehow accepted that my grandfather could put his arms around us, could pet our legs, could French kiss us when he greeted us, you know....This would be in public, and, yet, there was my mom smiling, there was my dad smiling, and his French kissing me in private wasn't far from that. Where did I draw the line? I didn't know.[48]

Practitioners need to be sensitive to the boundaries of touch both during and after treatments. For instance, when greeting or saying goodbye to a client do you shake hands, do you put your hand on the client's shoulder or back, or do you hug the client? These are all questions to think through and talk about when working with any client, and especially when working with a survivor. The boundaries of survivors have been so violated that they may be unaware of being violated, or don't protect themselves by saying no to unwanted touch, even if they're aware of it. The range of physical contact on and off the table must be handled very carefully with survivors.

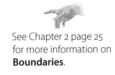

See Chapter 2 page 25 for more information on **Boundaries**.

Careful attention to boundaries helps to empower the client and protect against excessive, unmanageable transference reactions. The practitioner who works with survivors must maintain clear, consistent boundaries to both provide and model a relationship with good boundaries. An important part of the touch therapy work is to help the client rebuild boundaries and, thereby, empower the survivor to protect himself. The highest ethical standards on the practitioner's part are essential to the healing process.

Special Boundary Considerations

- List examples of how a practitioner can help a survivor rebuild physical and emotional boundaries during a session.
- Describe why a trauma survivor undergoing touch therapy should be in psychotherapy.
- Why is it important for the practitioner working with trauma survivors to understand transference and countertransference?
- Why is it unadvisable to engage in dual relationships with clients who are trauma survivors?
- Describe situations in working with a trauma survivor where supervision would be useful and necessary.
- Role-play the questions and concerns you would or could bring to a supervisor.

Protocol for Working with Self-Disclosed Survivors

We have discussed the nature of abuse, critical psychological concepts, and a number of prerequisites for working with survivors. The ethical practitioner attends not only to his treatment skills but his relational interactions and business practices as well. Nowhere is this more important than in working with a survivor of abuse or trauma.

A practitioner begins working with a survivor in a number of ways: a client is referred by her psychotherapist as part of the psychotherapy process; the practitioner is contacted by a survivor who has heard about the practitioner through a friend, or who has read about the benefits of hands-on therapy; or a current client discloses his status of previous abuse.

Initial Contact: The Phone Interview

The first contact with a new client begins when a practitioner talks with a client who has disclosed during a telephone call that he is a survivor of abuse. After asking for the caller's name and the name of the referring person or psychotherapist, an opportunity exists to create an appropriate context. The therapeutic relationship starts here by establishing boundaries, structure, and an initial sense of safety. Advance knowledge of the practitioner's approach to the initial and subsequent sessions benefits potential clients. Ask the person if she would like a brief description of an initial session. You might say something like:

> My first session is an hour and a half long. For the first half of the session I ask you for some information and give you a chance to ask me any questions. I see the first session as an exploration of whether we would like to work together. After 30-40 minutes of conversation you decide if you would like a short hands-on session.

Let the client know from the start that she is in charge. You might also say:

> If you aren't sure, if you want to think about it for a week, or if the match doesn't feel right to you, we can stop to give you time to decide.

At this point you could say something like:

> My fee for the first hour and a half session is $175 and for subsequent hour-long sessions it's $100. If you decide not to continue the session I don't charge anything for the initial 40 minutes (or, "I only charge $50"). If we do decide to work together and continue, I charge you for the full session.

NOTE: We recommend offering a reduced fee or not charging anything if the session stops at this point. The client shouldn't pay a practitioner to determine if the practitioner instills a sense of safety.

Always establish financial arrangements on the telephone to minimize the possibility of misunderstanding. Many practitioners also include additional information on the telephone such as clarifying that the client is in charge of where on the body the practitioner works and the amount of clothing the client removes for the treatment. The initial telephone call is a good time to mention if you have a sliding fee scale and how it's negotiated.

During the telephone conversation, also ask the client if there's anything she would like to ask you before the appointment. This invitation opens the door if the client feels hesitant. What you have done during this initial telephone conversation is begin the relationship. The client knows that she is free to interview you and shares control of the process.

Everything you discuss on the phone is to be repeated at the beginning of the first session. It is also best to put everything in writing for clarity, especially if the person's primary mode of processing information is visual. Sometimes the client is experiencing fear and anxiety just making the telephone call and most of what is discussed will be forgotten. Conducting telephone interviews along these lines gives a feeling of mutuality and respect, regardless of the specific arrangements.

> If you learn only methods you'll be forever tied to those methods. However, if you learn the principles behind those methods, you'll be free to devise your own methods.
>
> —Ralph Waldo Emerson

The Physical Environment

The physical environment of the practitioner's office should create a sense of safety and comfort. Some suggest making the office colors soft and neutral. If the practitioner works in a medical clinic, he might make it look less sterile by adding a few personal effects and some plants in the office. If the practitioner works in a home office, keep the treatment room separate from living space (if at all possible) and decorate it in a way that makes it feel professional. Minimize clutter in the waiting area and office. Be sure the windows are covered and there is a smock or a sheet laid out for the client. If possible, have a separate bathroom that's free of personal belongings. Before the client enters the office or treatment room, draw the curtains or blinds to ensure privacy.

Be sure the office is reasonably soundproof. Use a sleep sound machine or quiet music if the soundproofing isn't up to par. Choose music carefully; avoid songs with sexual lyrics, seductive instrumental music, or indistinct sounds. For instance, chants easily trigger flashbacks of cult abuse. Place literature (e.g., books, brochures, and articles that deal with abuse) in the waiting room. The practitioner might put a statement of policies in a small binder for clients to read (this statement can also be sent to the client prior to the first session). Exercise restraint with scents as they can be powerful flashback triggers, particularly flowery fragrances and incense.

First Session Preliminaries

As the client enters the treatment room or waiting area, greet the client in a friendly yet professional way. Shake hands only if the client extends a hand toward you first. If the client has to wait before you begin together, give him relevant literature to read or the written history form to fill out.

The Pre-Treatment Mutual Interview

After a client is settled in a chair, restate what was discussed on the telephone. As previously noted, it's very likely that the client was anxious during the initial phone conversation and doesn't remember everything that was said. Let the client know that the first half of the session is spent in conversation during which the client has an opportunity to ask questions.

Review Policies

After reviewing the structure of the first session, outline the policies for the client. Make sure that everything is understood. Have a written set of standard policies as well as a statement about survivors available for the client and go over those documents together. The following section highlights additional policy considerations for working with abuse survivors. Give the client opportunities to ask questions about your policies so that mutuality can be established. She has the right to ask questions about your approach, the ethical dimensions of the work, and any other questions about the treatment.

- CANCELLATION POLICY. When working with a survivor, as with any client, be clear about the cancellation policy. Some practitioners have a two-, five-, or 24-hour cancellation policy. Whatever your policy is, make the boundary clear and stick to it, allowing for the same flexibility you would give to any client if a situation arises where there is unusual distress or extraordinary circumstances.
- SUPERVISION. Inform the client of the kind of professional supervision you receive on all your clients and its function.
- CODE OF ETHICS. Tell the client that you follow a professional code of ethics developed by your profession or yourself and offer to give him a copy. Clearly state that you don't engage in social, intimate, sexual, or business relationships with your clients.
- CONFIDENTIALITY. Speak about the confidential nature of the therapeutic relationship. Affirm that while you must maintain confidentiality, *she* isn't bound to keep anything you say or do confidential. Let the client know that while you won't ask for any details about her abuse history, she is welcome to share any details that she feels is helpful to your work together.
- COLLABORATIVE NATURE OF YOUR WORK. Stress the importance of collaboration with the client and his psychotherapist or counselor. If the client isn't currently in psychotherapy, explain the benefits to consider it while receiving bodywork. Describe the possibility of opening up areas of memory, experience, and feelings, and the necessity of having a place to share and explore those experiences. It is assumed here that the treatment you undertake is specifically aimed at helping the client reconnect with her body—focused on dealing with the physical ramifications of the abuse.

- **Delayed Discovery of Sexual Abuse.** Sometimes a person comes for hands-on therapy and doesn't know he is a survivor, but figures it out after a period of treatment (this occurs with some frequency). If the client isn't in psychotherapy or his counselor isn't specifically trained to work with survivors, it's wise to delay treatment until the person settles into a supportive psychotherapy situation. Keep a list of referrals for such situations.
- **Level of Therapy.** After establishing that the client is in psychotherapy, ask the client if his psychotherapist agrees that he is in an appropriate stage of recovery for body therapy. When the client is referred by a psychotherapist, the appropriateness of treatment has probably been previously established.
- **Informed Consent.** As an addendum to the confidentiality agreement, inform the client that the only other persons who know about your work together are your supervisor (who won't know the client's name and identity), and the client's psychotherapist.
- **Disrobing.** A clear statement about disrobing is critical when working with survivors if the type of treatment you provide normally involves removal of clothing. Stress the importance of comfort for the client. Let the client know that she dresses and undresses in private. Make it clear that the client decides what she feels comfortable wearing: she can wear some or all of her clothing; take off shoes and socks only; or wear a smock. Let the client know it isn't at all unusual to leave clothes on for some time. It is recommended that a survivor not completely disrobe, even if completely covered under a sheet. Leaving underwear on helps create a safe boundary for the genital area. Tell the client that she is always covered with a sheet or towel except for the area you're working on. Give instructions such as, "I leave the room for you to change in private. Once you have had time to change, get on the table and cover yourself, I'll knock on the door before entering and ask if you're ready."

Take the Client History

After the mutual interview and policy discussion, review the client's history to build further rapport and gain valuable knowledge about the client's situation. Establish the survivor's strengths in creating strategies for his survival. Practitioners need to identify and build on the capacities and skills that helped the survivor get to where she is now. The history also assists the practitioner in finding out whether it's appropriate for the client to undertake bodywork at this time. When the client comes in, some practitioners have the client fill out a brief history form in the outer office before entering the treatment room; others just ask the questions verbally.

The history form, in addition to the normal details, should cover these questions:
- Are you seeing any other healthcare practitioners (e.g. medical doctor, psychotherapist) regularly?
- Have you had any type of body therapy before? If yes, was it a positive, negative, or neutral experience?
- What strategies help you manage some of the symptoms and stresses you have worked through?
- How are you feeling now in anticipation of this session?
- What would you like to accomplish from our work together?

At the end of the history form or on a separate form include the following statement:

I hereby give permission to (practitioner's name) and my psychotherapist (the psychotherapist's name) to exchange relevant information to help me in my healing process.

Have the client sign and date this statement. At the bottom of the history form you might add:

Please feel free to add additional comments below that might be helpful in our working together.

> Healing is a matter of time, but it is also a matter of opportunity.
>
> —Hippocrates

Follow-Up Questions

When reviewing the history you have the opportunity to build a connection, in addition to gaining some relevant new information. Ask the client about the following:

- **PAINS, INJURIES OR MEDICAL CONDITIONS**. This lets you know where to exercise caution. You don't want to cause the client any pain in the treatment.
- **MEDICATIONS AND DRUGS**. Certain medications affect the client's ability to feel sensations in the skin. Ask about the use of alcohol, recreational drugs, and smoking. These questions give you some idea if substance dependency is an issue for the client.
- **PERSONAL CARE**. This indicates how much the client takes care of himself physically, (e.g., exercise, diet, health care). Answers to these questions tell you the degree of care or abuse of his body.
- **BODY AWARENESS**. Obtain an idea of the degree to which the client is in touch with her body by asking where she carries stress and tension. Compare the client's assessment with your own after working on the client. If the client is fairly unaware, you may approach working with this client somewhat differently than if the client were more aware. For example, if a client thinks that her body is relaxed but in fact is quite tense, move gently and slowly in bringing that awareness to the client. Do not say, "Your back is really tense like a rock." On the other hand, you can speak more directly with a client who demonstrates keen awareness when telling you where she feels tension or deadness.
- **PREVIOUS BODYWORK**. If the client has had a bad experience or has never had bodywork before, you know to be careful and what needs more preparation. If the previous bodywork was a good experience, ask why the client didn't go back to that practitioner. This gives you information as to what the client is hoping to get from working with a new practitioner.

Ask a few open-ended questions after the history and follow-up to give the client an opportunity to offer additional information. At this time, it might be appropriate to ask if the client has ever experienced flashbacks. If so, ask what has been helpful in those experiences. You may ask, "Is there anything else you would like me to know?" but not "Have you had any particular abuse experiences that might impact our work?" In the second instance, the client might experience the question as intrusive—putting pressure on the client to reveal more than he initially wants to share.

Asking questions in a neutral manner shows care and interest. When clients feel comfortable and need to tell the practitioner about some aspect of their experience, they will. During one such open-ended conversation a client described being sexually molested and tortured around her face and neck. She had let the practitioner know when she was ready. The practitioner then knew to take special care when working near or on her face and neck. Another client revealed that a therapist had sexually abused him and that he was very anxious about the session. Others simply respond to this question by saying "No." Never push to elicit information from clients. When a client is ready, she will tell you what she wants you to know.

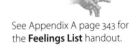

See Appendix A page 343 for the **Feelings List** handout.

Let the client know that sometimes survivors experience difficult emotional feelings or bodily sensations during or after a bodywork session, like a tingling feeling in the hands or feet, intense heat, or momentary dizziness. Give them the trauma survivor handout "Feelings List" found in Appendix A. You might also say, "If that happens, I will do my best to help you understand what's happening and refer you to additional sources of support if that appears necessary or appropriate."

Transition to Bodywork

In the first session, the mutual interview and history-taking requires about 30-40 minutes. After this phase is complete, it's time to ask the client, "Would you like to continue the session and have a hands-on treatment today, or would you prefer to stop now and think about whether you would like to work with me?" If the client isn't sure, suggest that he think about it and call to schedule a hands-on session when it feels right. Do not let anxiety or the desire to work with a particular client justify pressuring a client to continue. The treatment is more effective when you allow the client to be in charge.

If the client decides he wants to continue the session and try the hands-on work, move to the next phase which involves the specific work that the client and practitioner undertake together.

Set Goals Together

Ask the client what goals and expectations she has for the treatment. Discuss long-term goals and set short-term goals for the first session together. If the client has difficulty with this, give some examples of realistic goals such as: This treatment process helps me reduce the tension in my body so I feel positive and enjoyable sensations when touched; I remain present when being touched; I am not afraid when being touched; I feel connected with my body; I become more aware of how my body feels.

A short-term goal for the session might be to see if touch therapy is something he wants to do. Other short-term goals could be specific such as: I remain present while having my feet touched; I learn how to relax when touched on the foot; I allow work on my lower legs. Having the client establish a goal that the practitioner agrees can be accomplished in a session or two places a manageable limit or boundary on the session and puts the client in charge of the treatment options.

Empower the Client

Emphasize that you work as a team and that the client knows more about what he needs than the practitioner does. Consider saying something like, "I may make certain suggestions which you can decide to accept or reject." Invite the client to make suggestions. If you're uncertain about the appropriateness of the requests, discuss these with a supervisor or psychotherapist.

Tell the client, "You determine where on your body I work, how deeply I work, and how long I work in certain areas." Some clients like to use a body chart to identify zones where it's okay to be touched and zones where it isn't okay to be touched. The client is free to stop the session at any point. A technique that might make the client comfortable is citing examples of statements other clients made that relate to this situation such as: "One client asked me to work on her head and neck the first three months, and added the feet during the next two months; one client asked me to only insert acupuncture needles on the front of her body for the first few sessions; one client requested that I refrain from any direct manipulations to his neck for the first two months of treatments." It is reassuring for a client to know that it took someone else a bit of time to receive a standard treatment. The examples given must be real and truthful. Be careful to change details to protect the person's identity. Safeguard confidentiality when discussing another client's experience by changing details to protect the person's identity.

Develop with the client a one word cue that the client can say if he wants you to stop touching him. The simplicity helps when a client feels a rush of emotional overload. "Off" or "stop" can work, as can any word. In the first hands-on session, practice with the client by placing your hands on different areas and have the client say the chosen word. Then you remove your hands. Practicing in a non-activated moment encourages the client that it's okay to speak his needs and that you'll respect them.

Sometimes survivors see practitioners to receive the physical benefits of the work while others utilize the practitioner's work as a means to reconnect the survivor with her body and to gain control of that process. When the body is touched, many abuse survivors dissociate;

a major part of treatment is working with the client to stay with her body sensations while being touched. Other survivors become hypervigilant, or overfocus on the specifics of what is being done, and consequently don't relax. For these clients, the task is to defuse the narrowed concentration and to learn to focus on a wide area or on the entire body at once.

Create Emotional Safety

Ascertain what degree of safety has been established so far by asking how the client feels in anticipation of the physical part of the session. You might ask, "How would you like me to respond if you become upset—for instance, if you feel sad and begin to cry?" One client might request that you leave the room for a few minutes; another may ask you to just sit quietly for a moment and wait for him to finish. Remember that even though a client has expressed a preference beforehand, it's vital to check when feelings come up because the client may have a need that wasn't previously expressed.

During the initial discussion, a client may ask you to induce memories. If this happens, explain that memories come when the person feels safe enough to remember and that forcing memories to surface isn't useful. In fact, this can often be detrimental or harmful to the process and can derail your work together. Perhaps, share examples from this book. You can also say something like the following:

> Many clients experience emotional difficulty when trying to induce memories. Several clients related stories of being overwhelmed by memories that were forcefully induced in this way. One had to go to bed for weeks, another started a cycle of frequent uncontrollable flashbacks that took months of therapy to stabilize.[49]

Ask if the client has ever had a flashback or experienced being regressed to a frightening situation. Ask if this has ever occurred during a touch therapy session. Inquire as to what would be useful if a flashback occurred in a session. For instance, some clients might want the practitioner to immediately take her hands off the body and make eye contact; others would feel more comfortable if the practitioner's hand was placed on the client's arm or shoulder, or held the client's hand; and yet other clients might recommend that the practitioner cover them with a blanket and ask them to sit up or stand up to bring them back from the flashback.

The following exercise[50] assists to create safety, determine where to work, and to support the client in taking control of the bodywork. Some clients find the exercise helpful. After describing it, ask the client if he would be willing to try the exercise.

Practical Application: First Touch Exercise

1. Tell the client, "You have control of the treatment process with regard to the parts of the body I work on, the amount of pressure used, the types of work performed, and so forth. I would like to try something if you're willing." Then explain 2, 3 and 4.
2. With the client clothed and sitting in a chair say, "Tell me a part of your body where it would be comfortable to be touched while sitting here, for example your shoulder, hand, or back."
3. Say to the client, "Tell me when it's okay to touch you." When the client signals it's okay, touch firmly but gently.
4. Now tell the client, "Let me know when you would like me to remove my hand with a nod or a few words."

The Hands-On Treatment

When beginning the hands-on work, the practitioner demonstrates to the client that she intends that the client takes the lead in the process and starts the treatment on the area that the client requests.

Structure

Treatment structures create safety. It doesn't matter what the structure is as long as it's clear and establishes a routine that the client can count on. Do certain things the same way each week at each session. Pay special attention to being on time for the appointment. Whenever possible, schedule the appointment for the same time each week. Always ask the same one or two questions at the beginning of each treatment, for instance, "Is there anything about the last session or how you felt afterward that you want to tell me?" Then ask the client what he would like you to do today and where he would like you to work. Refrain from altering the routine unless the client is included in the process of making the change.

Set goals for each session and encourage the client to talk about the goals at the beginning of the session. *The Handbook on Sensitive Practice for Health Professionals* states, "Consent must be an ongoing, interactive process. Do not assume that consent given today applies to all successive days: ask for consent on each successive day of treatment."[51] At the beginning of each session, also repeat the statement that the client undress to her level of comfort. Do not allow interruptions during the session, including answering the telephone. Distractions interrupt attention and focus. Maintain clear touch boundaries; be careful not to touch the client's body casually when she isn't on the table.

Pace and Predictability of Touch

Move slowly from one part of the body to another. Before moving to the next part of the body to be touched, tell the client what will be done there, especially if it's different from the kinds of touch done just previously. For instance, when moving from the hand to the upper arm, or from the neck to the lower back, tell the client this is about to happen. Then, ask if it feels okay to proceed.

Create a kind of shorthand communication. If what you're doing is fine with the client, it may be suggested that the client say "okay" when asked. If not, he might say "no," which signals you to move on. This again puts direct control in the hands of the client. Every time the client says "okay" or "no," he is setting the boundaries. At first, you may ask rather frequently, "How's this?" "Is this movement all right?" As the work on a particular body part progresses over time, the frequency with which you ask questions may diminish. But as the work moves to another body part, the questioning process starts over again. If it becomes obvious that all the moves are okay, ask the client if he wants less "checking in" or for you to stop asking. The responses to this technique vary. Some find it very empowering, but after a while, it might become annoying.

Voice Quality

The tone of voice carries emotional messages such as warmth, kindness, professional distance, boredom, impatience, and condescension. Be conscious of the messages created through your voice. The quality and presence of voice is important. When a practitioner feels empathic, accepting, and positively disposed toward the client, she is gentle, genuine, concerned, and present in the feeling tone of the voice. When this isn't occurring (it isn't easy to recognize in oneself), the practitioner may want to work with a teacher, supervisor, or colleague to get some feedback on empathic abilities and what is coming through in the quality of her voice.

Be aware that some clients may react to a hypnotic voice by going into a trance state that encourages dissociation. Check out how your voice is being received by the client.

Language

Practitioners must have a feel for appropriate language when working with trauma survivors. Language should be warm and professional, not intimate, yet not so formal as to be distancing. Practitioners who use language that is too familiar, too critical, or contains a sexual overtone inevitably violate a client's boundary. For instance, making unsolicited positive, negative, or even neutral comments about the person's body (i.e., not in the treatment contract) is a violation of a client's boundary if the client hasn't asked for this feedback. Comments like, "Boy, your spine is kind of twisted, it needs work!" or "Was it hard for you to lose weight?" are inappropriate boundary crossings even if these issues were part of the reason the client came to see the practitioner.

Being Present

Being present is the most important factor in treating survivors. This means that the practitioner needs to be attentive moment by moment to where the client is in relation to the work being done. Because it's common for survivors to dissociate or become hypervigilant, the practitioner needs to find ways to frequently check in to see if the client is present, and if not, bring the client more into contact with himself. The practitioner can explore creative ways to help the client remain present to his experience of touch as it occurs. If the client is dissociating, one helpful technique is to instruct the client to focus attention on the point being worked on, or to imagine breathing into that part of the body. If the person becomes hypervigilant and overfocused, suggest releasing that focus onto a broader, more general area. If this is a problem, try frequently switching the area of the body being worked.

Suggest visual images, or request that the client brings a favorite piece of music to listen to . during the session. Sometimes having the eyes open allows the client to feel more present, while others prefer their eyes closed. Actively working together to find what assists the client continues to build trust and a sense of safety. The more present the practitioner is, the more possible it is for the client to be present as well.

Throughout a session, a practitioner can bring his attention to his own inner experience. Taking deep breaths or slowing the pace can give him space to shift any uncomfortable feelings, sensations, or thoughts flowing within him. If a practitioner's inner experiences become intense, one option is to excuse himself briefly from the room to re-focus, re-center, and re-ground before returning. If a practitioner zones out from his own or his client's experiences, there is a greater risk that the client will become triggered or dissociated.

> If you can learn from hard knocks, you can also learn from soft touches.
>
> —Carolyn Gilmore

Continuous Communications

Working with survivors of abuse requires a special type of communication during the treatment. Actively track the client as the session proceeds to prevent disassociation. For instance, it's helpful to regularly ask, "How are you doing?" or "Where are you?" This brings the client's attention and awareness into the body. Another possibility is to say something like, "I am focusing on your foot," and then begin to make positive affirming statements from time to time, like, "Are you experiencing your foot relaxing?" or "I think your foot is letting go, but I'm not sure. Tell me what you feel."

Clients frequently withdraw or lose connection to their experience and have no idea how or why this happened. By exploring these reactions together, over time, awareness develops that helps a client begin to understand her own behavior. These kinds of interactions encourage the client's collaboration with the practitioner in the exploration of her body.

Closure

As you move toward the last two or three minutes of the hands-on portion of the session, tell the client that the hands-on part of the session is close to finishing. As this segment ends always fully re-drape the client or re-adjust the clothing (this may seem obvious, but many practitioners forget this simple act). Tell the client that the bodywork portion of the session is over and then leave the room. After you leave, the client dresses (or rests awhile before dressing). Knock before returning or instruct the client to indicate he is ready by opening the door.

Leave time to talk with the client at the end of the session. After returning to the room, ask how the client is feeling and how the session went. Ask if the client wants to talk about anything specific that happened during the session, and if anything could've been done differently, which would be helpful in the future. Encourage the client to tell you if any boundaries were inadvertently crossed. Because this is usually difficult for the client, consider an opening like: "Did I work too hard on any part of your body?" or "Did I move too quickly?" Use your judgment as to when such questions are appropriate. Often, the first or second session is too soon.

Figure 11.3 Checklist for Somatic Therapy with Trauma Survivors

1. Conduct a thorough intake interview.
2. Assess the recovery stage before consenting to work with a self-disclosed survivor.
3. Spend time connecting with the client.
4. Consider using subtle, gentle, non-invasive body therapy techniques.
5. Invest in education about trauma and shock, and understanding their somatic impact. There are resource centers that offer such training.
6. Always remember to ask permission to touch. Be willing and ready to wait and not to touch.
7. Remind a client that she can change her mind and revoke permission at any time in the session.
8. Establish a relational connection first. Never touch mechanically.
9. If a flashback occurs, bring the person back to the present immediately.
10. Keep in regular contact with the client's psychotherapist. Have clear, written permission from your client for these conversations.
11. Be gentle but clear about boundaries.
12. Behave as a team and set goals together.
13. Allow the client to control the pace of the treatment.
14. Allot a time for closure at the end of each session.
15. Be present, inquire and never assume. Do not hesitate to check with your client, asking about her experience.
16. Develop a referral list of psychotherapists and counselors. Establish personal connections with these therapists before you refer them clients.
17. Develop the skills that allow you to distinguish shock from trauma and to identify them when they're activated.
18. Receive bodywork or energy medicine treatment yourself to clear your own system of fatigue and repression, thereby preventing secondary traumatization and burnout.
19. Consider volunteering at a local safehouse for survivors of domestic violence or joining the bodywork team at an AIDS service agency. These organizations usually provide a volunteer training that is excellent education about the treatment of trauma.
20. Cultivate a supervisory relationship and bring issues to your supervisor or peer supervision group.

This checklist is adapted with permission from Stephanie Mines, PH.D.[52]

Feelings

Feelings often surface after touch therapy. Discuss this with your client at the end of the first session. The "Feelings List" handout briefly describes common after-effects that may be experienced after the session. Supplying the client with this information, either verbally or in writing (or both), is quite useful to the survivor, especially given that in the first few weeks of bodywork many of these sensations and feelings occur. Knowledge of these possible responses helps create client safety and comfort. You have permission to freely copy the Feelings List and give it to your clients.

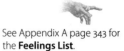

See Appendix A page 343 for the **Feelings List**.

▌ Conclusion

Touch therapy is a powerful adjunct in the recovery from abuse. With this power comes the need for great responsibility on the part of the practitioner. The practitioner who provides ethical treatment for abuse survivors comes from a place of sensitivity, caring, and the desire to help, as well as from one of detailed education, extensive training, and ongoing supervision. Bodywork might be the first experience of pain relief or nurturing that survivors have on the physical level. It may be the path home.

Appendix A
Forms

Boundary Clarification Activity Answer Key

Client Bill of Rights

Sample Massage Therapy Center Policies

Sample Asian Medicine Office Policies

Sample Massage Therapy Informed Consent

Sample School Clinic Informed Consent

Trauma Survivor Handout: Feelings List

Boundary Clarification Activity Answer Key

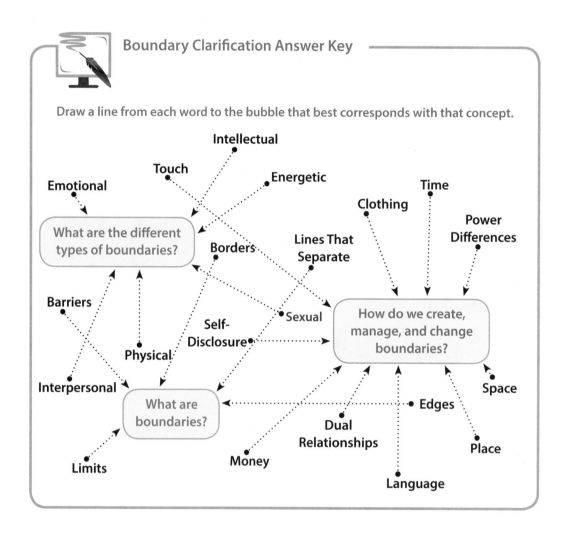

Boundary Clarification Answer Key

Draw a line from each word to the bubble that best corresponds with that concept.

Intellectual

Touch

Emotional

Energetic

Time

Clothing

Power
Differences

What are the different
types of boundaries?

Borders

Lines That
Separate

Barriers

Self-
Disclosure

Sexual

How do we create,
manage, and change
boundaries?

Interpersonal

Physical

Space

What are
boundaries?

Dual
Relationships

Edges

Place

Limits

Money

Language

▦ Client Bill of Rights

An informational handout for consumers of healthcare services

This handout has been prepared to better inform you about sexual misconduct in the health and wellness field. It delineates your rights as a consumer and tells you how to protect yourself if your rights are violated.

In this brochure, the client is defined as anyone who receives services for any therapy or health care. Sexual misconduct is defined as including sexual touching of the client by the practitioner and/or any activity or verbal behavior that is sexual in nature. Sexual contact includes a wide range of behaviors besides intercourse; it includes any behaviors that aim to arouse sexual feelings. They range from suggestive verbal remarks to erotic hugging and kissing, in addition to direct sexual contact. The behavior does not have to be coercive to be inappropriate.

Broken Boundaries

Within the therapeutic relationship, it is always the responsibility of the therapist, doctor, or health professional to set and maintain a professional boundary. It is not unusual or abnormal for a client to feel attracted to a healthcare practitioner who has treated them with kindness, care, and attention. However, for a practitioner to take advantage of this special vulnerability and to move the relationship into a social or sexual one, even if the client wants it, is always inappropriate and unethical. At this point, we can say that a practitioner is abusing his/her power within the relationship and is no longer able to put the needs and rights of the client first.

All types of therapy and healthcare services can be of invaluable help to many people. The vast majority of therapists and health professionals practice in an ethical manner. Unfortunately, sometimes sexual misconduct does occur in treatment relationships. A sexually intimate relationship between a client/patient and a therapist, physician, or healthcare professional is never appropriate and is a violation of professional ethics.

Consumer Rights

You have a right to:
- safe treatment, free from physical, sexual, or emotional abuse.
- refuse treatment and not be pressured to continue.
- question any action that you experience as invasive or sexual.
- terminate treatment if you feel threatened.
- discuss your therapy/health care with friends outside of the therapy relationship.
- professional consultation with other practitioners to discuss your situation.
- report unethical and illegal behavior.

Warning Signs of Sexual Inappropriateness

- The practitioner makes sexual jokes or references that are inappropriate to treatment.
- You have any concern that a treatment relationship is moving from the professional to the inappropriately personal.
- The practitioner tells you his or her intimate personal problems.
- You are asked to go outside the bounds of a professional relationship such as going on a dinner date or a social meeting outside the office.
- The practitioner tells you that having a sexual relationship with him or her is good treatment and/or the only way you can get well.
- The practitioner offers you recreational drugs or alcohol.
- The practitioner suggests that you be secretive about your relationship with him or her and that you do not discuss it with anyone.
- The practitioner suggests to you that forms of touching you consider to be intimate have been proven to be therapeutic for your condition.
- You feel that something is not right in the practitioner's behavior toward you, but you cannot quite pinpoint what is happening.

If you experience any of these warning signs, trust your own feelings and intuition. Talk to a friend or neutral third party, or talk directly to the practitioner if you feel comfortable doing so. Otherwise, talk to his or her supervisor, consult a different practitioner, or if you get no satisfactory response, call the appropriate licensing board or professional association to check on and report the practitioner's behavior.

Common Experiences

If sexual behavior occurs with a health professional, a client may experience feelings that include, but are not limited to:

- confusion about the experience that sometimes encompasses protective, loving, and angry feelings about the abuser, and/or feelings that the client's mind is being controlled.
- fear, isolation, and distrust because the client believes that there is no one to tell, that no one will believe what happened, and/or that he/she is the only one to whom this has happened.
- indecision and/or a temporary inability to make decisions, to work at a job, or to tend to personal needs.
- guilt, shame, and feelings of responsibility (a sexual relationship with a practitioner is always the health professional's responsibility, not the client's).
- depression, feeling out of control or suicidal because the client's trust has been betrayed.
- recurrent nightmares, fears or images of intrusion and/or flashbacks about the experience, and difficulty concentrating in other areas of life.

Options for Recovery

Talk to someone you trust about your experience. There are other clients who have been survivors of sexual misconduct in every state. Many of these individuals have sought and received help from therapy and support groups.

Therapy: Subsequent psychotherapy or body therapy is difficult for many victims to consider, yet it is often vital in providing the necessary support for someone who has been through the trauma of sexual misconduct. Choose a therapist carefully by finding someone who is appropriately outraged by what has happened, someone who has experience in this type of case, or someone who can help think through an effective course for recovery and/or recourse.

Networking: Contacting other individuals who have experienced sexual abuse or misconduct—individually or through support groups—can be extremely helpful. Breaking the silence can be liberating and may help prevent the victimization of others.

Therapist Responsibility: Accept that the therapist is responsible for what has occurred. Understand that most people who have experienced sexual abuse feel that they are at fault or should have behaved differently in some way. These feelings are natural but do not change the fact that the therapist is responsible for his/her misconduct.

Reporting Misconduct: It is important to report abusive therapists. Most people who abuse others do so with many of their clients. Stopping them is essential, whether it takes psychological help, professional censure, revocation of a license, education, or action by the courts.

Possible Actions

The first step, if the situation was not overtly abusive or dangerous, is to speak directly to the therapist and tell him/her what you are feeling. If this is not possible or is unsuccessful, try to talk with the offending practitioner about what happened in the presence of a neutral third party.

This kind of session can be very helpful. If the practitioner fears a lawsuit, he/she is less likely to be willing to do this with you, since the neutral third party could become a witness in a trial. The practitioner that realizes that he/she has made a big mistake and wants an opportunity to apologize may consent to meet with you in the hopes of avoiding legal action. You can often find psychotherapists willing to serve as the third party through a professional therapy association or local advocacy group, such as a Rape Crisis Center. If you choose this option, make sure you are very comfortable with the person you find to be the third party.

If the offending practitioner is willing to meet with a third party, you might want an additional fourth person to be present. Choose someone close to you who is level-headed and could support you and help you talk about this confrontation afterward.

If you choose to approach the practitioner or the organization where you were treated directly, and are satisfied with the response, you may wish to leave it at that. For example, a satisfactory response, depending on the violation, might be that you are given a sincere apology by the practitioner, have your money refunded, and feel assured that appropriate educational measures and psychotherapy for the practitioner will occur or that disciplinary action by the place of employment is being taken. If you are not satisfied with the response you get, you might consider registering a complaint or taking legal action.

Registering Complaints

When ready, and with appropriate support, filing a complaint can be an important phase of the healing process. There are state government agencies called Licensing Boards that receive and investigate complaints. Licensing Boards have the authority to discipline an individual (for example, revoke a license) if that person violates the law. No matter how serious your complaint may be, the Boards have no legal authority to award money damages or to criminally prosecute someone.

Professional organizations also receive complaints about members of their societies. The ethical codes of most professional organizations specifically prohibit sexual contact between therapists/ health professionals and their clients/patients.

Legal Recourse

Another course of action is through the legal system. Be aware that there are time limitations for civil and criminal actions.

Civil Action: A civil lawsuit may be a way to derive some monetary compensation for losses incurred and damages suffered. Attorneys specializing in these cases may be located through victim advocacy groups.

Criminal Action: Criminal prosecution may be pursued through the Office of the District Attorney in the abuser's county. The District Attorney's Office may also have a victim advocate who can assist you and answer questions.

Remember, if you feel that you have been sexually abused in a therapy or healthcare relationship, you can get help. We encourage you to seek help as an important part of your healing process. Please feel free to photocopy, adapt and distribute this article. It is important that this information be available to all consumers of healthcare services.

*This handout was prepared and edited by Ben Benjamin, PH.D., with materials obtained from: The Education Subcommittee of the Massachusetts Committee on Sexual Misconduct by Physicians, Therapists and Other Health Professionals; and materials provided by Estelle Disch, clinical sociologist.

▌ Sample Massage Therapy Center Policies

Background and Training

I have been practicing massage therapy since 1985. I was trained at the Montana School of Massage Therapy in a 750 hour program. The style of bodywork that I practice incorporates Swedish massage, Shiatsu, and a therapy called deep frictioning, which reduces scar tissue caused by injuries. I specialize in working with people of all ages who are athletic and suffer from various types of tension and pain problems. My style of bodywork focuses in two directions:

1. Stress reduction and relaxation
2. Pain reduction and injury recovery

Massage therapy is useful for a variety of pain, injury, and tension problems, but does not address serious medical conditions. After assessing a client, I may refer you to an osteopath, chiropractor, nutritionist, orthopedic surgeon, or an Alexander teacher, among other possibilities.

Who Can Benefit

Massage therapy is successful in working with problems related to excess tension build up, chronic pain, and musculoskeletal injuries. In addition to working with pain and tension problems in the neck, back, ankle, knee, shoulder, and so forth, massage therapy is very effective with people who suffer from chronic headaches, insomnia, and problems of fatigue. These are the areas in which I feel competent.

Massage therapy is also beneficial for pregnant women, and is often used as an adjunct to certain medical conditions on the recommendation of a physician (e.g., high blood pressure, anxiety, stress).

Others that may benefit greatly from massage are people in psychotherapy who would like to be more in touch with their bodies.

Client/Practitioner Expectations

The first session begins with an interview and health history. You are asked a series of questions and an assessment is performed. Keep in mind that privacy and confidentiality are maintained at all times. Clients may wear a smock and may leave on their underwear if they wish. During the session, clients are covered and draped with sheets and towels, uncovering only the body part to be worked on. The genitals are never exposed or massaged.

Massage sessions may start with the client lying face up or face down, depending on the purpose of the session. If the session focuses on a particular injury, that body part is generally worked on first. For a regular stress-reduction session, the back and neck are worked on first, followed by the legs, feet and arms. Clients can ask for different parts of the body to be worked on, or not worked on, and are encouraged to discuss this with me at the beginning of the session.

Some kinds of massage sessions use oil or lotion, and others do not. When Swedish massage is employed, oil/lotion is used. When Shiatsu or friction therapy is performed to eliminate scar tissue, oil/lotion is not used. When oil/lotion is used, clients may request that it be cleaned off with alcohol to keep their clothes clean, as I do not have shower, sauna, or whirlpool facilities at the office.

During the session, clients are encouraged to relax, and inform me if anything makes them uncomfortable, either physically or psychologically. Talking may occur during the session, but often I will ask you to talk with me before or after, as the massage session may take a good deal of concentration. If something feels uncomfortable during the session, please speak up immediately. I want to know as soon as possible.

The sessions do not vary much in length. They last between 50 and 60 minutes. If you are receiving massage related to an injury, you might be sore for one to two days. Be sure to tell me if this occurs. If you are sore for longer than two days, the massage needs to be adjusted to be gentler.

I reserve the right to refrain from working on a person who is under the influence of alcohol or drugs.

Sexual harassment is not tolerated. If the practitioner's safety feels compromised, the session is stopped immediately.

Appointment Policies

- Each session is 60 minutes long.
- The first appointment, which includes a history and an assessment, lasts approximately 90 minutes.
- If a client is late for a treatment session, the session still falls within the 60 minute allotted time slot.
- If I am late, the session lasts the full 60 minutes or the treatment rate is discounted.
- If you wish to cancel an appointment, you must do so 24 hours in advance, or you are charged for the full amount of the session unless the appointment can be filled. Someone answers the telephone from 9:00 a.m. until 6:00 p.m., but if you get an answering machine, please leave a message on the machine, including the date and time of the call. At the practitioner's discretion, you may not be charged for an emergency cancellation. If I need to cancel an appointment, I do so within 24 hours whenever possible. If I cannot do so, your next session is at no charge.
- All of the appointments occur at 122 Mellon St.
- I do not do house calls.
- I see clients Monday through Friday from 10:00 a.m. to 6:00 p.m. with extended hours on Thursday evening until 9:00 p.m.
- I return calls within 24 hours unless I am out of town.

Fees

- If, during my assessment, I determine with reasonable certainty that my work cannot help you, we end the session at that time and you are not charged for the initial appointment.
- Massage therapy sessions are $60.
- If you would like a double session, the charge is $100.
- Payment is due at the time of service unless other arrangements have been made prior to treatment. I accept cash, checks, and credit cards. I do not bill clients nor provide direct billing for insurance.
- Individuals who have financial constraints are welcome to discuss this with me to see what can be worked out, such as a sliding fee scale, referral to a practitioner with a fee you can afford, or referral to a student clinic at a nearby massage school.
- Sometimes private insurance companies reimburse clients for my services. It is best to get a prescription from a doctor if you wish to submit to your insurance company. I provide you with a receipt but cannot guarantee that your visits will be covered by insurance. In many cases they will be covered, but that is at the discretion of the insurance company.
- Fees increases are generally not implemented more than once per year.

Professionalism

- Our profession ascribes to a code of ethical behavior, which is available upon request. I follow all of the statements in this ethical code and have strong beliefs that practitioners and clients should not engage in intimate social relationships.
- Personal and professional boundaries are respected at all times.
- I perform services for which I am qualified (professionally, physically, and emotionally) and able to do, and refer to appropriate specialists when work is not within my scope of practice or not in the client's best interest.
- I customize my treatment to meet the client's needs.
- I keep accurate records and review charts before each session.
- I respect all clients regardless of their age, gender, race, national origin, sexual orientation, religion, socio-economic status, body type, political affiliation, state of health, and personal habits.

Recourse Policy

If you are dissatisfied with the massage session, you receive a full refund for that session or a complimentary treatment. You may return for refund any unused products (in salable condition) within 10 days of purchase.

▌ Sample Asian Medicine Office Policies

The purpose of these policies is to assure that your care is as effective and efficient as possible. We have found that patients who adhere to these policies get the best results.

Timeliness

It is important that you are on time for all appointments. A certain amount of time is allotted for each patient visit. If you are late, your remaining time may not be sufficient for your full treatment. We do our best to make accommodations, nevertheless, the full session fee is charged.

During your first visit, you may agree to a course of treatment, designed specifically for you. If a certain number of treatments in a set period is required to get the results we both desire and you need to change the time of an appointment, please plan to come at another time that same day. If the same day is not possible, please be sure to make it up within one week.

We request 24-hour notice for cancellations. If we do not receive this, we will have to charge you $50 for reserving the space/time for you. (True emergencies are exempted.)

Payment

Payment for all services is due at the time of your visit. Many insurance carriers now cover acupuncture, including Workers' Compensation, auto accident policies, and other private carriers. If you have insurance, you must still pay for your visits. We provide you with a receipt that you can submit to your insurance company for reimbursement. We highly recommend that you call your insurance company to find out if Asian Medicine services are covered and if there are any restrictions, such as needing a prescription from your primary care physician.

We accept MasterCard and Visa.

_____   _____

Patient's Signature   Date

▌ Sample Massage Therapy Informed Consent

I, _____ (client's name), understand that massage therapy provided by,
_____ (therapist's name), is intended to enhance relaxation, reduce pain caused by
muscle tension, increase range of motion, improve circulation and offer a positive experience of touch. Any other
intended purposes for massage therapy are specified below:

The general benefits of massage, possible massage contraindications, and the treatment procedure have been
explained to me. I understand that massage therapy is not a substitute for medical treatment or medications, and
that it is recommended that I concurrently work with my Primary Care Provider for any condition I may have. I am
aware that the massage therapist does not diagnose illness or disease, does not prescribe medications, and that spinal
manipulations are not part of massage therapy.

I have informed the massage therapist of all my known physical conditions, medical conditions and medications,
and I will keep the massage therapist updated on any changes. I understand that there shall be no liability on the
practitioner's part due to my forgetting to relay any pertinent information.

If I experience any pain or discomfort during the session, I immediately communicate that to the therapist so the
treatment can be adjusted.

I have received a copy of the therapist's policies, I understand them and agree to abide by them.

_____   _____
Client's Name (Print)   Date

_____
Client's Signature

▌ Sample School Clinic Informed Consent

I, _____ (patient's name), HEREBY voluntarily request to receive clinical services from _____ (school clinic name). I consent that these services may include acupuncture, moxabustion, nutritional / dietary counseling, herbology, Bach flower essences, TuiNa therapeutic massage, and lifestyle counseling, among other related services. I acknowledge that no guarantees have been made to me as to the effect of such care.

I further acknowledge that none of the above services is meant to be construed by me as the diagnosis or treatment of disease, but rather as an aid to balancing my energy and to improving my general wellness.

I understand that the acupuncture clinic holds traditional Oriental medicine to be complementary to orthodox medical treatment, unless contrary medical advice is given. I am advised that if I am sick, I should consult my doctor.

I understand that prior to the beginning of any procedure, I will receive an explanation of its nature and purpose and any probable risks involved. I understand that I may refuse any and all services at any time.

I understand that the clinic is part of the acupuncture school and that, as such, its main purpose is the training of acupuncture interns. Interns are supervised by a faculty member who is a Board Certified Acupuncturist. Interns do not receive compensation.

I recognize that I am responsible for my health and wellbeing, and that it is my duty to myself to be an informed partner in the care I receive at the clinic. To this end, I will secure the self-knowledge that I need in order fully to work with my intern.

In the event that I am not able to keep my appointment, I will try to give at least 48 hours notice so that someone else can use the time. I will pay the fee of $25 for any cancellation that is made within 24 hours from the appointment time. If I do not show up for the appointment as scheduled, then I will pay the fee of $30.

I understand that payment by cash, check, or credit card is due at the time of service. Should I have a complaint or grievance regarding services, I will speak with the clinic coordinator.

Finally, I understand that all records will be kept confidential.

_____
Witness

_____
Date

_____
Patient's Signature

_____
Date

We are a fragrance-free facility.

▍Feelings List

There is no "right" way to feel after a treatment. Listen to your body. Feel your own experience—that is what is right for you.

1. **A SENSE OF ALIVENESS OR PLEASURE IN YOUR BODY OR A FEELING OF PHYSICAL WELLBEING.** This may include a sense of connectedness in your whole body, awareness of sexual energy, or feelings and a sense of deep relaxation. You may find that you sleep more restfully that evening.

2. **LESS NUMBNESS IN SPECIFIC AREAS OF YOUR BODY.** You may experience a sense of "letting go," "thawing," or "melting" in those areas that felt "frozen." Those areas may actually become warmer to the touch. On the other hand, you may experience trembling or shakiness. Keep warm by covering yourself with a blanket, applying a heating pad, or wearing additional layers of clothing.

3. **AWARENESS OF MORE TENSION IN PARTS OF YOUR BODY.** You may notice tension in areas you were previously unaware that held stress, or it may be in other areas. If this occurs, think of things that helped you reduce tension in the past. Some people find it helpful to imagine breathing into those areas to relax them and give your attention to any feelings that have been held in those muscles and are now more accessible.

4. **INCREASED EMOTIONAL AWARENESS.** Being more in touch with your body brings awareness of new and different emotions. You may start to feel things that you knew about before but were disconnected from emotionally. Unexpected memories may surface, you might feel fear or sadness or a sense of emptiness. For instance, you may experience feelings of deprivation, stimulated by the nurturing touch that you did not get enough of as a child. Grieving for the nurturing touch you never received, or never received enough of, is appropriate. Feelings of anger about your deprivation may also be part of your experience.

5. **APPREHENSION ABOUT RETURNING.** It is common to feel apprehensive about returning for another session. This reluctance stems from feelings of exposure and vulnerability with the practitioner. Realize that this experience is different from your past experiences with touch. If the session feels good, you do not need to feel guilty for wanting, even longing for, safe nurturing touch. It is what you always deserved—even when you did not get it. Let yourself take it in now. If you continue to feel apprehension about returning, this may be a signal to take a pause in receiving bodywork. It may not be the right time in your recovery process, or it may be that the practitioner is not a good fit for your current needs.

6. **SHUTTING DOWN.** Another natural reaction to experiencing increased sensation in your body is for your body to contract and shut down temporarily. If this happens, be patient with yourself and ask your therapist to go slower with you. Everyone needs to move at their own pace. Respect your own body's rhythm.

Adapted with permission from a client handout developed by Krishnabai.

Appendix A

Appendix B
Codes of Ethics

Alexander Technique International (ATI)

American Chiropractic Association (ACA)

American Holistic Nurses Association (AHNA)

American Massage Therapy Association (AMTA)

American Naturopathic Medical Association (ANMA)

American Nursing Association (ANA)

American Organization for Bodywork Therapies of Asia™ (AOBTA)

American Physical Therapy Association (APTA)

American Reflexology Certification Board (ARCB)

Associated Bodywork & Massage Professionals (ABMP)

College of Massage Therapists of Ontario (CMTO)

Complementary Therapists Association (CTHA)

International Council of Nurses (ICN)

Massage Association of Australia Ltd (MAA)

The National Certification Board for Therapeutic Massage and Bodywork (NCBTMB)

National Certification Commission for Acupuncture and Oriental Medicine (NCCAOM)

Ontario College of Reflexology (OCR)

Yoga Alliance (YA)

Alexander Technique International (ATI)

Code of Ethics for Teaching Members

This Code of Ethics sets forth ethical principles for Alexander Technique teachers. The public has the right to expect that all ATI teaching members are properly evaluated and qualified to teach the F.M. Alexander Technique. ATI members act in a constructive, non-sectarian, non-discriminatory manner with colleagues, associates, students and the public.

1. The Teacher-Student Relationship

1.1 It is the responsibility of the Alexander Technique teacher to maintain a professional attitude throughout the period of time during which the Alexander Technique teacher/ student are working together.

1.2 An Alexander Technique teacher does not use their authority for personal gain, whether that gain be cultural, emotional, political or religious in nature. An Alexander Technique teacher does not enter into a sexual relationship with a student.

1.3 Students retain the right of confidentiality, and no information regarding the pupil is released to a third party without the consent of the pupil.

1.4 While the use of the principles of the F.M. Alexander Technique may produce effects that are beneficial or therapeutic, an Alexander Technique teacher informs all students that the F.M. Alexander Technique is an educational process, which improves the general level of functioning of the individual. In cases where professional medical assistance is indicated, Alexander Technique teachers encourage their students to seek such help. At no time does an Alexander Technique teacher make medical diagnoses or prescribe medical remedies. An Alexander Technique teacher does not proffer claims that the F.M. Alexander technique is a cure for any malady.

1.5 Any policy regarding payment, cancellation, lateness, or proper attire is fully explained to the student prior to the commencement of lessons and put in writing.

1.6 F.M. Alexander Technique lessons do not require the student to disrobe. Special projects requiring special dress are to be explained and agreed upon beforehand by all participants.

1.7 Students have the right to register a complaint with the ATI Ethics Committee. Their Alexander Technique teacher informs them of the process for doing so.

2. The Teacher-Teacher Relationship

2.1 ATI Teaching Members interact with each other and all Alexander Technique Teachers with professional and collegial respect. Differences of professional opinion are addressed without personally attacking or devaluing another's work.

2.2 ATI Teaching Members assist, support and encourage each other and all Alexander Technique Teachers in acquiring and maintaining the integrity, competency and highest standards of the profession.

2.3 ATI Teaching Members do not use their authority for personal gain over any colleague, whether that gain be cultural, emotional, financial, political or religious in nature.

2.4 ATI Teaching Members do not intentionally solicit or canvas known pupils, students, or trainees of any Alexander Technique Teacher without the permission of those teachers. Mailings to the general public, or the publicizing of specific courses, lecture, or workshops are not included in this provision.

2.5 Respecting the confidentiality of other ATI Teaching Members, ATI Teaching Members do not communicate to a third party any information that may be damaging to another Alexander Technique Teacher's reputation. If a third party's safety is at risk, ATI Teaching Members act upon their best judgement, taking into account the urgency of the situation and the laws of the country where the parties reside.

2.6 ATI Teaching Members who perceive a breach of The Code of Professional Conduct by a colleague speak directly to the colleague or teacher, before taking further action. If the ATI Member experiences difficulty approaching a colleague or teacher directly, the member may request an Advocate be appointed by the Ethics Advisory Committee Chair (for further clarification see Procedures for filing a complaint). If at all possible the Advocate speaks the language of the member with a complaint.

2.7 ATI Teaching Members may seek support from the ATI Ethics Advisory Committee to resolve any ethical concern.

2.8 ATI Members (both Teaching and Trainee), receiving a complaint about a third party from a colleague or a teacher, respectfully encourage and support the colleague in addressing the complaint directly to the third party or to the Ethics Advisory Committee.

2.9 Members who serve on the ATI Ethics Advisory Committee or who are Sponsoring Members may discuss information about ATI Teaching Members only within the jurisdiction of their committees, and the Board Members informed of decisions made within these committees are also bound by the same rule of confidentiality. If a member of the board or committee is involved directly or indirectly with the issue that member shall withdraw.

2.10 ATI committee and board members inform their committees and board members of possible conflicts of interest which might affect their functioning within the committee or board. The committee or board decides the extent to which that member should be involved in the discussion or decision making in that particular matter before the committee or board. Conflicts of interest might be personal, professional, legal or financial in nature.

2.11 ATI Teaching members maintain clearly defined boundaries in all dealings with each other. ATI strongly recommends that when entering into business relationships, members clarify expectations in a written contract agreed upon by all parties, defining roles and spelling out clearly any financial arrangements.

3. Teacher-Professional Responsibility

3.1 ATI Teaching Members continue to deepen their knowledge and understanding of the F.M. Alexander Technique and to improve their teaching skills. ATI Teaching Members participate regularly in professional interactions, workshops, research and publications.

3.2 ATI Teaching Members recognize the labor necessary to run ATI and contribute their time and expertise to ATI on committees or other positions of leadership when possible.

3.3 ATI Teaching Members accurately represent their professional qualifications and experience and describe the F.M. Alexander Technique without false or exaggerated claims.

3.4 Public advertisement of the F.M. Alexander Technique does not include any false, fraudulent, misleading or deceptive statements or claims by ATI Teaching Members.

3.5 ATI Teaching Members maintain the integrity of the F. M. Alexander Technique. When other modalities are introduced within the context of a lesson or workshop, they are clearly identified as being distinct from the Alexander Technique.

3.6 In their teaching ATI Teaching Members acknowledge appropriately the work or ideas of others.

3.7 ATI Teaching Members understand and respect personal boundaries, and accept the responsibility to hold inviolate the well-being of self, students and associates within the Alexander Technique community and the community at large.

3.8 ATI Teaching Members establish respectful and cooperative professional relationships with other practitioners and other professions.

3.9 ATI Teaching Members maintain a high level of personal integrity, bearing in mind that their behavior and how they represent themselves within the community is a reflection on ATI.

http://www.ati-net.com/atiethic.php

American Chiropractic Association (ACA)

Code of Ethics

Preamble

This Code of Ethics is based upon the acknowledgment that the social contract dictates the profession's responsibilities to the patient, the public, and the profession; and upholds the fundamental principle that the paramount purpose of the chiropractic doctor's professional services shall be to benefit the patient.

Tenets

I. Doctors of chiropractic should adhere to a commitment to the highest standards of excellence and should attend to their patients in accordance with established best practices.

II. Doctors of chiropractic should maintain the highest standards of professional and personal conduct, and should comply with all governmental jurisdictional rules and regulations.

III. Doctor-patient relationships should be built on mutual respect, trust and cooperation. In keeping with these principles, doctors of chiropractic shall demonstrate absolute honesty with regard to the patient's condition when communicating with the patient and/or representatives of the patient. Doctors of chiropractic shall not mislead patients into false or unjustified expectations of favorable results of treatment. In communications with a patient and/or representatives of a patient, doctors of chiropractic should never misrepresent their education, credentials, professional qualification or scope of clinical ability.

IV. Doctors of chiropractic should preserve and protect the patient's confidential information, except as the patient directs or consents, or the law requires otherwise.

V. Doctors of chiropractic should employ their best good faith efforts to provide information and facilitate understanding to enable the patient to make an informed choice in regard to proposed chiropractic treatment. The patient should make his or her own determination on such treatment.

VI. The doctor-patient relationship requires the doctor of chiropractic to exercise utmost care that he or she will do nothing to exploit the trust and dependency of the patient. Sexual misconduct is a form of behavior that adversely affects the public welfare and harms patients individually and collectively. Sexual misconduct exploits the doctor-patient relationship and is a violation of the public trust.

VII. Doctors of chiropractic should willingly consult and seek the talents of other health care professionals when such consultation would benefit their patients or when their patients express a desire for such consultation.

VIII. Doctors of chiropractic should never neglect nor abandon a patient. Due notice should be afforded to the patient and/or representatives of the patient when care will be withdrawn so that appropriate alternatives for continuity of care may be arranged.

IX. With the exception of emergencies, doctors of chiropractic are free to choose the patients they will serve, just as patients are free to choose who will provide healthcare services for them. However, decisions as to who will be served should not be based on race, religion, ethnicity, nationality, creed, gender, handicap or sexual preference.

X. Doctors of chiropractic should conduct themselves as members of a learned profession and as members of the greater healthcare community dedicated to the promotion of health, the prevention of illness and the alleviation of suffering. As such, doctors of chiropractic should collaborate and cooperate with other health care professionals to protect and enhance the health of the public with the goals of reducing morbidity, increasing functional capacity, increasing the longevity of the U.S. population and reducing health care costs.

XI. Doctors of chiropractic should exercise utmost care that advertising is truthful and accurate in representing the doctor's professional qualifications and degree of competence. Advertising should not exploit the vulnerability of patients, should not be misleading and should conform to all governmental jurisdictional rules and regulations in connection with professional advertising.

XII. As professions are self-regulating bodies, doctors of chiropractic shall protect the public and the profession by reporting incidents of unprofessional, illegal, incompetent and unethical acts to appropriate authorities and organizations and should stand ready to testify in courts of law and in administrative hearings.

XIII. Doctors of chiropractic have an obligation to the profession to endeavor to assure that their behavior does not give the appearance of professional impropriety. Any actions which may benefit the practitioner to the detriment of the profession must be avoided so as to not erode the public trust.

XIV. Doctors of chiropractic should recognize their obligation to help others acquire knowledge and skill in the practice of the profession. They should maintain the highest standards of scholarship, education and training in the accurate and full dissemination of information and ideas.

The ACA's Code of Ethics was revised and ratified by the ACA House of Delegates September 2007.
http://www.acatoday.org/content_css.cfm?CID=719

American Holistic Nurses Association (AHNA)

Code of Ethics

We believe that the fundamental responsibilities of the nurse are to promote health, facilitate healing, and alleviate suffering. The need for nursing is universal. Inherent in nursing is the respect for life, dignity, and the rights of all persons. Nursing care is given a context mindful of the holistic nature of humans, understanding the body-mind-spirit. Nursing care is unrestricted by considerations of nationality, race, creed, color, age, sex, sexual preference, politics, or social status. Given that nurses practice in culturally diverse settings, professional nurses must have an understanding of the cultural background of clients in order to provide culturally appropriate interventions.

Nurses render services to clients who can be individuals, families, groups, or communities. The client is an active participant in health care and should be included in all nursing care planning decisions.

To provide services to others, each nurse has a responsibility towards the client, co-workers, nursing practice, the profession of nursing, society, and the environment.

Nurses and Self

The nurse has a responsibility to model health care behaviors. Holistic nurses strive to achieve harmony in their own lives and assist others striving to do the same.

Nurses and the Client

The nurse's primary responsibility is to the client needing nursing care. The nurse strives to see the client as whole and provides care that is professionally appropriate and culturally consonant. The nurse holds in confidence all information obtained in professional practice and uses professional judgment in disclosing such information. The nurse enters into a relationship with the client that is guided by mutual respect and a desire for growth and development.

Nurse and Co-workers

The nurse maintains cooperative relationships with co-workers in nursing and other fields. Nurses have a responsibility to nurture each other and to assist nurses to work as a team in the interest of client care. If a client's care is endangered by a co-worker, the nurse must take appropriate action on behalf of the client.

Nursing and Nursing Practice

The nurse carries personal responsibility for practice and for maintaining continued competence. Nurses have the right to use all appropriate nursing interventions and have the obligation to determine the efficacy and safety of all nursing actions. Wherever applicable, nurses use research findings in directing practice.

Nurses and the Profession

The nurse plays a role in determining and implementing desirable standards of nursing practice and education. Holistic nurses may assume a leadership position to guide the profession towards holism. Nurses support nursing research and the development of holistically oriented nursing theories. The nurse participates in establishing and maintaining equitable social and economic working conditions in nursing.

Nurses and Society

The nurse, along with other citizens, has the responsibility for initiating and supporting actions to meet the health and social needs of the public.

Nurses and the Environment

The nurse strives to manipulate the client's environment to become one of peace, harmony, and nurturance so that healing may take place. The nurse considers the health of the ecosystem in relation to the need for health, safety, and peace of all persons.

September 1992, AHNA
http://www.ahncc.org/images/AHNACodeofethics.pdf

American Massage Therapy Association (AMTA)

Code of Ethics

This Code of Ethics is a summary statement of the standards of conduct that define ethical behavior for the massage therapist. Adherence to the Code is a prerequisite for admission to and continued membership in the American Massage Therapy Association (AMTA).

Principles of Ethics

The Principles of Ethics form the first part of the Code of Ethics. They are aspirational and inspirational model standards of exemplary professional conduct for all members of the association. These Principles should not be regarded as limitations or restrictions, but as goals for which members should constantly strive.

Massage therapists/practitioners shall:

1. Demonstrate commitment to provide the highest quality massage therapy/bodywork to those who seek their professional service.
2. Acknowledge the inherent worth and individuality of each person by not discriminating or behaving in any prejudicial manner with clients and/or colleagues.
3. Demonstrate professional excellence through regular self-assessment of strengths, limitations, and effectiveness by continued education and training.
4. Acknowledge the confidential nature of the professional relationship with clients and respect each client's right to privacy within the constraints of the law.
5. Project a professional image and uphold the highest standards of professionalism.
6. Accept responsibility to do no harm to the physical, mental and emotional well-being of self, clients, and associates.

Rules of Ethics

The Rules of Ethics are mandatory and direct specific standards of minimally-acceptable professional conduct for all members of the association. The Rules of Ethics are enforceable for all association members, and any members who violate this Code shall be subject to disciplinary action.

Massage therapists/practitioners shall:

1. Conduct all business and professional activities within their scope of practice and all applicable legal and regulatory requirements.
2. Refrain from engaging in any sexual conduct or sexual activities involving their clients in the course of a massage therapy session.
3. Be truthful in advertising and marketing, and refrain from misrepresenting his or her services, charges for services, credentials, training, experience, ability or results.
4. Refrain from using AMTA membership, including the AMTA name, logo or other intellectual property, or the member's position, in any way that is unauthorized, improper or misleading.
5. Refrain from engaging in any activity which would violate confidentiality commitments and/or proprietary rights of AMTA or any other person or organization.

Effective Date May 1, 2010
http://www.amtamassage.org/About-AMTA/Core-Documents/Code-of-Ethics.html

American Naturopathic Medical Association (ANMA)

Code of Ethics

I will

- First do no harm. *Primum no nocere*;
- Practice the healing power of nature. *vis medicatrix naturae*;
- Identify and treat the cause. *tolle causam*;
- Treat the whole person. The multi-factorial nature of health and disease;
- Practice prevention. Prevention is the best "cure";
- Not discriminate against clients or professionals based on race, religion, age, sex, handicaps, national ancestry, sexual orientation or economic conditions;
- Promise to abide by all state and local laws;
- Promise not to exceed my scope of practice, either in abilities or by law;
- Strive to be objective in the treatments of clients and performance of duties, recognizing the rights of all persons, and my limitations;
- Distinguish clearly, in public between my statements and actions as an individual and as a representative of Naturopathy;
- Encourage policy, procedures and personal practices which will enable others to conduct themselves in accordance with the values, goals and objectives of the American Naturopathic Medical Association;
- Constantly strive to achieve these objectives and ideals, dedicating myself to my chosen profession.

http://www.anma.org/codeofethic.html

American Nursing Association (ANA)

Code of Ethics

Provision 1. The nurse, in all professional relationships, practices with compassion and respect for the inherent dignity, worth, and uniqueness of every individual, unrestricted by considerations of social or economic status, personal attributes, or the nature of health problems.

    1.1 Respect for human dignity
    1.2 Relationships to patients
    1.3 The nature of health problems
    1.4 The right to self-determination
    1.5 Relationships with colleagues and others

Provision 2. The nurse's primary commitment is to the patient, whether an individual, family, group, or community.

    2.1 Primacy of the patient's interests
    2.2 Conflict of interest for nurses
    2.3 Collaboration
    2.4 Professional boundaries

Provision 3. The nurse promotes, advocates for, and strives to protect the health, safety, and rights of the patient.

    3.1 Privacy
    3.2 Confidentiality
    3.3 Protection of participants in research
    3.4 Standards and review mechanisms
    3.5 Acting on questionable practice
    3.6 Addressing impaired practice

Provision 4. The nurse is responsible and accountable for individual nursing practice and determines the appropriate delegation of tasks consistent with the nurse's obligation to provide optimum patient care.

    4.1 Acceptance of accountability and responsibility
    4.2 Accountability for nursing judgment and action
    4.3 Responsibility for nursing judgment and action
    4.4 Delegation of nursing activities

Provision 5. The nurse owes the same duties to self as to others, including the responsibility to preserve integrity and safety, to maintain competence, and to continue personal and professional growth.

    5.1 Moral self-respect
    5.2 Professional growth and maintenance of competence
    5.3 Wholeness of character
    5.4 Preservation of integrity

Provision 6. The nurse participates in establishing, maintaining, and improving health care environments and conditions of employment conducive to the provision of quality health care and consistent with the values of the profession through individual and collective action.

    6.1 Influence of the environment on moral virtues and values
    6.2 Influence of the environment on ethical obligations
    6.3 Responsibility for the health care environment

Provision 7. The nurse participates in the advancement of the profession through contributions to practice, education, administration, and knowledge development.

    7.1 Advancing the profession through active involvement in nursing and in health care policy
    7.2 Advancing the profession by developing, maintaining, and implementing professional standards in clinical, administrative, and educational practice
    7.3 Advancing the profession through knowledge development, dissemination, and application to practice

Provision 8. The nurse collaborates with other health professionals and the public in promoting community, national, and international efforts to meet health needs.

    8.1 Health needs and concerns
    8.2 Responsibilities to the public

Provision 9. The profession of nursing, as represented by associations and their members, is responsible for articulating nursing values, for maintaining the integrity of the profession and its practice, and for shaping social policy.

    9.1 Assertion of values
    9.2 The profession carries out its collective responsibility through professional associations
    9.3 Intraprofessional integrity
    9.4 Social reform

http://nursingworld.org/MainMenuCategories/EthicsStandards/CodeofEthicsforNurses/Code-of-Ethics.pdf

American Organization for Bodywork Therapies of Asia™ (AOBTA)

Code of Ethics

AOBTA Members pledge to honor the ethical and professional requirements set forth in this AOBTA Code of Ethics.

1. Social/Ecological Concern

   Members recognize their intrinsic involvement in the total community of life on the planet Earth.

2. Professional Conduct

   AOBTA members conduct themselves in a professional and ethical manner, performing only those services for which they are qualified, and represent their education, certification, professional affiliations and other qualifications honestly. They do not in any way profess to practice medicine or psychotherapy, unless licensed by their State or Country to do so.

3. Health History and Referrals

   AOBTA members keep accurate client records, including profiles of the body/mind health history. They discuss any problem areas that may contraindicate use of Asian Bodywork techniques, and refer clients to appropriate medical professionals when indicated.

4. Professional Appearance

   AOBTA members pay close attention to cleanliness and professional appearance of self and clothing, of linens and equipment, and of the office environment in general. They endeavor to provide a relaxing atmosphere, giving attention to reasonable scheduling and clarity about fees.

5. Communication and Confidentiality

   AOBTA members maintain clear and honest communications with their clients, and keep all information, whether medical or personal, strictly confidential. They clearly disclose techniques used, appropriately identifying each in the scope of their professional practice.

6. Intention and Trust

   AOBTA members are encouraged to establish and maintain trust in the client relationship and to establish clear boundaries and an atmosphere of safety.

7. Respect of Clients

   AOBTA members respect the client s physical/emotional state and do not abuse clients through actions, words or silence, nor take advantage of the therapeutic relationship. They, in no way, participate in sexual activity with a client. They consider the client s comfort zone for touch and for degree of pressure, and honor the client s requests as much as possible within personal, professional and ethical limits. They acknowledge the inherent worth and individuality of each person and therefore do not unjustly discriminate against clients or colleagues.

8. Professional Integrity

   AOBTA members present Asian Bodywork in a professional and compassionate manner representing themselves and their practice accurately and ethically. They do not give fraudulent information, nor misrepresent AOBTA or themselves to students or clients, nor act in a manner derogatory to the nature and positive intention of AOBTA. They conduct their business honestly.

9. Professional Courtesy

   AOBTA members respect the standards set by the various AOBTA modalities, and they respect service marks, trademarks and copyright laws. Professional courtesy includes respecting all ethical professionals in speech, writing, or otherwise, and communicating clearly with others.

10. Professional Excellence

    AOBTA members strive for professional excellence through regular assessment of personal and professional strengths and weaknesses, and by continued education and training.

Copyright 2008

http://www.aobta.org/index.php?option=com_content&view=article&id=50:aobta-code-of-ethics&catid=29:about-menu-articles&Itemid=143

American Physical Therapy Association (APTA)

Code of Ethics (Abbreviated)

Preamble

This Code of Ethics of the American Physical Therapy Association sets forth Principles for the ethical practice of physical therapy. All physical therapists are responsible for maintaining and promoting ethical practice. To this end, the physical therapist shall act in the best interest of the patient/client. This Code of Ethics shall be binding on all physical therapists.

Principle 1

Physical therapists shall respect the rights and dignity of all individuals and shall provide compassionate care.

Principle 2

Physical therapists shall be trustworthy and compassionate in addressing the rights and needs of patients/clients.

Principle 3

Physical therapists shall be accountable for making sound professional judgments.

Principle 4

Physical therapists shall demonstrate integrity in their relationships with patients/clients, families, colleagues, students, research participants, other health care providers, employers, payers, and the public.

Principle 5

Physical therapists shall fulfill their legal and professional obligations.

Principle 6

Physical therapists shall enhance their expertise through the lifelong acquisition and refinement of knowledge, skills, abilities, and professional behaviors.

Principle 7

Physical therapists shall promote organizational behaviors and business practices that benefit patients/clients and society.

Principle 8

Physical therapists shall participate in efforts to meet the health needs of people locally, nationally, or globally.

http://www.apta.org/uploadedFiles/APTAorg/About_Us/Policies/Ethics/CodeofEthics.pdf

American Reflexology Certification Board (ARCB)

Code of Ethics

A Reflexologist communicates with an open mind and a peaceful presence while recognizing that his/her relationship to the client is a serious responsibility. The art and science of Reflexology is an honorable one.

Therefore, as a professional reflexologist I shall:

- Conduct myself in a professional, honest, and ethical manner at all time.
- Adhere to the ARCB Professional Business Standards.
- Not infringe on any other professions' scope of practice, and perform only those services for which I am qualified and licensed to provide.
- Not present myself as a medical practitioner. I shall refer clients to appropriate medical or other healthcare professionals when appropriate.
- Treat other reflexologists and healthcare professionals in a courteous and respectful manner at all times.
- Establish and maintain trust in the client-practitioner relationship.
- Treat every client with the same kind, ethical attitude.
- Keep all client information and conversations strictly confidential.
- Work within the client's comfort zone and pain tolerance.
- Keep the standard of my professional work current and as high as possible by continuing my education and training and attending conferences.
- Ensure that anyone employed by me or working in my office shall also adhere to this Code of Ethics.

http://arcb.net/cms/?page_id=165

Associated Bodywork & Massage Professionals (ABMP)

Professional Code of Ethics

As a member of Associated Bodywork & Massage Professionals (ABMP), I pledge my commitment to the highest principles of the massage and bodywork profession as outlined here:

Commitment to High-Quality Care

I will serve the best interests of my clients at all times and provide the highest quality of bodywork and service possible. I recognize that the obligation for building and maintaining an effective, healthy, and safe therapeutic relationship with my clients is my responsibility.

Commitment to Do No Harm

I will conduct a thorough health history intake process for each client and evaluate the health history to rule out contraindications or determine appropriate session adaptations. If I see signs of, or suspect, an undiagnosed condition that massage may be inappropriate for, I will refer that client to a physician or other qualified health-care professional and delay the massage session until approval from the physician has been granted. I understand the importance of ethical touch and therapeutic intent and will conduct sessions with the sole objective of benefitting the client.

Commitment to Honest Representation of Qualifications

I will not work outside the commonly accepted scope of practice for massage therapists and bodywork professionals. I will adhere to my state's scope of practice guidelines (when applicable). I will only provide treatments and techniques for which I am fully trained and hold credible credentials. I will carefully evaluate the needs of each client and refer the client to another provider if the client requires work beyond my capabilities, or beyond the capacity of massage and bodywork. I will not use the trademarks and symbols associated with a particular system or group without authentic affiliation. I will acknowledge the limitations of massage and bodywork by refraining from exaggerating the benefits of massage therapy and related services throughout my marketing.

Commitment to Uphold the Inherent Worth of All Individuals

I will demonstrate compassion, respect, and tolerance for others. I will seek to decrease discrimination, misunderstandings, and prejudice. I understand there are situations when it is appropriate to decline service to a client because it is in the best interests of a client's health, or for my personal safety, but I will not refuse service to any client based on disability, ethnicity, gender, marital status, physical build, or sexual orientation; religious, national, or political affiliation; social or economic status.

Commitment to Respect Client Dignity and Basic Rights

I will demonstrate my respect for the dignity and rights of all individuals by providing a clean, comfortable, and safe environment for sessions, using appropriate and skilled draping procedures, giving clients recourse in the event of dissatisfaction with treatment, and upholding the integrity of the therapeutic relationship.

Commitment to Informed Consent

I will recognize a client's right to determine what happens to his or her body. I understand that a client may suffer emotional and physical harm if a therapist fails to listen to the client and imposes his or her own beliefs on a situation. I will fully inform my clients of choices relating to their care, and disclose policies and limitations that may affect their care. I will not provide massage without obtaining a client's informed consent (or that of the guardian or advocate for the client) to the session plan.

Commitment to Confidentiality

I will keep client communication and information confidential and will not share client information without the client's written consent, within the limits of the law. I will ensure every effort is made to respect a client's right to privacy and provide an environment where personal health-related details cannot be overheard or seen by others.

Commitment to Personal and Professional Boundaries

I will refrain from and prevent behaviors that may be considered sexual in my massage practice and uphold the highest professional standards in order to desexualize massage. I will not date a client, engage in sexual intercourse with a client, or allow any level of sexual impropriety (behavior or language) from clients or myself. I understand that sexual impropriety may lead to sexual harassment charges, the loss of my massage credentials, lawsuits for personal damages, criminal charges, fines, attorney's fees, court costs, and jail time.

Commitment to Honesty in Business

I will know and follow good business practices with regard to record keeping, regulation compliance, and tax law. I will set fair fees and practice honesty throughout my marketing materials. I will not accept gifts, compensation, or other benefits intended to influence a decision related to a client. If I use the Associated Bodywork & Massage Professionals logo, I promise to do so appropriately to establish my credibility and market my practice.

Commitment to Professionalism

I will maintain clear and honest communication with clients and colleagues. I will not use recreational drugs or alcohol before or during massage sessions. I will project a professional image with respect to my behavior and personal appearance in keeping with the highest standards of the massage profession. I will not actively seek to take someone else's clients, disrespect a client or colleague, or willingly malign another therapist or other allied professional. I will actively strive to positively promote the massage and bodywork profession by committing to self-development and continually building my professional skills.

http://www.abmp.com/about/code_of_ethics.php

College of Massage Therapists of Ontario (CMTO)

Code of Ethics (Abbreviated)

Principle I - Respect For Persons

Meaning:

To value the dignity and worth of all persons regardless of age, race, culture, creed, sexual identity, gender, ability and/or health status.

Application:

Client autonomy is demonstrated by:

a. Ensuring that clients are as fully involved as possible in the planning and implementation of their own health care

b. Providing complete and accurate information in a sensitive and timely fashion to enable clients, or when necessary a client's substitute decision maker, to make informed choices

c. Listening to and respecting a client's values, opinions, needs, and cultural beliefs

d. Encouraging and being responsive to a client's choice to accept, augment, modify, refuse or terminate treatment

e. Being informed about moral and legal rights of a client

f. Advocating for and supporting a client in exercising his/her moral and legal Rights

g. Safeguarding the client's right to privacy and confidentiality by holding all personal and health information in confidence unless otherwise required by law.

Principle II - Responsible Caring

Meaning:

Providing sensitive, compassionate and empathetic quality massage therapy.

Application:

Responsible care of a client is demonstrated by:

a. Listening to and respecting the client's values, opinions, needs, and cultural beliefs

b. Promoting the client's best interest and well-being, through the highest possible standard professional practice

c. Seeking assistance when conflicts arise between the value systems of the practitioner and the client

d. Recognizing and referring the client to other health care providers when it is in the client's best interest to do so

e. Being alert to and reporting, as required, any unethical practice by any member of the regulated health professions

f. Approaching and co-operating with substitute decision makers in assessing the client's wishes and best interests in the event of incapacity

g. Protecting the client's physical and emotional privacy

h. Collecting only that information which is relevant to the provision of health care.

Principle III - Integrity in Relationships

Meaning:

To practice with integrity, honesty and diligence in our professional relationships with ourselves, our clients, our professional colleagues and society.

Application:

Commitments to Clients are demonstrated by:

a. Ensuring that we always act in our client's best interest as defined by the client's wishes and consistent with the standards of practice of the profession

b. Informing the client about health care services available to support them

c. Referring to other health care providers as necessary and appropriate

d. Obtaining assistance when value conflicts arise which threaten to impede client autonomy

e. Providing client-centered health care which includes the following:

i. Explaining to the client and advocating for his/her right to receive information about, and take control of his/her health care

ii. Providing information about the proposed treatment, alternative courses of action, the material effects, risks and side effects in each case and the consequences of not having the treatment

iii. Assisting the client to comprehend information

iv. Responding to questions about our client's health care/treatment

Commitments to Self are demonstrated by:
a. Being pro-actively committed to our own health and personal and professional development
b. Being competent, conscientious and empathetic practitioners
c. Being aware of our personal values and being able to identify when value conflicts interfere with client care
d. Keeping our professional commitment by integrating massage values and principles in our daily practice

Commitments to our Professional Colleagues are demonstrated by:
a. Respecting our colleagues and working co-operatively with them
b. Intervening in situations where the safety and well being of a client is in jeopardy
c. Reporting to appropriate authorities any regulated health care practitioner who abuses a client physically, verbally, sexually or financially
d. Referring to other health care providers when necessary and appropriate
e. Co-operating with regulatory functions of the profession
f. Contributing to continuous quality improvement initiatives
g. Upholding standards and guidelines of the profession
h. Advocating with other health care providers to promote and support social changes that enhance individual and community health and well-being
i. Representing ourselves honestly, and performing only those services for which we are qualified.

Principle IV - Responsibility to Society

Meaning:
To be accountable to society and conduct our selves in a manner that fosters and promotes high ethical standards.

Application:
Ethical practice is demonstrated by:
a. Pursuing continued career-long, professional learning
b. Advocating for and supporting a client's ethical and moral rights
c. Participating in the promotion of the profession of massage therapy through advocacy, research and maintenance of the highest possible standards of practice
d. Being committed to promoting the welfare and well-being of all persons in society
e. Making every reasonable effort to ascertain that our clinical environment will permit provision of care consistent with the values in the Code of Ethics
f. Committing to continuous improvement and implementation of standards of massage practice
g. Collaborating with members of the other health professions to meet the health needs of the public
h. Continuing to develop ways to clarify massage therapist's accountability to society.

http://www.cmto.com/cmto-wordpress/assets/codeethics.pdf

Complementary Therapists Association (CTHA)

Code of Practice

1. Members shall have respect for the religious, spiritual, political and social views of any individual irrespective of race, colour, creed, sexual orientation or gender.

2. Members shall at all times conduct themselves in an honourable and courteous manner and with due diligence in their relations with their clients and the public. They should seek a good relationship and shall work in a co-operative manner with other healthcare professionals and recognise and respect their particular contribution within the healthcare team, irrespective of whether they perform from an allopathic or alternative/complementary base.

3. The relationship between a member and her/his client is that of a professional with a client. The client places trust in a member's care, skill and integrity and it is the member's duty to act with due diligence at all times and not to abuse this trust in any way.

4. Proper moral conduct must always be paramount in members' relations with clients. They must behave with courtesy, respect, dignity, discretion and tact. Their attitude must be competent and sympathetic, hopeful and positive, thus encouraging an uplift in the client's mental outlook and belief in a progression towards good health practices.

5. In furtherance of 4. above, members must not enter into a sexual relationship of any kind with a client and must be diligent in guarding against any act, suggestion or statement that may be interpreted, mistakenly or otherwise, as having a sexual implication.

6. Hypnotherapists may only make home visits to clients subject to there being a friend, relative or independent witness on the premises at all times. Stage and entertainment hypnosis is not permitted.

7. All members working within hospitals, hospices and any other medical establishment will comply with the protocols and guidelines in force at such establishments.

8. Members must never claim to 'cure'. The possible therapeutic benefits may be described; 'recovery' must never be guaranteed.

9. Members should ensure that they themselves are medically, physically and psychologically fit to practise.

10. Discretion must be used for the protection of the member when carrying out private treatment with clients who are mentally unstable, addicted to drugs or alcohol, or severely depressed, suicidal or hallucinated. Such clients must be treated only by a member with relevant competency. A member must not treat a client in any case which exceeds her/his capacity, training and competence. Where appropriate, the member must seek referral to a more qualified person.

11. Registered medical practitioners and members of other health care professions remain subject to the general ethical codes and disciplinary procedures of their respective professions.

12. The aim of CTHA membership is to offer a service to clients as well as a service and therapeutic modalities to, and with, the medical profession. Members must recognise that where a client is delegated to them by a registered medical practitioner, that person remains clinically accountable for their patient and for the care offered by the member.

13. Members must guard against the danger that a client without previously consulting a doctor may come for therapy for a known disorder and subsequently be found, too late, to be suffering from another serious disorder. To this end new patients/clients must be asked what medical advice they have received. If they have not seen a doctor, they must be advised to do so. Since it is legal to refuse medical treatment, no client can be forced to consult a doctor. The advice must be recorded for the member's protection. It is not a breach of ethics to treat a client who gives informed consent to receive a therapy.

14. Members must not countermand instructions or prescriptions given by a doctor.

15. Members must not advise a particular course of medical treatment, such as to undergo an operation or to take specific drugs. It must be left to the client to make her/his own decision in the light of medical advice.

16. Members must never give a medical diagnosis to a client in any circumstances, unless medically qualified to do so; this is the responsibility of a registered medical practitioner. However, many members have a 'gift' of diagnosis and of discovering dysfunctions in the physical, emotional, mental and spiritual aspects. In this case the member may make mention of any disorder which he may discover, and advise the client to see her/his doctor for a medical diagnosis and record this action on the client's records.

17. Members must not use titles or descriptions to give the impression of medical or other qualifications unless they possess them and must make it clear to their clients that they are not medical doctors and do not purport to have their knowledge or skills.

18. Members are forbidden to diagnose, perform tests on or treat animals in any way, unless specifically qualified, or give advice following diagnosis by a registered veterinary surgeon or to countermand her/his instructions.

19. Members must not attend women in childbirth or treat them for ten days thereafter unless they hold an appropriate qualification approved by CTHA. This does not preclude treatment given with the permission of the client's midwife, doctor or medical team.

20. Members must not practise dentistry unless they hold an appropriate qualification.

21. Members must not treat any venereal disease as defined in the 1917 Act.

22. Clients suffering from AIDS may be treated at the discretion of the member.

23. Members must not use manipulation or vigorous massage unless they possess an appropriate professional qualification.

24. Members must not prescribe or administer remedies, herbs, supplements, essential oils or other products unless their training and qualifications entitle them to do so.

25. At the present time, no alternative or complementary therapy is approved as 'medical aid' under the law. It is a criminal offence for a parent or guardian not to seek 'medical aid' for a child under the age of 16. The member should secure a signed statement from a parent or guardian who refuses to seek medical aid as defined under the law in the following format: "I have been warned by (enter name of member) that according to law I should consult a doctor concerning the health of my child (enter name of the child) Signed (signed by parent or guardian) Signed (by person witnessing the parent's or guardian's signature).

26. Advertising must be dignified in tone and shall not contain named testimonials or claim to cure any disease etc. It shall be confined to drawing attention to the therapy available, the qualifications of the member and offer a general service together with necessary details.

27. Members will display their certificate of membership of CTHA in their normal place of work. Members working in several locations and/or offering visiting services will have available at all times a copy of their current membership certificate issued by CTHA.

28. Before treatment members must explain fully either in writing or verbally all the procedures involved in the treatment including such matters as questionnaires, likely content and length of consultation, number of consultations, fees etc. Where a client has an existing medical condition members must ensure that they have the client's informed consent in writing to perform the treatment or that of the client's medical practitioner.

29. Members must act with consideration concerning fees and justification for treatment. Members should not be judgmental and they should recognise the client's right to refuse treatment or ignore advice. It is the client's prerogative to make their own choices with regard to their health, lifestyle and finances.

30. Members must ensure they keep clear and comprehensive records of their treatments including the dates, advice given and all consent forms. This is especially important for the defence of any negligence actions for at least 7 years, as well as for efficient and careful practice.

31. In determining whether or not any record of the nature of any treatment administered is reasonable, it shall be for the member compiling the record to show that on the basis of her/his notes he/she can demonstrate what treatment was undertaken and whether that treatment was competently and reasonably undertaken and that the client consented to the treatment.

32. Confidentiality. Members, their assistants and receptionists have an implicit duty to keep attendances, all information, records and views formed about clients entirely confidential. No disclosure may be made to any third party, including any member of the client's own family, without the client's consent unless it is required by due process of the law, whether that be by Statute, Statutory instrument, order of any court of competent jurisdiction or howsoever otherwise.

33. Members must ensure that they comply with the Data Protection Act.

34. No third party, including assistants and members of the client's family, may be present during the course of a consultation with an adult without the client's express consent, which should be recorded.

35. All members must be adequately insured to practise. Normally this will be through CTHA's scheme but private insurance is permitted and if adopted, members must provide evidence of this to CTHA. The insurance policy must state provision for public liability and indemnity as well as the provision for professional treatments.

36. All members shall ensure that their working conditions are suitable for the practice of their therapy.

37. Members will follow and abide by decisions made under the disciplinary, complaints and appeals procedures appended to this Code.

http://www.ctha.com/CodeOfPractice/

International Council of Nurses (ICN)

Code of Ethics

Preamble

Nurses have four fundamental responsibilities: to promote health, to prevent illness, to restore health and to alleviate suffering. The need for nursing is universal. Inherent in nursing is a respect for human rights, including cultural rights, the right to life and choice, to dignity and to be treated with respect. Nursing care is respectful of and unrestricted by considerations of age, colour, creed, culture, disability or illness, gender, sexual orientation, nationality, politics, race or social status.

Nurses render health services to the individual, the family and the community and coordinate their services with those of related groups.

The Code

The ICN Code of Ethics for Nurses has four principal elements that outline the standards of ethical conduct.

Elements of the Code

1. Nurses and people
    i. The nurse s primary professional responsibility is to people requiring nursing care.
       In providing care, the nurse promotes an environment in which the human rights, values, customs and spiritual beliefs of the individual, family and community are respected.
    ii. The nurse ensures that the individual receives accurate, sufficient, and timely information in a culturally appropriate manner on which to base consent for care and related treatment.
    iii. The nurse holds in confidence personal information and uses judgement in sharing this information.
    iv. The nurse shares with society the responsibility for initiating and supporting action to meet the health and social needs of the public, in particular those of vulnerable populations.
    v. The nurse advocates for equity and social justice in resource allocation, access to health care and other social and economic services.
    vi. The nurse demonstrates professional values such as respectfulness, responsiveness, compassion, trustworthiness and integrity.
2. Nurses and practice
    i. The nurse carries personal responsibility and accountability for nursing practice, and for maintaining competence by continual learning.
    ii. The nurse maintains a standard of personal health such that the ability to provide care is not compromised.
    iii. The nurse uses judgement regarding individual competence when accepting and delegating responsibility.
    iv. The nurse at all times maintains standards of personal conduct which reflect well on the profession and enhance its image and public confidence.
    v. The nurse, in providing care, ensures that use of technology and scientific advances are compatible with the safety, dignity and rights of people.
3. Nurses and the profession
    i. The nurse assumes the major role in determining and implementing acceptable standards of clinical nursing practice, management, research and education.
    ii. The nurse is active in developing a core of research-based professional knowledge that supports evidence-based practice..
    iii. The nurse, acting through the professional organisation, participates in creating and maintaining safe, equitable social and economic working conditions in nursing.
    iv. The nurse practices to sustain and protect the natural environment and is aware of its consequences on health.
    v. The nurse contributes to an ethical organisational environment and challenges unethical practices and settings.
4. Nurses and co-workers
    i. The nurse sustains a collaborative and respectful relationship with co-workers in nursing and other fields.
    ii. The nurse takes appropriate action to safeguard individuals, families, and communities when their care is endangered by a co-worker or any other person.
    iii. The nurse takes appropriate action to support and guide co-workers to advance ethical conduct.

Revised 2012

http://www.icn.ch/about-icn/code-of-ethics-for-nurses/

Massage Association of Australia Ltd (MAA)

Code of Conduct

The objective of the Massage Association of Australia's (MAA) Code of Conduct is to provide its practitioners with a basis for professional and self reflection, and evaluation on ethical conduct. This document defines and identifies acceptable behaviour, promotes high standards of practice, and establishes a framework for professional behaviour and responsibilities. The MAA is a professional organisation and has an obligation to its members, the general public and the industry as a whole.

The Public Interest

- Members shall ensure that within their chosen fields they have appropriate knowledge and understanding of relevant legislation; Federal, State, Territory and local council laws and regulations; and that they comply with such requirements.
- Members shall in their professional practice have regard to basic human rights, compassion and respect for others and shall avoid any actions that adversely affect such rights.

Duty of Client Care

- Members shall practice within the boundaries of their qualification/s and shall cause no harm to clients either of a physical or emotional nature.
- Members shall carry out treatment with due care and diligence in accordance with the requirements of the client and will treat according to the client's informed consent.
- Where a client is unable to give informed consent for any reason (for example medical condition, psychological state of mind, age), informed consent must be obtained from the client's legal guardian.
- When treating minors (under 16 years of age) the client must be accompanied for treatment by a parent or guardian and have permission for any treatment.
- Uphold client confidentiality.
- Members must maintain accurate clinical records in a secured environment, for the duration necessary to meet legal requirements.
- Members must recognise their professional limitations and be prepared to refer a client to other health service practitioners as appropriate.
- Members shall not engage in services that are sexual in nature with the client.

Duty to the Profession

- Members shall uphold the reputation of the profession and shall seek to improve professional standards through participation in personal development and will avoid any action, which will adversely affect the good standing of the MAA.
- Members shall seek to advance public knowledge and to counter false or misleading statements, which are detrimental to the profession.
- Members shall act with integrity toward fellow therapists/practitioners and to members of other professions with whom they are concerned in a professional capacity.

Professional Competence and Integrity

- Members shall maintain professional skills to represent themselves at a professional standard, seeking to continue or maintain personal and professional development skills.
- Members shall accept professional responsibility for their work.
- Members shall not lay claim to any level of competence which they do not possess, or provide services which are not within their professional competence.

Advertising

- Members must not advertise in a false, misleading or deceptive manner.
- Members must not abuse the trust or exploit the lack of knowledge of consumers.
- Members must not make claims of treatments that can not be substantiated.
- Members must not encourage excessive or inappropriate use of services.

Privacy

- Members will abide by the requirements of Federal, State and Territory privacy and patient record law.
- Members shall honour the information given by a client in the therapeutic relationship.
- Members shall ensure that there will be no wrongful disclosure, either directly or indirectly, of personal information.
- Records must be securely stored, archived, passed on or disposed of in accordance with Federal, State and Territory record law.
- The client has a right to be adequately informed as to their treatment plan and have access to their information as far as the law permits.

Disciplinary Procedures

This Code sets out certain basic principles that are intended to help members maintain the highest standards of professional conduct. All members must accept professional, legal and ethical responsibilities in order to protect themselves and the public's interest. Should a case arise where a member is in breach of the Code of Conduct, MAA has the right to cancel a practitioner's membership or take other action in accordance with Section 11 of the Constitution. Further information can be found in the MAA's Constitution and in the Complaints, Disputes and Disciplinary Procedures.

March 2011

http://www.maa.org.au/LinkClick.aspx?fileticket=XcZaRs3ZEyA%3d&tabid=2287&language=en-US

The National Certification Board for Therapeutic Massage and Bodywork (NCBTMB)

Code of Ethics

NCBTMB certificants and applicants for certification shall act in a manner that justifies public trust and confidence, enhances the reputation of the profession, and safeguards the interest of individual clients. Certificants and applicants for certification will:

I. Have a sincere commitment to provide the highest quality of care to those who seek their professional services.

II. Represent their qualifications honestly, including education and professional affiliations, and provide only those services that they are qualified to perform.

III. Accurately inform clients, other health care practitioners, and the public of the scope and limitations of their discipline.

IV. Acknowledge the limitations of and contraindications for massage and bodywork and refer clients to appropriate health professionals.

V. Provide treatment only where there is reasonable expectation that it will be advantageous to the client.

VI. Consistently maintain and improve professional knowledge and competence, striving for professional excellence through regular assessment of personal and professional strengths and weaknesses and through continued education training.

VII. Conduct their business and professional activities with honesty and integrity, and respect the inherent worth of all persons.

VIII. Refuse to unjustly discriminate against clients and/or health professionals.

IX. Safeguard the confidentiality of all client information, unless disclosure is requested by the client in writing, is medically necessary, is required by law, or necessary for the protection of the public.

X. Respect the client's right to treatment with informed and voluntary consent. The certified practitioner will obtain and record the informed consent of the client, or client's advocate, before providing treatment. This consent may be written or verbal.

XI. Respect the client's right to refuse, modify or terminate treatment regardless of prior consent given.

XII. Provide draping and treatment in a way that ensures the safety, comfort and privacy of the client.

XIII. Exercise the right to refuse to treat any person or part of the body for just and reasonable cause.

XIV. Refrain, under all circumstances, from initiating or engaging in any sexual conduct, sexual activities, or sexualizing behavior involving a client, even if the client attempts to sexualize the relationship unless a pre-existing relationship exists between an applicant or a practitioner and the client prior to the applicant or practitioner applying to be certified by NCBTMB.

XV. Avoid any interest, activity or influence which might be in conflict with the practitioner's obligation to act in the best interests of the client or the profession.

XVI. Respect the client's boundaries with regard to privacy, disclosure, exposure, emotional expression, beliefs, and the client's reasonable expectations of professional behavior. Practitioners will respect the client's autonomy.

XVII. Refuse any gifts or benefits that are intended to influence a referral, decision, or treatment, or that are purely for personal gain and not for the good of the client.

XVIII. Follow the NCBTMB Standards of Practice, this Code of Ethics, and all policies, procedures, guidelines, regulations, codes, and requirements promulgated by the National Certification Board for Therapeutic Massage & Bodywork.

2008

http://www.ncbtmb.org/download/ncbtmb-code-ethics-2-page

National Certification Commission
For Acupuncture and Oriental Medicine (NCCAOM)

Code of Ethics

All practitioners certified by the National Certification Commission for Acupuncture and Oriental Medicine must be committed to responsible and ethical practice, to the growth of the profession's role in the broad spectrum of American health care, and to their own professional growth. All Diplomates, Applicants, and Candidates for certification agree to be bound by the NCCAOM Code of Ethics.

Commitment to the Patient

I will:
- Respect the rights and dignity of each person I treat.
- Accept and treat those seeking my services in a nondiscriminatory manner.
- Keep the patient informed by explaining treatments and outcomes.
- Protect the confidentiality of information acquired in the course of patient care.
- Maintain professional boundaries in relationships with patients and avoid any relationships that may exploit practitioner/patient trust.
- Keep accurate records of each patient's history and treatment.
- Treat only within my lawful scope of practice.
- Render the highest quality of care and make timely referrals to other health care professionals as may be appropriate.
- Avoid treating patients if I am unable to safely and effectively treat due to substance abuse, physical or psychological impairment.
- Bill patients and third party payers accurately and fairly.
- Not engage in sexual contact with a current patient if the contact commences after the practitioner/patient relationship is established.
- Not engage in sexual contact with a former patient unless a period of six (6) months has elapsed since the date that the professional relationship ended.
- A sexual relationship must not exploit the trust established during the professional relationship.

Commitment to the Profession

I will:
- Continue to work to promote the highest standards of the profession.
- Provide accurate, truthful, and nonmisleading information in connection with any application for licensure, certification, NCCAOM disciplinary investigation or proceeding or recertification.
- Report any changes to the information on my application regarding professional ethics and my on-going fitness to practice, including but not limited to reporting to the NCCAOM any disciplinary action taken by a school or regulating agency against me, and any criminal charges or civil actions that may be relevant to my health care practice or fitness to practice.
- Comply with NCCAOM Examination Policies.
- Report to NCCAOM or appropriate licensing authorities information about any violations by me or by my peers of the Code of Ethics or Grounds for Professional Discipline.

Commitment to the Public

I will:
- Provide accurate information regarding my education, training and experience, professional affiliations, and certification status.
- Refrain from any representation that NCCAOM certification implies licensure or a right to practice unless so designated by the laws in the jurisdiction in which I practice.
- Use only the appropriate professional designations for my credentials.
- Advertise only accurate, truthful, nonmisleading information and refrain from making public statements on the efficacy of Oriental medicine that are not supported by the generally accepted experience of the profession.
- Respect the integrity of other forms of health care and other medical traditions and seek to develop collaborative relationships to achieve the highest quality of care for individual patients.
- Comply with all public health and public safety reporting duties imposed on licensed health care professionals.

Effective October 14, 2008
http://www.nccaom.org/regulatory-affairs/code-of-ethics

Ontario College of Reflexology (OCR)

Code of Ethics

A Reflexologist's primary purpose is the promotion of health, prevention of disease and to restore, maintain and optimize health and well-being through individualized client care and public education. Each Reflexologist shall act, at all times, in a manner as to justify public trust and confidence, to uphold and enhance the good standing and reputation of the profession, to serve the interest of society, and above all to safeguard the interests of individual clients. Every Reflexologist is accountable for his/her practice, and, in the exercise of professional accountability, shall:

A: Service To The Public:

1. Consider first the well-being of the client.
2. Practise Reflexology competently, with integrity, and without impairment.
3. Do no harm.
4. Give the highest possible qualify of care.
5. Not discriminate.
6. Create firm financial, emotional and sexual boundaries with all clients.
7. Recognize their own limitations (when known) and refer their clients to other practitioners or health professionals when required.
8. Maintain a safe and supportive environment.
9. Maintain a clean work environment and practise proper disinfection procedures.
10. Not diagnose, prescribe or treat specific conditions unless accredited in another profession allowing the legal right to do so.
11. Avoid making inappropriate claims for reflexology in advertising or while in service to clients.
12. Maintain client privacy and confidentiality. The reflexologist will disclose personal information only with the express permission of the client or if there is a risk of harm to the client or other person.
13. Be sensitive when providing information or feedback to the client.
14. Respect the client's autonomy and respect their decisions according to the number and frequency of sessions.

B: Service to the Profession:

1. Recognize that self-regulation of the profession is a privilege and that each Reflexologist has an ongoing responsibility to merit the retention of that privilege.
2. Behave in a manner that is beyond reproach.
3. Respect other legal health care providers and treat colleagues with dignity and respect.
4. Maintain proper client records and documentation.
5. Maintain proper business practices and records particularly as it pertains to billing and taxes.
6. Maintain memberships in applicable professional organizations.
7. Continue their professional development through continuing education.
8. Seek out current research.
9. Share the results of their own research.
10. Maintain professional malpractice insurance for the protection of the Reflexologist and the client.

C. Service to the Self:

1. Recognize their own personal biases.
2. Strive to maintain personal health and well-being.
3. Maintain an acceptable level of health and well-being for themselves.
4. Seek help from colleagues and appropriately qualified professionals for personal problems that might adversely affect service to clients, society or the profession.

D. Service to the Ontario College of Reflexology:

1. Comply with all governing legislation, Standards of Practice, policies, by-laws and guidelines approved by the Ontario College of Reflexology.
2. Report to the College any conduct of a colleague which may generally be considered unprofessional or unbecoming to the profession.
3. Cooperate and assist the college in its work.
4. Accept censure amongst their peers through the disclosure of their name (in OCR Footnotes) should they be found guilty of any client complaint.

June 17, 2013

http://www.ocr.edu/ethics.htm

Yoga Alliance (YA)

Code of Conduct

Our code of conduct is a declaration of acceptable ethical and professional behavior by which all registrants agree to conduct the teaching and business of yoga. It is not intended to supersede the ethics of any school or tradition but is intended to be a basis for yoga principles. As a RYT, E-RYT or representative of a RYS, I agree to uphold the following ethical principles:

- Conduct myself in a professional and conscientious manner.
- Acknowledge the limitations of my skills and scope of practice and where appropriate, refer students to seek alternative instruction, advice, treatment or direction.
- Create and maintain a safe, clean and comfortable environment for the practice of yoga.
- Encourage diversity by respecting all students regardless of age, physical limitations, race, creed, gender, ethnicity, religion or sexual orientation.
- Respect the rights, dignity and privacy of all students.
- Avoid words and actions that constitute sexual harassment.
- Adhere to the traditional yoga principles as written in the yamas and niyamas.
- Follow all local government and national laws that pertain to my yoga teaching and business.

http://www.yogaalliance.org/ya/a/Policy_Docs/Code_of_Conduct.aspx

Glossary

Abandonment: To withdraw support, especially in spite of duty, allegiance, or responsibility.

Abuse: The improper use, handling, or treatment, often to unfairly or improperly gain benefit.

Accountability: An obligation or willingness to accept responsibility or to account for one's actions and consequences.

Aggressive Language: Communicates undertones of anger through the words, the voice tone, or both.

Ambiguity: When a communication is not clear, the message received by the listener can be very different from the message the speaker intended to send.

Apprenticeship: A system of training practitioners in a structured competency-based set of skills that combines on-the-job training with academic instruction. Apprenticeships often last many years.

Arbitration: This is an alternative form of dispute resolution that takes place out of court. All parties in the dispute select an impartial third party (arbitrator), agree in advance to comply with the arbitrator's award, and participate in a hearing where evidence and testimonies are presented. The arbitrator's decision is usually final, and courts rarely reexamine it.

Arousal: A physiological and psychological state of being awake, reactive to stimuli, or ready for activity. It involves the brain stem, the autonomic nervous system, and the endocrine system.

Assertion Sequence: A communication process designed to minimize misunderstandings in boundary discussions and to help in the skillful responses to any challenges. It consists of four stages of increasingly forceful conversations.

Assertive Language: Communicates clearly, with minimal emotional content. The voice tone is neutral—not a monotone, but a natural intonation free from hostility, whining, hesitation, and anything else that might potentially distract or upset the person who's listening.

Assessment: A systematic method or approach to gathering information about a client's condition and symptoms.

Attitude: A feeling, disposition, or expression of a positive or negative evaluation of people, objects, event, activities, or ideas.

Autonomy: The ability to make one's own decisions.

Benchmarking: The process of comparing one's performance metrics to industry best practices.

Beneficence: The principle of "do good." Beneficence is action that is done for the benefit of others.

Benevolence: A disposition to do good to others.

Body Language: Nonverbal communication in which people reveal clues to unspoken intentions or feelings through their physical behaviors, such as posture, gestures, facial expressions, and eye movements.

Body Memories: Body sensations that symbolically or literally capture some aspect of trauma. Sensory impulses are recorded in the brain, and these remembrances of bodily sensations can be felt when similar occurrences or cues stimulate the stored memories.

Boundary: Border or limit that separate people from their environment and from other people.

Boundary Crossing: A transgression that may or may not be experienced as harmful.

Boundary Violation: A harmful transgression of a boundary.

Burnout: A psychological term that refers to long-term physical or emotional exhaustion.

Business Association: A legal business formation in which individual practitioners under one roof each maintain their own separate businesses, while contributing to common expenses.

Business Page: Business information entered when registering on social media websites designated for promoting products and services.

Care Coordination: The planned organization of patient care activities between multiple practitioners.

Case Management: See *Care Coordination*.

Case Manager: A designated person whose exclusive role is to coordinate care and services among providers.

Certification: A voluntary regulatory method which offers the use of vocational titles to distinguish professional services. It refers to the confirmation of certain characteristics that is often, but not always, provided by some form of external review, education, assessment, or audit. In some states, certification is used as the designation for practitioners rather than licensure.

Change Agents: Factors that influence the ways we establish, maintain, and change boundaries (e.g., location of service, interpersonal space, appearance, self-disclosure, language, touch, time, and money).

Client-Centeredness: The principle that practitioners always act in the best interest of the client.

Clinical Supervision: A process of meeting regularly with a person who is trained in the skills of supervision, to discuss casework and other professional issues in a structured way.

Coaching: A group or individual process that helps participants set and reach goals. Usually there is one leader directing the activities and guiding the person(s) to finding their own inner strength to follow through on their dreams.

Code of Conduct: A set of rules designed to address applicable state and federal laws as well as established business and professional ethical standards.

Code of Ethics: Operating principles and behavioral guidelines that members of a profession are expected to uphold.

Competency: Having requisite or sufficient skill, knowledge, ability, or qualities.

Complex Posttraumatic Stress Disorder (CPTSD): A term for those subjected to prolonged, repeated trauma.

Compliance: Adherence to applicable laws and standards.

Confidentiality: The client's guarantee that what occurs in the therapeutic setting remains private and protected.

Conflict: A state of disharmony between incompatible or antithetical persons, ideas, or interests; a clash.

Conflict of Interest: Circumstances wherein personal interests may conflict with business interests.

Confrontation: The act of facing and dealing with a problematic situation.

Consent: Approve, permit, agree, or comply.

Consistency: Harmony of conduct or practice; reliability or uniformity of successive results or events.

Contradictory Communication: Sending two conflicting messages at the same time.

Copyright Infringement: Using someone's words or ideas as if they were your own works; reproducing, displaying, distributing, or performing another's work without the permission of the copyright holder.

Countertransference: Transference occurring in the direction from practitioner to client.

Defamation: A general term to describe intentional false communication, either written or spoken, that harms a person's reputation.

Defense Mechanisms: Psychological strategies of relating to the world that are developed unconsciously to protect people from shame, anxiety, and other emotionally painful experiences that they are unable to handle.

Demeanor: The way in which a person behaves toward others, including body language.

Denial: A defense mechanism that involves active refusal to recognize or acknowledge the full implications of an unpleasant reality. Denial bears some similarity to repression, but requires the collaboration of the conscious mind.

Desexualize: Steps taken to ensure that the treatment is not turned into a sexual experience for either the practitioner or the client.

Diagnosis: The identification of the underlying cause, etiology, pathology, or nature of a set of signs and/or symptoms.

Discriminate: To distinguish by noting differences. To unfairly treat a person or group of people differently from others, because of characteristics such as, personal beliefs, race, religion, or intelligence.

Dissociate: Separate ideas, feelings, information, identity, or memories that normally go together. Dissociation involves a detachment from reality (as opposed to a loss of reality) and exists on a continuum of mild (e.g., daydreams) to severe disorders.

Dual Relationships: The overlapping of professional and social roles and interactions between two people.

Duties: The practitioner's obligations to her clients to act in a particular manner.

Duty of Care: A legal requirement that a practitioner adheres to a standard of reasonable care while performing any acts that could possibly be harmful. If a practitioner's actions don't meet this standard of care, then the acts are considered negligent, and any damages resulting may be claimed in a lawsuit for negligence.

Empathy: The action of understanding, being sensitive to, and identifying with another person's situation, feelings, thoughts, and motives.

Ethical Congruence: Making decisions that are consistent, or in alignment with the ethical values that apply to each situation.

Ethical Dilemma: A situation in which two or more duties, rights, or a combination of duties and rights are in conflict. As a result, regardless of what action is taken, something of value will be compromised.

Ethics: The study of ethics is the study of right and wrong conduct, of how we should and should not behave.

Etiquette: A code of behavior that delineates expectations. Professional etiquette concerns behaviors that fall under the heading of good manners: cancellation notification and being punctual; hygiene; and personal habits.

Externship: Learning programs similar to internships, offered by educational institutions to give students short practical experiences in their field of study. They are generally shorter than internships and last approximately a few weeks to months.

Fair Use: A doctrine that allows limited reproduction of copyrighted works for educational and research purposes.

Feedback: The transmission of evaluative or corrective information about an action, event, or process.

Fiduciary: A fiduciary is a legal or ethical relationship of trust between two or more parties.

Flashback: The experience of reliving or re-experiencing a traumatic event as if it is occurring or is imminent.

Franchise Systems: Business models in which a company with a successful product or business system allows other businesses to operate in a particular territory under their trade name for a fee.

Fraud: A criminal act of intentional deception by false representation of a matter of fact, made for personal gain or to damage another individual.

Gender Identity: The personal concept of self as male, female, or neither. Most people develop an identity that matches their biological sex. However, some experience their gender identity as different from their biological or assigned sex.

Geotagging: The process of adding location-based metadata to any media, such as photos or videos, to social networking posts.

Gestalt Theory: This psychological theory emphasizes the organized character of human experience and

behavior. It views boundaries from an interactive perspective that are described as existing in relationships between individuals.

Harassment: The act of systematic and/or continued unwanted and disturbing actions of one party or a group, including threats, pressure, intimidation, and demands.

Health Insurance Portability and Accountability Act (HIPAA): This act addresses the use and disclosure of individuals' health information, the rights granted to individuals, and breach notification requirements.

Hyperarousal: A state of constant alertness to danger experienced by the survivor of trauma. It is also described as a chronic state of fight or flight.

Hypervigilance: An enhanced state of sensory sensitivity accompanied by an exaggerated intensity of behaviors or an overfocused narrowing of attention onto one idea, one part of the body, or a particular sensation or feeling. This is usually accompanied by increased anxiety.

Informed Consent: The process of getting a client's permission before proceeding with a healthcare treatment. The client must have a clear understanding of the procedures, alternative approaches, benefits, and potential consequences. This information must be presented in a form the client can understand and consent must be given without coercion.

Insider Trading: Financial gains that individuals may make based on information about company stock not available to the public.

Integrated Memory: A memory that may have been painful at one time but has been remembered, understood, and accepted.

Integrity: The quality or state of being complete; unbroken condition; wholeness; honesty; and sincerity. People who possess integrity behave ethically, honor confidences, and keep their word. The three major levels of integrity are: keeping one's agreements; being true to one's principles; and the highest level is being true to oneself.

Intellectual Property: A legal concept which refers to creations of the mind (e.g., inventions, literary works, artistic works, designs, images) for which exclusive rights are recognized. Common types of intellectual property rights include copyright, trademarks, patents, and industrial design rights.

Interactive Boundary: The theory that views boundaries as existing in relationships between individuals.

Interactive Speaking: A three-step communication process of speak, invite, and reflect.

Internship: A short-term program (usually less than one year) that combines on-the-job training with academic instruction for those entering the field.

Intervention Model: A communication model developed by Daphne Chellos, for practitioners to use when verbal or nonverbal communication from a client is unclear or when practitioners feel their boundaries are being violated.

Intimacy: A close association with, detailed knowledge of, or deep understanding of, a person.

Intrusion: When information that is related to the theme of a certain memory, but wasn't actually a part of the original episode, becomes associated with the event.

Kickback: A form of negotiated bribery in which a commission of money, goods, or services is paid to the bribe-taker in return for a business favor.

Laws: Codified rules of conduct set forth by a society, generally based on shared ethical or moral principles.

Learning Styles: A person's preferred method to take in information. The three most common are visual, auditory, and kinesthetic.

Legal Entity: In business, a legal entity is a legal construct through which the law allows a group of people to act as if they are a single person.

Libel: Defamation by written/printed words, images, pictures, or broadcast via radio, television, or film.

Licensure: The most restrictive form of regulation, yet it provides the greatest level of public protection. Licensing programs typically involve the completion of a prescribed educational program, passing an examination that measures a minimal level of competency, and usually requires the licensee to adhere to a code of ethics or professional conduct.

Malpractice: Improper, negligent treatment, or incompetent treatment of a patient/client resulting in injury, damage, or loss.

Mastermind Groups: A focused group setting where the individuals in the group create specific goals for their business/career and provide each other with support and inspiration for achieving those goals.

Maturity: The ability to respond in an appropriate manner and be accountable for one's actions.

Mediation: This has become a very common form of dispute resolution where a third party (mediator) works with disputants to agree on a fair result. It is less costly and less time consuming over the long term and can be the way to finding innovative, mutually beneficial solutions. However, mediation does not always result in a settlement.

Mentoring: A professional relationship in which a more experienced practitioner shares information, skills, and insights with a less-experienced practitioner to provide encouragement and support.

Mind-Reads: The communication process in which one talks as though knowing what another person thinks or feels, thus acting on assumptions rather than reality.

Morals: Standards by which behaviors and character traits are judged as right or wrong.

Multiple Intelligences: Howard Gardner's theory that people possess a variety of different intellectual capacities (9) that operate relatively independently of one another.

National Provider Identifier (NPI): Under HIPAA guidelines, each practitioner who transmits electronically must obtain an assigned a NPI.

Negligence: Careless, not intentional, harm caused by conduct that falls below the standards of behavior established by law for the protection of others against unreasonable risk of harm.

Noise: The interference of the transfer of information.

Non-Fraternization: The prohibition of certain relationships between teachers/students, employers/employees, and co-workers. These policies are developed to avoid favoritism, coercion, or sexual harassment.

Nonmaleficence: The principle of "do no harm." The pertinent ethical issue is whether the benefits outweigh the burdens.

Nonverbal Communication: See *Body Language*.

Online Discussion Forums: There are many free online discussion and support groups (e.g., Facebook, LinkedIn) for various practitioners wherein you can ask questions and get answers from many others in the same or similar careers.

Partnership: A legal relationship between two or more persons in which each agrees to furnish a part of the capital and labor for a business enterprise, and by which each shares a fixed proportion of profits and losses.

Passive Language: Communicates a lack of self-confidence or self-esteem. The tone of voice may be whiny, hesitant, or self-deprecating. Passive statements are generally ambiguous, failing to clearly specify what the practitioner wants or expects to have happen and what the consequences will be if the client does not comply.

Payer Discrimination: Charging insurance companies higher rates than clients who do not utilize insurance coverage.

Peer Support Groups: The process of working with a group of practitioners whose main goal is to listen to each other in a way that provides support for the many challenges that arise during the course of dealing with clients.

Perception: The ability to see, hear, or become aware of something through the senses.

Permeable Boundary: A permeable boundary allows information and feelings to flow easily in and out without barriers.

Personal Boundary Model: The theory that views the nature of boundaries as a continuum of permeable to rigid. The degree of permeability also represents vulnerability.

Personal Profile: Personal information used to register on social media websites.

Pin: Common term used to describe posts on the social media site Pinterest (https://www.pinterest.com/).

Policy: A statement of intent that defines expectations and is implemented as a procedure or protocol.

Post: A public display or notice, can also commonly be referred to as status updates when sharing information on the Internet.

Posttraumatic Stress Disorder (PTSD): A mental health condition that's triggered by a terrifying event. Symptoms may include flashbacks, nightmares, and severe anxiety.

Power Differential: The role difference between a practitioner and client, in which the client is vulnerable and the practitioner has more power by virtue of training and experience.

Prejudice: An adverse, preconceived judgment or opinion formed without sufficient knowledge or examination of the facts. It is usually not based on reason or actual experience.

Principles: An individual's rules or laws of behavior that enable her to behave with integrity.

Privacy: The expectation that the collection and sharing of personal data is safeguarded.

Pro Bono: A Latin phrase meaning work done without compensation for the public good.

Proactive Discussions: Conversations where boundaries are set in the initial phases of working with clients, with the objective of preventing boundary crossings and violations from occurring.

Professionalism: The behaviors and qualities that mark an individual as a reliable, competent, trustworthy, and polished professional person.

Projection: A defense mechanism in which a person unconsciously rejects his or her own unacceptable attributes, thoughts, or feelings by ascribing them to objects or other people.

Protected Health Information (PHI): Under the HIPAA Privacy Rule, PHI refers to any information about health status, provision of health care, or payment for health care that can be linked to a specific individual.

Protocol: A detailed plan of a therapeutic treatment or procedure.

Psychosexual: The mental, emotional, and behavioral aspects of sexual development.

Psychosocial: Involving both psychological and social environment aspects.

Psychotherapy: The treatment of mental, emotional, or behavioral disorders by psychological methods.

Quid Pro Quo: A Latin term meaning an equal exchange or substitution; "this for that."

Rapport: A harmonious relationship marked by trust, openness, and mutual understanding.

Recovery: The process of regaining strength, composure, and balance. Combating a disorder.

Redundant Messages: Communication that is so repetitious that the people on the receiving end tend to stop listening.

Reflection: A communication method in which the essence of a message is captured and relayed back by rephrasing what the other person said, rather than repeating it verbatim.

Registration: A regulatory method by which a government agency keeps track of practitioners by informational recordkeeping. These types of programs can entail title protection and practice exclusivity.

Repression: A defense mechanism in which feelings or memories that are too painful to bear are blocked from conscious awareness.

Rights: What clients are entitled to receive.

Rigid Boundary: A boundary which is very firm and distinct. A rigid boundary severely limits the flow of information and feelings moving in or out.

SAVI®: A System for Analyzing Verbal Interaction developed by Anita Simon and Yvonne Agazarian.

Scope of Practice: The where, when, and how a practitioner may provide services or function as a professional.

Secondary Traumatization: The stress resulting from empathic engagement with traumatized clients.

Self-Accountability: Holding oneself responsible for one's actions.

Self-Awareness: The ability to perceive aspects of one's personality, traits, behaviors, feelings, motivations, and thought processes.

Self-Determination: Freedom from interference in regards to one's life and autonomy.

Self-Disclosure: The act of revealing professional or personal information about oneself.

Self-Esteem: A psychological term that reflects an overall emotional evaluation of one's own worth, abilities, and self-respect.

Semi-Permeable Boundary: This boundary indicates a flexible relationship with the outside world. It is characterized by allowing closeness if appropriate and keeping someone at a distance when necessary.

Sensuality: The quality or state of being sensual. Connection with the senses, as opposed to the intellect. The awareness of bodily sensation, taking pleasure in sensation and utilizing sensation to be more fully present in our bodies.

Sequential Relationships: When one set of roles completely ends before a different set of roles begins.

Sex: A term relating to gender, biology, reproduction, and sexual activity.

Sexual Harassment: Unwelcome sexual advances, bullying or coercion of a sexual nature. It can also include the promise of rewards in exchange for sexual favors, or the threat of consequences for non-compliance.

Sexual Misconduct: A continuum of behavior from sexual impropriety to sexual violation. Sexual misconduct occurs when the fiduciary aspect of a therapeutic relationship is compromised, and is the result of the disregard of ethics, boundaries, and genuine care for the client.

Sexual Orientation: Refers to which gender(s) a person is attracted to sexually.

Sexual Response Cycle: A four-phase cycle in men and women, with distinct, gender-specific physiological changes that occur in each phase.

Sexuality: The emotional, physical, cultural, or spiritual actions or reactions to sexual arousal. Sexuality is greater than the sum of its parts. Sexuality encompasses biological (anatomy and physiology), psychological (thoughts, feelings, and values) and cultural (family, society, and religious) influences.

Sexualization: Making an event, procedure, conversation, or experience into something that is sexual or could be interpreted as sexual.

Share: A term commonly used on social networking site when you like a comment and want to share it on your own account, or make a comment and share it publicly.

Slander: A fleeting oral defamation by methods such as spoken words or sounds, sign language, and gestures. Note: Due to their broad reach, words broadcasted on television, radio, and video is considered libel.

Social Media Policy: A code of conduct that provides guidelines to those who post content on the Internet either as part of a business or as a private individual.

Standards of Practice: Statements that describe the underlying principles of a given field, the expectations of professional conduct and the quality of care provided to clients.

Sublimation: The psychological term of diverting the energy of a primitive impulse (especially a sexual one) into activities that are considered to be more acceptable socially, morally, or aesthetically.

Supervision: The process of working with a more experienced practitioner or counselor for the purpose of dealing with day-to-day challenges, ethical dilemmas, and setting boundaries.

Survivor: A person who perseveres despite hardships or trauma.

Therapeutic Constellation: This term is used when working with minors. It refers to the caretakers involved in making decisions for a minor. These may be one or both biological parents, adoptive parents, foster parents, social workers, or healthcare providers.

Title Protection: The lowest levels of regulation. Only those who satisfy certain requirements may use the relevant prescribed title. Practitioners are not required to register or notify the state. Thus, anyone may engage in the particular practice, but only those who satisfy the prescribed requirements may use the specific title.

Touch: The sensation produced by pressure receptors in the skin. Touch is a basic human need, as well as a sensory process through which we communicate.

Transference: A normal psychological phenomenon characterized by unconscious redirection of feelings from client to practitioner.

Trauma: A serious injury or shock to the body, as from violence or an accident. An emotional wound or shock that creates substantial, lasting harm.

Trigger: An experience that sets off a traumatic memory in someone who has experienced trauma. The trigger itself may not be traumatic, including things such as a person, place, sound, image, smell, body position, or vocal tone.

Tweet: A term used to describe posted materials on Twitter.

Unintegrated Memory: A memory that is so painful that parts of the memory are blocked and many of the details missing.

Values: Beliefs about what is intrinsically worthwhile or desirable, rather than what is right and correct.

Vicarious Traumatization: The cumulative effect of working with survivors of traumatic life events. (See *Secondary Traumatization*.)

Work Ethic: A set of values based on the moral virtues of hard work and diligence.

Endnotes

Chapter 1

1. P. Susan Penfold, *Sexual Abuse by Health Professionals* (Toronto: University of Toronto Press, 1998) 112-131.
2. Steven B. Bisbing et al., *Sexual Abuse by Professionals: A Legal Guide* (Charlottesville, Virginia: The Michie Company, 1995) 482-483.
3. Kylea Taylor, *The Ethics of Caring*, (Santa Cruz, CA: Hanford Mead Publishers, 1995) 35-72
4. Albert Schweitzer, "The Ethics of Reverence for Life" *Christendom*, 1 (1936): 225-39
5. Dan Ariely, *The (Honest) Truth about Dishonesty*, (New York, NY: HarperCollins Publishers 2012)
6. Mark Annett, *The Scruples Methodology*, June 16, 2002 http://www.scruplestore.com/TheScruplesMethodology/thebook.html.
7. Marianne Corey, Gerald Corey and Patrick Callanan, *Issues and Ethics In the Helping Professions* (Pacific Grove, CA: International Thomson Publishing Inc., 1998) 16-17.

Chapter 2

1. Jane Bluestein, PH.D., *Parents, Teens and Boundaries* (Deerfield, FL: Health Communications, Inc., 1993).
2. Ronan M. Kisch, *Beyond Technique: The Hidden Dimensions of Bodywork* (Dayton, OH: BLHY Growth Publications, Inc., 1998) 331-332.
3. Ernst Hartmann, M.D., *Boundaries in the Mind: a New Psychology of Personality*, New York, NY: Basic Books, 1991) 4-9.
4. Salvador Minuchin, *Families and Family Therapy* (Cambridge, MA: Harvard University Press, 1974).
5. Sonia Nevis, personal interview, 1995.
6. Hartmann 113.
7. Charles Whitfield, M.D.., Boundaries and Relationships: Knowing, Protecting and Enjoying the Self (Deerfield, FL: Health Communications, Inc., 1993).
8. Thomas Guthiel, M.D., and Glen Gabbard, M.D., "The Concept of Boundaries in Clinical Practice: Theoretical and Risk-Management Dimensions," *American Journal of Psychiatry* Feb. 1993.
9. Kisch 325.
10. Estelle Disch, PH.D., "Are You in Trouble with a Client," *Massage Therapy Journal* Volume 31, Number 3 (Summer 1992).

Chapter 3

1. Mary Jo Bennett and Katy Butler, "Can We Tell the Truth: Let's End Our Conspiracy of Silence about our Ambiguous Boundaries," *Psychotherapy Networker* (March/April 2002): 32-77.
2. Daphne Chellos and Ben Benjamin, "Dual Roles and Other Ethical Considerations," *Massage Therapy Journal* (Spring 1992): 23.
3. Nanette Gartrell et al., "Psychiatrist-Patient Sexual Contact: Results of a National Survey, I: Prevalence," *American Journal of Psychiatry* 143 (1986): 1126. (See also: Judith Herman et al., "Psychiatrist-Patient Sexual Contact: Results of a National Survey, II: Psychiatrists' Attitudes," *AJP* 44 (1987): 164..
4. Jean. C. Holroyd and Annette M. Brodsky, "Psychologists' Attitudes and Practices Regarding Erotic and Nonerotic Physical Contact with Patients," *American Psychologist* 32 (1977): 843.
5. Chellos and Benjamin 22.
6. http://www.aclu-mn.org/legal/casedocket/commissionerofhealthvfjell/, Commissioner of Health v. Fjellman, November 15, 2007
7. Dr. Sonia Nevis, personal consultation, January 2006.
8. Gary Schoener, PH.D., *Personal Relationships with Former Clients* (a monograph), The Walk-In Counseling Center, September 2006.
9. Schoener, September 2006.
10. Nina McIntosh, *The Educated Heart*, Third Edition (Maryland: Lippincott, Williams & Wilkins, 2011), 116-117.
11. Peter Rutter, M.D., *Sex in the Forbidden Zone* (London: Mandala, 1991) 87-88.
12. http://www.apa.org/topics/ethics/potential-violations.aspx
13. Nina McIntosh, 116.
14. Chellos and Benjamin

Chapter 4

1. Albert G. Mulley, Chris Trimble, and Glyn Elwyn, "Stop the Silent Misdiagnosis: Patients' Preferences Matter," *BMJ* Volume 345, Issue 7883 (2012): e6572.
2. Yvonne M. Agazarian and Susan P. Gantt, *Autobiography of a Theory: Developing the Theory of Living Human Systems and Its Systems-Centered Practice* (London: Jessica Kingsley Publishers Ltd, 2000)
3. Anita Simon and Yvonne M. Agazarian, *SAVI: Sequential Analysis of Verbal Interaction* (Philadelphia: Research for Better Schools, 1967)
4. Anita Simon and Yvonne Agazarian, "SAVI — the System for Analyzing Verbal Interaction," *The Process of Group Psychotherapy: Systems for Analyzing Change*, Ariadne P. Beck and Carol M. Lewis, Editors (Washington, D.C., American Psychological Association, 2000), 357–380.
5. Claude Shannon and Warren Weaver, *The Mathematical Theory of Communication* (University of Illinois Press, Urbana, Il, 1971).
6. Ben Benjamin, Amy Yeager, and Anita Simon, *Conversation Transformation: Recognize and Overcome the 6 Most Difficult Communication Patterns* (New York, McGraw Hill, 2012).
7. Carol D. Tamparo and Wilburta Q. Lindh, *Therapeutic Communications for Health Care*, 3rd ed. (Clifton Park, NY: Cengage Learning, 2008).
8. Ronan M. Kisch, *Beyond Technique: The Hidden Dimensions of Bodywork* (Dayton, OH: BLHY Growth Publications, Inc., 1998), 325.
9. Yvonne M. Agazarian, *Systems Centered Therapy for Groups* (London: Karnac Books, 2004) 153
10. Benjamin, Yeager, and Simon, 178–180.
11. Sheldon Kopp, *Back to One: A Practical Guide for Psychotherapists* (Palo Alto, CA: Science of Behavior Books, 1977).
12. Ben E. Benjamin and Amy Yeager, "Communication Challenges for MTs: Giving and Getting Effective Feedback," *Massage & Bodywork* (December/January 2007) 116–120. (*excerpted and adapted).
13. Matthew D. Lieberman, Naomi I. Eisenberger, Molly J. Crockett, Sabrina M. Tom, Jennifer H. Pfeifer, and Baldwin M. Way, "Putting Feelings Into Words: Affect Labeling Disrupts Amygdala Activity in Response to Affective Stimuli," *Psychological Science* Volume 18, Issue 5 (2007): 421–428.

Chapter 5

1. Robert Bolton, PH.D., *People Skills: How to Assert Yourself, Listen to Others and Resolve Conflicts* (New York: Simon & Schuster, Inc., 1979). 7
2. Howard Gardner, *Multiple Intelligences: The Theory in Practice* (New York: Basic Books, 1993).
3. Ellen Langer, Arthur Blank, and Benzion Chanowitz, "The Mindlessness of Ostensibly Thoughtful Action: The Role of "Placebic" Information in Interpersonal Interaction," *Journal of Personality and Social Psychology*, Volume 36, Number 6 (1978), 635-42.
4. Bolton 137-176.

Chapter 6

1. William Greenburg of the AMTA Grievance Board, personal interview, 11 October 1995.
2. June M. Reinisch and Ruth Beasley, *The Kinsey Institute New Report on Sex: What You Must Know to be Sexually Literate* (New York: St. Martin's Press, 1990) xviii.
3. A. P. Stern, "The feeling we can't do without," *McCall's* (November 1992): 84+, 86.
4. Tiffany Field, *touch* (Cambridge, MA: A Bradford book, MIT Press, 2001) 59.
5. Phyllis Davis, PH.D., *The Power of Touch* (Carlsbad, CA: Hay House, Inc., 1999) 6.
6. Ashley Montagu, *Touching* (New York: Harper & Row Publishers, 1971) 34, 46.
7. Montagu 198-203.
8. Montagu 198-203.
9. Montagu.
10. Laurel Catherine Bentsen, "Women and Touch Deprivation," *Massage Therapy Journal* Volume 33, Number 4 (Fall 1994): 54-106, 60.
11. Stern 84+, 90.
12. T. Field, M. Hernandez-Reif, O. Quintino, et. al., *Journal of Applied Gerontology* Volume 17 (1998) 229-239.
13. Grant Jewell Rich, ed., Ruth Remington, "Hand massage in the agitated elderly," *Massage Therapy: The Evidence for Practice*, (New York: Mosby, Harcourt Publishers Limited, 2002) 165-185).
14. Jeffrey D. Fisher et al., "Hands Touching Hands: Affective and Evaluative Effects of an Interpersonal Touch." *Sociometry* Volume 39, Number 4 (1976): 417.
15. Richard Heslin and Tari Alper, "Nonverbal Communication," *Sage Annual Reviews of Communications Research* Volume 11 (1982).
16. Helen Colton, *Touch Therapy* (New York: Kenshington Publishing Corp., 1983) 159.
17. *Webster's New Universal Unabridged Dictionary*, 2nd ed., (New York: Simon and Schuster, 1981).
18. Stephen Thayer, "Close Encounters," *Psychology Today* (March 1988).
19. Susan Forward and Craig Buck, *Betrayal of Innocence: Incest and It's Devastation* (New York: St. Martin's Press, 1978).
20. *Sexual Health Magazine*, http://www.sexualhealth.com, 1.
21. Ruth Brecher and Edward Brecher, *An Analysis of Human Sexual Response* (New York: New American Library, 1966).
22. *Sexual Health Magazine*.
23. William H. Gotwald Jr.and Gale Holtz Golden, *Sexuality: The Human Experience* (New York: Macmillan Publishing, 1981) 295.
24. Gotwald and Golden, 297-298.
25. *Sexual Health Magazine*.
26. Alfred C. Kinsey et al., *Sexual Behavior in the Human Male* (Philadelphia, PN: W. B. Saunders, 1948).
27. Kinsey et al.
28. Elizabeth Glaeser, *Aspects of Gender Identity Development: Searching for an Explanation in the Brain* (NYU Applied Psychology OPUS Spring 2011).
29. The American Association of Sex Educators, Counselors and Therapists, *Contemporary Sexuality* Volume 33 (March 1999).

30. Miriam Ehrenberg and Otto Ehrenberg, *The Intimate Circle: The Sexual Dynamics of Family Life* (New York: Simon and Schuster, 1988).

31. *Fowler's Modern English Usage*, 2nd Ed. (New York: Oxford University Press, 1985).

32. Carol D. Tamparo, B.S., PH.D., CMA-A and Wilburta Q. Lindh, CMA, *Therapeutic Communications for Health Professionals* (Clifton Park, NY: Delmar Thomson Learning, 2000) 72.

33. Daphne Chellos, *Creating Boundaries Handbook*, (Boulder, CO, 1993).

34. Pamela R. Fletcher and Martha Roth, eds., *Transforming a Rape Culture* (Minneapolis, MN: Milkweed Editions, 1995) 130.

35. From "The Hippocratic Oath," a translation by Ludwig Edelstein, *Supplements to the Bulletins of the History of Medicine*, no.1 (Baltimore, MD: John Hopkins University Press, 1943).

36. Steven B. Bisbing, Linda Mabus Jorgenson, and Pamela K. Sutherland, *Sexual Abuse by Professionals: A Legal Guide* (Charlottesville, VA: Michie, 1995).

37. North Carolina Board of Massage & Bodywork Therapy http://www.bmbt.org/downloads/Rules%20%20 Regulations%20Revised%2003-11.pdf .0508, 12-13.

38. John C. Gonsiorek, *Breach of Trust: Sexual Exploitation by Health Care Professionals and Clergy* (Thousand Oaks, CA: Sage Publications 1995).

39. Department of Health, Board of Massage Therapy, Petitioner, vs. Miodrag Visacki, LMT, Respondent. Case No. 01-2257PL, State of Florida Division of Administrative Hearings, 2001 Fla. Div. Adm. Hear. LEXIS 3131, September 18, 2001, Recommended Order.

40. Dr. Melvin Mashner v. W. Pennington, Jr. 1970738, Supreme Court of Alabama, 729 So. 2D 262; 1998 Ala. LEXIS 301, November 20, 1998; Released.

41. Marie M. Fortune, *Love Does No Harm: Sexual Ethics for the Rest of Us* (New York: The Continuum International Publishing Group, 1995) 85-86.

42. Peter Rutter, M.D., *Sex in the Forbidden Zone* (London: Mandala, 1991) 87.

43. Angelica Redleaf, D.C., *Behind Closed Doors: Gender, Sexuality & Touch in the Doctor/Patient Relationship*. (Westport, CT: Auburn House, 1998). 129-133.

44. Linda Greenhouse, "Same-Sex Harassment Ruled Illegal," *The Providence Journal-Bulletin* sec. A-1, 11 (Tuesday, 5 March 1998).

45. From the schedule of conference events published by organizers of "It's Never O.K., The Third International Conference on Sexual Exploitation by Health Professionals, Psychotherapists and Clergy," held in Toronto, Ontario, Canada, Oct. 13-15, 1994.

Chapter 7

1. Noah Webster, *Webster's New Universal Unabridged Dictionary* (Cleveland, OH: Dorset & Baber, 1983) 1436-1437.

2. Jerry Buley, PH.D., "What Is a Professional?," *Arizona Communication Association*, The Hugh Downs School of Human Communication (2000).

3. Patricia M. Holland and Sandra K. Anderson, *Communication & Ethics for Bodywork Practitioners* (Philadelphia, PA: F.A. Davis Company, 20012) 167-169.

4. Webster 953.

5. George F. Sheldon, M.D., FACS, *Bulletin of the American College of Surgeons*, Volume 83, Number 12 (Chicago, IL, 1998) 16.

6. Sandy Fritz, *Mosby's Fundamentals of Therapeutic Massage* (St. Louis, MO: Van Hoffmann Press, 1995) 435.

7. Whitney Lowe, LMT, "Exploring Orthopedic Assessment," *Massage Today* Volume 1, Number 1 (January 2001) 7.

8. Donald Veres, M.D., M.S.J., ed., *Taber's Cyclopedic Medical Dictionary* (Philadelphia, PA: F.A. Davis Company, 1997).

9. Sandy Fritz, James M. Grosenbach, and Kathy Paholsky, "Ethics and Professionalism: Scope of Practice," *Massage Magazine* March/April 1997.

10. Patricia J. Benjamin, "Paper Tiger Credentials," *Massage Therapy Journal* Volume 29, Number 3 (Summer 1990) 9.

11. Nina McIntosh, *The Educated Heart: Professional Guidelines for Massage Therapists, Bodyworkers, and Movement Teachers* (Memphis, TN: Decatur Bainbridge Press, 1999) 97.

12. G. Corey, M.S. Corey, and P. Callanan, *Issues and Ethics in the Helping Professions* 5th ed., (Pacific Grove, CA: Brooks/Cole Publishing Company, 1998) 16-17.

13. Tara Roehl, M.S. CCC-SLP, *HIPAA: Double Lock Rule*, http://www.speechykeenslp.com/blog/hipaa-double-lock-rule/

Chapter 8

1. Case Management Society of America, *Standards of Practice for Case Management* (Little Rock, AK: Case Management Society of America, 1995).

2. Cindy Ling, *Why and What you Should Know about Case Management* http://www.NurseWeek.com.

3. Cherie M. Sohnen-Moe, *Business Mastery* (Tucson, AZ: Sohnen-Moe Associates, Inc., 2008) 127-184.

4. Sohnen-Moe 159-159, 272-277.

5. CG Funk, personal interview, May 2013.

6. Funk, May 2013.

Chapter 9

1. Kenneth Blanchard and Norman Vincent Peale, *The Power of Ethical Management* (New York: William Morrow and Company, Inc., 1988).

2. 1 Timothy 6:10.

3. Lu Bauer, "Clean Up Your Money Operating System," *Massage Therapy Journal* Volume 39, Number 1 (Spring 2000).

4. Suze Orman, *9 Steps to Financial Freedom: Practical and Spiritual Steps So You Can Stop Worrying* (New York: Three Rivers Press, 2001).

5. Cherie M. Sohnen-Moe, *Business Mastery* (Tucson, AZ: Sohnen-Moe Associates, Inc., 2008) 214.

6. Sohnen-Moe 214.

7. Sohnen-Moe 309-311.

8. Sohnen-Moe 397-400.

9. The California Codes, Civil Code Section 1749.5 states:

   1749.5. (a) On or after January 1, 1997, it is unlawful for any person or entity to sell a gift certificate to a purchaser containing an expiration date. Any gift certificate sold after that date shall be redeemable in cash for its cash value, or subject to replacement with a new gift certificate at no cost to the purchaser or holder. (b) A gift certificate sold without an expiration date is valid until redeemed or replaced.

10. Sohnen-Moe 263-265.

11. Sohnen-Moe 265.

12. Gary Wolf, personal interview, June 2001.

13. Cherie Sohnen-Moe, "Copyright," *Massage Therapy Journal* Volume 40, Number 4 (Winter 2002).

14. Sohnen-Moe 250-253.

15. Stewart Levine, *Getting to Resolution: Turning Conflict into Collaboration* (San Francisco, California: Berrett-Koehler Publishers, Inc., 1998).

16. Joan C. Calcagno, "Mediation is the Best Way to End a Dispute," *Massage Therapy Journal* Volume 38, Number 4 (Winter 2000).

17. Massachusetts Continuing Legal Education, Inc., Jury Instructions for Civil Trials (MA: Massachusetts Continuing Legal Education, Inc., 1995) 36 (95-05.34);

18. Brine v. Belinkoff, 235 N.E.2d 23, 26 (Wis. 1987).

19. Sohnen-Moe 272-277.

20. Internal Revenue Service, Employer's Tax Guide (Publication 15, Circular E).

Chapter 10

1. Marianne Schneider Corey, Jerald Corey, *Becoming a Helper* (Brooks/Cole, Cengage Learning 2010).
2. Nancy Bridges, "Psychodynamic perspective on therapeutic boundaries: Creative clinical possibilities," *Psychotherapy Practice and Research* Volume 8, Number 4 (1999): 1-9.
3. Nancy Bridges, "The role of supervision in managing intense affect and constructing boundaries in therapeutic relationships," *Journal of Sex Education and Therapy* Volume 24, Number 4 (2000): 218-225.
4. Bridges, "Psychodynamic perspective on therapeutic boundaries."
5. Ann Alonso, *The Quiet Profession* (New York: Macmillan Publishing Company, 1985).
6. Les Kertay, "Ethical considerations for bodyworkers who counsel," *Massage Magazine* (July/August 1998).
7. Bridges, "Meaning and management of attraction."
8. Bridges, "Psychodynamic perspective on therapeutic boundaries."
9. George J. Allen, Sandor J. Szollos, and Bronwen E. Williams, "Doctoral students comparative evaluations of best and worst psychotherapy supervision," *Professional Psychology: Research and Practice* Volume 17, Number 2 (1986): 91-99.
10. Christine H. Hutt, Judith Scott, and Mark King, "A phenomenological study of supervisees= positive and negative experiences in supervision," *Psychotherapy: Theory, Research and Practice* Volume 20, Number 1 (1983): 118-122.
11. Allen, Szollos, and Bronwen.
12. Hutt, Scott, and King.
13. Jeannette Milgrom, *Boundaries in Professional Relationships* (Minneapolis, MN: Walk-In Counseling Center, 1992).
14. Glen O. Gabbard, "Can patients sexually harass their physicians?" *Archives of Family Medicine* Volume 4 (1995): 261-265.
15. Redleaf and Baird.
16. Redleaf and Baird.
17. Redleaf and Baird.
18. Allen, Szollos, and Bronwen.
19. Hutt, Scott, and King
20. Napoleon Hill, *Think & Grow Rich* (Fawcett Crest Books, NY, 1960) 168-169.
21. International Coach Federation http://www.coachfederation.org/need/landing.cfm?ItemNumber=978&navItemNumber=567

Chapter 11

1. Melissa Soalt, personal interview, 1994.
2. Stephanie Mines, PH.D., "Secrets: Healing Triumphs over Domestic Violence," *Massage and Bodywork* (Oct/Nov 2001): 18.
3. Karrie Mowen, "Trauma Touch Therapy: An Interdisciplinary Approach to Trauma," *Massage and Bodywork* (Oct/Nov 2001): 28-36.
4. Janet Yassen, personal interview, 1994.
5. Janet Yassen, personal interview, 1991.
6. Maryanna Eckberg, PH.D., *Victims of Cruelty: Somatic Psychotherapy in the Treatment of Posttraumatic Stress Disorder* (Berkeley, CA: North Atlantic Books, 2000) 3.
7. Eckberg 45.
8. Tiffany Field, *touch* (Cambridge, MA: A Bradford book, MIT Press, 2001) 136.
9. Patricia Tjaden and Nancy Thoennes, "Prevalence, Incidence and Consequences of Violence Against Women: Findings From the National Violence Against Women Survey," *NCJ* (Washington DC: U.S. Department of Justice, Bureau of Justice Statistics, November 1998): 172837.
10. U.S. Department of Health and Human Services, Administration for Children, Youth and Families, "Child Maltreatment," 2002, *Reports from the States to the National Child Abuse and Neglect Data Systems,* (Washington, D.C.: 2004).

11. R. Badgley, "Report of the federal committee on sexual offenses against children and youth," *Canadian Government Publishing Centre* (Ottowa 1984).

12. Judith Herman, *Trauma and Recovery* (New York: Harper Collins Publishers, 1992) 6-32.

13. Mines 22.

14. Herman 6-32.

15. Steven Hassan, *Releasing the Bonds: Empowering People to Think for Themselves* (Sommerville, MA: Freedom of Mind Press, 2000).

16. Herman 168.

17. Herman 195.

18. Herman 207.

19. American Psychiatric Association, *Diagnostic and Statistical Manual of Mental Disorders*, 4th ed. (Washington DC: American Psychiatric Association, 1994).

20. Herman 6-32.

21. Eckberg.

22. Herman 6-32.

23. *Incest: The Victim No One Believes*, film, Motorola Teleprogram Information (MTI), Deerfield IL, (1978).

24. Herman 121.

25. Herman 121.

26. Kirtland C. Peterson, Maurice F. Prout, and Robert A. Schwartz, *Post Traumatic Stress Disorder: A Clinician's Guide* (New York: Plenum Press, 1992).

27. Candace Pert, "Neuropeptides: The Emotions and Bodymind," *Massage Therapy Journal* Volume 26, Number 4 (Fall 1987): 39.

28. Wilhelm Reich, *Character Analysis* (London, England: Vision Press, 1950) 55, 357-365.

29. *Incest: The Victim No One Believes*.

30. Soalt.

31. Eckberg 41-48.

32. Eckberg 48-58.

33. Survivor Interviews, videotape, Ben Benjamin, Boston, MA, 1992.

34. Eckberg 58-61.

35. Survivor Interviews.

36. Robert. Timms and Patrick Connors, *Embodying Healing* (Brandon, VT: The Safer Society Press, 1992) 24.

37. Timms and Connors 38.

38. Soalt.

39. Mines 24.

40. Eckberg 63.

41. Mowen 32.

42. Yassen 1994.

43. Eckberg 216-218.

44. Herman 196-213.

45. Herman 175-195.

46. Yassen 1991.

47. Soalt.

48. *Incest: The Victim No One Believes*.

49. Judith Herman, M.D., lecture, Bunting Institute of Radcliffe College, Harvard, Cambridge, MA, May 1994.

50. Clyde Ford, D.C., adapted from a seminar, 1991.

51. Candice Schachter, Carol Stalker and Eli Teram, *Handbook on Sensitive Practice for Health Professionals: Lessons from Women Survivors of Childhood Sexual Abuse* (Ottawa, Canada: Health Canada, 2001) 20.

52. Mines 24.

Index

Interactive Speaking 113, 118, 119
Internet 207, 261
Internship 298
Interpersonal Space 56
Intervention Model 151-153
Intimacy 67, 138, 139
Intrusion Errors 309

K

Kickback 253, 254

L

Law(s) 12, 13, 20, 71, 74, 220, 262, 263, 265
   Competency 178
   Compliance 207
   Confidentiality 186, 187
   Employment 211
   Scope of Practice 171-177
   Standards 181
   Violation 72
Lawsuit 61, 210, 220, 267-272, 303
Learning Styles 118, 119
Legal Entity 220
Legal Liability 71, 223
Libel 263-264
Licensure 171, 172, 177
   loss of 263, 271
Limbic System 141, 142
LinkedIn 257, 262, 293. *See also Social Media*
Location 56, 163, 207

M

Malpractice 263, 267-271
Marketing 221, 254, 264
   Materials 165-166, 254-257
Mastermind Groups 296, 297
Mature/Maturity 9, 11, 69, 183, 202
Media 33, 34, 48, 63, 132, 143, 154, 257. *See also Social Media*
Mediation 266, 267
Memory 307, 308, 310, 315. *See also Integrated Memory, Unintegrated Memory*
Mentor 294, 296, 298
   Mentoring 294-296, 298
Mind-Read 84, 86, 115
Minors 164, 193-195
Misleading Ploy 225. *See also Marketing*
Money 56, 64, 202, 203, 210, 236-247. *See also Fees, Finances*
Morals 14, 15, 262
Motivate/Motivation 148, 168, 280, 295, 318
Multiple Intelligences 118, 119

N

National Provider Identifier (NPI) 188, 189
Negligence 208, 268, 270, 272
Network 179, 180, 198, 201, 292, 294, 316
Noise 82, 85, 107
Nonmaleficence 3, 20
Nonverbal Communication 115-117, 136, 149, 151. *See also Body Language*
Nutritional Supplements 170, 173, 174, 251-252

O

Online Discussion Forums 298

P

Parasympathetic Nervous System 134, 141, 142, 150, 314
Partnership 70, 72, 219-222
Passive Language 96, 97
Payer Discrimination 276
Peer Supervision 44, 282, 283, 330. *See also Supervision*
Peer Support Groups 291-293
Perception 68, 83, 131
Permeable Boundary 35, 36, 39. *See also Boundaries*
Personal Boundary 27, 35, 36, 314. *See also Boundaries*
Personal Profile 63, 257, 258, 260. *See also Social Media*
Pin 257, 260, 261. *See also Social Media*
Policies 14, 19, 47, 55-57, 169, 224, 323, 324
   Client 200-203
   Insurance 263, 267, 271, 275
   Manuals 208-209
   Non-fraternization 78
   Reinforcing 122
   Sample Statements 338-340
   Social Media 258-260
   Statements 55, 165, 200-203
   See also Change Agents
Post 49, 257-262. *See also Social Media*
Posttraumatic Stress Disorder (PTSD) 307, 308, 316, 318
Power Differential 5-8, 56, 60, 118, 203, 250, 254
   Complications 6-8
   Employment 211
   Friendship 63
   Impact of 68
   In Communication 87, 88
   In Retail 250
   Misconduct 156
   Power Dynamics 41, 72
   Romantic Relationships 74
   Schools 78
Prejudice 36
Primary Care Provider (PCP) 189, 221, 232, 276
Principles 11-15

Continuing Education Series

The Ethics of Touch Continuing Education Series takes an in-depth look at ethical issues through reading materials and reflective exercises. The modules are designed per the NCBTMB Standards of Practice requirements using *The Ethics of Touch* book (purchased separately) as the reading material. Each module is 3 Contact Hours and meets the NCBTMB Ethics Standard V: Roles and Boundaries.

Sohnen-Moe Associates is approved by the National Certification Board for Therapeutic Massage and Bodywork (NCBTMB) as a continuing education provider (No. 031932-00) and our courses are accepted by the AMTA, ABMP, Florida State Department of Health (Provider No.MCE477-05), and many other healthcare practitioners' national and state boards. Please check with your board(s) for details and certification guidelines.

Chapter One: Ethical Foundations   E6001Z   3 hours $35

Being ethical is not limited simply to knowing and following ethical codes, laws, and regulations. Ethical behavior also involves striving to bring the highest values into your work and aspiring to do your best in all interactions. This module introduces the basic concepts necessary in discussing ethics for hands-on practitioners. It includes reading chapter One of *The Ethics of Touch* and answering 20 test questions.

Chapter Two: Boundaries   E6002Z   3 hours $35

The foundation of an ethical practice is built upon establishing, maintaining, and respecting personal and professional boundaries. By increasing your awareness of your clients' boundaries, as well as your own, you can improve the therapeutic relationship and avoid many inadvertent slips into unethical behavior. This module introduces the basic concepts relevant to the discussion of boundaries. It includes reading chapters One and Two of *The Ethics of Touch* and answering 20 test questions.

Chapter Three: Dual and Sequential Relationships   E6003Z   3 hours $35

Dual and sequential relationships commonly consist of many layers, and encompass a number of professional and social components. Some dual relationships evolve easily and naturally, and initially seem relatively simple. Upon closer examination, their dynamics can be surprisingly complex with ramifications ranging from vital and stimulating to tragically harmful. The work of a helping professional often occurs within complex sets of relationships where boundaries and matters of authority take on shades of gray. This module examines the fundamental concepts of dual and sequential relationships and how to address them within the context of the therapeutic relationship. It gives solid guidelines for the ethical practitioner to safeguard the therapeutic relationship. It includes reading chapters One and Three of *The Ethics of Touch* and answering 20 test questions.

Chapter Four: Dynamics of Effective Communication   E6004Z   3 hours $35

Human communication can be a complex process, subject to misunderstanding and confusion. The challenges are intensified in the therapeutic relationship. You enhance your relationships with clients by understanding the dynamics of communication and using proven tools to clarify and maintain professional boundaries. This module introduces common communication tools necessary for the hands-on practitioner. It includes reading chapters One and Four of *The Ethics of Touch* and answering 20 test questions.

Chapter Five: Communication Techniques & Strategies E6005Z 3 hours $35

The time invested in enhancing your communication skills promotes mutual understanding, strengthens the therapeutic relationship, and helps you overcome any challenges you may encounter. This module covers five types of interactions that are essential for practitioners to manage effectively: reflecting, inviting input, responding to body language, educating, and asserting boundaries. It includes reading chapters One, Four, and Five of *The Ethics of Touch* and answering 20 test questions.

Chapter Six: Sex, Touch, and Intimacy E6006Z 3 hours $35

Awareness of the physical, social, and cultural dynamics, and a knowledge of behavioral strategies, helps practitioners increase their effectiveness as a safe, healing presence. This module introduces many issues practitioners need to address in regards to sex, touch, and intimacy. It includes reading chapters One and Six of *The Ethics of Touch* and answering 20 test questions.

Chapter Seven: Practice Management E6007Z 3 hours $35

Ethical practice management calls for high standards and personal integrity on the part of every somatic practitioner. Respecting the responsibilities of belonging to a profession, you can feel confident in interactions with governing bodies, colleagues, and clients. This module introduces issues necessary for consideration and includes reading chapters One and Seven of *The Ethics of Touch* and answering 20 test questions.

Chapter Eight: The Team Approach E6008Z 3 hours $35

Developing the structure for practice alliances is of significant importance. This module helps identify the issues relevant to working in a situation such as a group practice, clinic, hospital, or spa. It includes reading chapters One and Eight of *The Ethics of Touch* and answering 20 test questions.

Chapter Nine: Business Ethics E6009Z 3 hours $35

Business ethics covers the major ethical issues that relate to managing a successful business: general finances; setting fees; tips; barter; gift certificates; taxes; product sales; referrals; marketing materials; complying with local, state, and federal laws; regulating bodies; insurance coverage; slander/libel; contracts; civil lawsuits; employees; client custody; and insurance reimbursement. This module includes reading chapters One and Nine of *The Ethics of Touch* and answering 20 test questions.

Chapter Ten: Support Systems E6010Z 3 hours $35

Identifying and understanding intense, sometimes objectionable, feelings in professional relationships is central to the management of professional boundaries. Support systems can assist you with identifying and managing your feelings around these boundary dilemmas; as well as, sorting out clinical and interpersonal dilemmas. This module introduces you to the various support systems and includes reading chapters One and Ten of *The Ethics of Touch* and answering 20 test questions.

Chapter Eleven: Working with Trauma Survivors E6011Z 3 hours $35

On average, one of every five clients a practitioner sees has a history of some kind of trauma or abuse. Whether or not you are aware of it, in a large percentage of your sessions, the client in your treatment room may be a survivor. To avoid ethical complications, every practitioner who uses touch needs basic knowledge about trauma and abuse survivors and a clear protocol to safely support these particular clients. This module introduces the issues relevant to working with trauma clients. It doesn't train you in how to work with survivors, rather it brings awareness to the special considerations you must make with these clients. It includes reading chapters One and Eleven of *The Ethics of Touch* and answering 20 test questions.

To order: visit www.TheEthicsOfTouch.com or call 520-743-3936

Other Offerings

Free Resources

SMA Community Site: sohnenmoe.customerhub.net

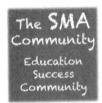

The SMA Community site contains free ebooks, posters, reproducible forms, and other practice-building resources. Your personal FileBox is available 24 hours a day. It maintains all the free files you download, as well as any digital products you purchase from our online store.

SMA Blog: blog.sohnen-moe.com

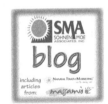

Our blog contains hundreds of free, informative articles written by experts and successful practitioners in the wellness fields. Topics include marketing, technology, treatment planning, overall success strategies, and more.

Marketing Mastery: sohnen-moe.com/marketingmastery

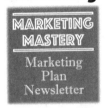

The *Marketing Mastery Newsletter* is a free subscription service to a year-long overall marketing plan. The plan includes monthly goals and weekly activity reminders delivered directly to your inbox. Use all or part of this plan to expand your marketing efforts, elevate your visibility in the community, and increase your client base.

Consulting Services

Coaching with Cherie Sohnen-Moe: sohnen-moe.com/services

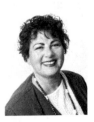

Coaching provides support for you in resolving problems and provides suggestions to implement change for a more efficient, vital, and flourishing practice. Being as consummate in business as you are in technique requires learning an entirely different set of skills. Mastering these skills can take a long time, particularly if you work alone. Direction in acquiring these skills and knowledge, along with consistent support and encouragement, can help you create the business/career you envision.

Publications

Business Mastery, 5th edition

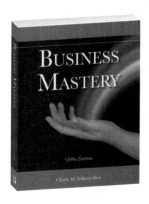

For the past 3 decades, the *Business Mastery* text has served as a trusted guide for people seeking to live their career dreams. This book is specifically designed to support you on your journey to a fulfilling and financially rewarding career. Within the pages of this classic, time-tested book, you will find everything you need to launch and effectively manage a thriving practice, or successfully work for a company. You will also find practical, innovative tools and tips on how to market your skills, work smarter, develop alliances through networking, fine-tune your communications skills, increase profits, and create a dynamic online presence. The 5th edition is fully revised and updated throughout, with new information for today's somatic practitioner. **www.BusinessMastery.us**

Present Yourself Powerfully

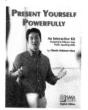

Public speaking is one of the best ways to build your business. *Present Yourself Powerfully* is a kit designed to alleviate the hassles of public speaking. This PDF is a toolbox of ideas, techniques, and reproducible materials for helping practitioners to give talks, workshops, and demonstrations.

Marketing Communications

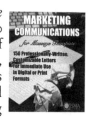

Marketing Communications for Massage Therapists is filled with more than 100 professionally written examples of marketing emails, announcements, letters, and press releases. The pages of this PDF can be copied and pasted into your preferred word processing or email application for easy editing.

Build Your Business Plan

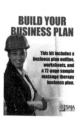

A business plan is an essential road map for a successful practice. *Build Your Business Plan* simplifies the planning, writing, and finalizing of this process. This kit is a PDF that includes a business plan outline, worksheets, and a 70-page sample massage therapy business plan to use as your guide.

Marketing Tools

These marketing templates are digital files that you download, customize, and print as often as needed.

Gift Certificates

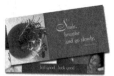

Richly illustrated, customizable gift certificates to offer your clients for their friends, family, and any one else.

Postcards

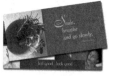

Richly illustrated cover art, designed specifically for the healing arts practitioner. Use for all your direct mail or email marketing efforts: announcements, wvents, reminders, birthdays, and other special occasions.

Client Education Brochures

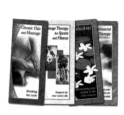

Educate your clients about a variety of products, modalities, and specialties available in your practice. These elegantly written and illustrated brochures have extensive information on a large number of subjects.

Business Cards

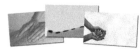

Choose from richly illustrated cover art designs, specifically created with the healing arts practitioner in mind.

www.Sohnen-Moe.com/products